Smart Healthcare Systems

Smart Healthcare Systems

Edited by
Adwitiya Sinha and Megha Rathi

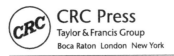

CRC Press
Taylor & Francis Group
Boca Raton London New York

CRC Press is an imprint of the
Taylor & Francis Group, an **informa** business

CRC Press
Taylor & Francis Group
6000 Broken Sound Parkway NW, Suite 300
Boca Raton, FL 33487-2742

© 2020 by Taylor & Francis Group, LLC
CRC Press is an imprint of Taylor & Francis Group, an Informa business

No claim to original U.S. Government works

Printed and bound by CPI Group (UK) Ltd, Croydon, CR0 4YY on acid-free paper

International Standard Book Number-13: 978-0-367-03056-8 (Hardback)

Library of Congress Cataloging-in-Publication Data

Names: Sinha, Adwitiya, editor. | Rathi, Megha, editor.
Title: Smart healthcare systems / edited by Adwitiya Sinha and Megha Rathi.
Description: Boca Raton : CRC Press, [2019] | Includes bibliographical references and index.
Identifiers: LCCN 2019010019 | ISBN 9780367030568 (hardback)
Subjects: LCSH: Artificial intelligence—Medical applications. | Medical informatics.
Classification: LCC R859.7.A78 S63 2019 | DDC 610.285—dc23
LC record available at https://lccn.loc.gov/2019010019

Visit the Taylor & Francis Web site at
http://www.taylorandfrancis.com

and the CRC Press Web site at
http://www.crcpress.com

Contents

Preface

With the rapid development of advanced data mining techniques and bioinformatics sensor, advent of smart mobile technologies and web-based medical support systems have enabled the development of smart healthcare systems which are used to improve clinical and health practices. Basically, smart healthcare models are data-oriented models with intensive data collected in the form of electronic health records (EHRs); EHR plays a vital role in the development of smart healthcare model and keeps health information in one single repository. Advanced mobile technologies and biomedical sensors enable us to collect medical data, contributing to developing smart models in the healthcare sector. Health monitoring models are still not so advanced, as most of them are stand-alone applications that need to be merged with mobile technologies to discard the constraint of stand-alone applications. Health Service provider, policy, and decision maker need correct, accurate, and timely data to improve healthcare systems and the quality of services rendered by them. Mobile and sensors bridge the gap of timely data collection in healthcare industry so that smart medical models need to be developed by researchers. The expected benefits of merging all three fields together include high-quality medical services, reduced treatment and diagnosis cost, reduced mortality rate due to early disease detection, and effective decision making. Integrating valuable information, knowledge, and Internet of Things (IoT) technologies in healthcare sector ensures medical data and patient security, provides better health policies, and facilitates the use of smart healthcare models by government healthcare sector. Healthcare informatics is gaining attention these days, both by researchers and by government healthcare organizations.

Data produced within healthcare sector has grown tremendously, and analysis of medical data is required, as it leads to providing best healthcare models for practitioners and aids effective decision making. Many challenges are associated with healthcare records, for example, managing and analyzing this data in an effective, secure, and reliable manner. Healthcare informatics helps in gaining insight to medical data so that quality of services produced by healthcare is improved. Accurate, precise, and timely data is the foundation of smart healthcare models. Nowadays, mobile-based data collection is gaining popularity for improving the quality of healthcare services. Also, biomedical sensors have enabled a new advanced generation of health information systems. Mobile medical technology and biomedical/body sensors can reduce the overall cost and improve the quality of services offered by smart healthcare models, such as continuously monitoring health indicators using body sensors on mobile screen, tracking real health data when a patient undergoes any surgery or therapy, or recommending exercises or diet based on patient profile. Smartphone is the basic need of everyone, so by integrating healthcare system into a mobile, many patients are able to manage their health needs. Telemedicine is integrated with these devices and mobile apps via advanced medical devices. Body sensors and mobile apps support fitness, calculate calories, detect disease, suggest treatment options, suggest drugs based on patient history, and manage disease collaboratively. Insight gained from data mining and machine learning will drive telemedicine for creation of smart healthcare systems. Modern medical advancement and data mining motivate and advance the need and progress of smart healthcare models for better healthcare quality.

Audience and Prerequisites

This book is mainly targeted at researchers, undergraduate and postgraduate students, academicians, and scholars working in the area of data science and its application to health sciences. Also, this book is beneficial for engineers who are engaged in developing actual healthcare solutions. This book helps the readers to have an acquaintance toward open-source software for data analysis, data processing, and data mining. Moreover, in several sections of this book, different datasets are used, thereby exploring real case studies related to medical informatics. This book will also be a useful resource for the learners to have some prior ideas regarding machine learning, data analytics, computer vision, and sustainable computing.

Editors

Dr. Adwitiya Sinha has completed Ph.D. from School of Computer & Systems Science (SCSS), Jawaharlal Nehru University (JNU) New Delhi, India. She was also awarded with *Senior Research Fellowship* (SRF) from *Council of Scientific & Industrial Research* (CSIR), New Delhi, India. She is presently working as assistant professor (senior grade) in the Department of Computer Science, Jaypee Institute of Information Technology (JIIT), Noida, Sector 62, Uttar Pradesh, India. She has been organizing and conducting special sessions in several international conferences as chairperson and session chair for invited sessions. She has also delivered lectures series in *The Consortium for Educational Communication* (CEC), University Grants Commission (UGC), and gave several invited talks in *The Human Resource Development Centre* (HRDC), JNU, New Delhi, India, on sensor networks and social media sciences. She has been promoted to IEEE Senior Member in 2019 by *The Institute of Electrical and Electronics Engineers* (IEEE), New York, USA. Her major research interest lies in sustainable computing, social networking, large-scale graph algorithms, and wireless sensor networks.

Megha Rathi is presently working as assistant professor (Senior Grade) in the Department of Computer Science, JIIT, Noida, Sector 62, Uttar Pradesh, India. She has ten years of teaching experience and worked on a research project of Xform generator at National Informatics Centre (NIC), Delhi, India. She has experience in software development and worked as a project associate at Indian Institute of Technology (IIT), Delhi, India. She has organized several special sessions in international conferences and also delivered invited talk. Her research areas include sustainable computing, data mining, data science analytics, health science, and machine learning.

Contributors

Harshit Agarwal
Department of Computer Science
Jaypee Institute of Information
  Technology
Noida, Uttar Pradesh, India

Urvi Agarwal
Department of Computer Science
Jaypee Institute of Information
  Technology
Noida, Uttar Pradesh, India

Uday Aggarwal
Department of Computer Science
Jaypee Institute of Information
  Technology
Noida, Uttar Pradesh, India

Siddharth Agrawal
Department of Computer Science
Jaypee Institute of Information Technology
Noida, Uttar Pradesh, India

Niyati Baliyan
Department of Computer Science
Indira Gandhi Delhi Technical University
  for Women
Delhi, India

Rakhi Bansal
Department of Biotechnology
Jaypee Institute of Information Technology
Noida, Uttar Pradesh, India

Priti Bhardwaj
Centre for Development of Advanced
  Computing
Indira Gandhi Delhi Technical University
  for Women
Delhi, India
and
Centre for Development of Advanced
  Computing
Noida, Uttar Pradesh, India

Prantik Biswas
Department of Computer Science
Jaypee Institute of Information Technology
Noida, Uttar Pradesh, India

Arjun Singh Chauhan
Department of Computer Science
Jaypee Institute of Information Technology
Noida, Uttar Pradesh, India

Nisha Chaurasia
Department of Computer Science
Jaypee Institute of Information Technology
Noida, Uttar Pradesh, India

Shweta Dang
Department of Biotechnology
Jaypee Institute of Information Technology
Noida, Uttar Pradesh, India

Suma Dawn
Department of Computer Science
Jaypee Institute of Information Technology
Noida, Uttar Pradesh, India

Asmita Dixit
Department of Computer Science
Jaypee Institute of Information Technology
Noida, Uttar Pradesh, India

Reema Gabrani
Department of Biotechnology
Jaypee Institute of Information Technology
Noida, Uttar Pradesh, India

Muskan Garg
Department of Computer Science
Jaypee Institute of Information Technology
Noida, Uttar Pradesh, India

Siddharth Gaur
Department of Computer Science
Jaypee Institute of Information Technology
Noida, Uttar Pradesh, India

Abhinav Gautam
Department of Computer Science
Jaypee Institute of Information Technology
Noida, Uttar Pradesh, India

Ritu Ghildiyal
Department of Biotechnology
Jaypee Institute of Information and
  Technology
Noida, Uttar Pradesh, India

Charu Goyal
Department of Computer Science
Jaypee Institute of Information
  Technology
Noida, Uttar Pradesh, India

Shilpa Gundagatti
Department of Computer Science
Deewan Group of Institutions
Meerut, Uttar Pradesh, India

Sonal Gupta
Department of Biotechnology
Jaypee Institute of Information Technology
Noida, Uttar Pradesh, India

Chetan Jadon
Department of Computer Science
Jaypee Institute of Information Technology
Noida, Uttar Pradesh, India

Samyak Jain
Department of Computer Science
Jaypee Institute of Information Technology
Noida, Uttar Pradesh, India

Atinderpal Kaur
Department of Biotechnology
Jaypee Institute of Information Technology
Noida, Uttar Pradesh, India

Raghav Maheshwari
Department of Computer Science
Jaypee Institute of Information Technology
Noida, Uttar Pradesh, India

Aparajita Nanda
Department of Computer Science
Jaypee Institute of Information Technology
Noida, Uttar Pradesh, India

Mahima Narang
Department of Computer Science
Jaypee Institute of Information Technology
Noida, Uttar Pradesh, India

Charu Nigam
Department of Computer Science
Jaypee Institute of Information Technology
Noida, Uttar Pradesh, India

Sanchi Prakash
Department of Computer Science
Jaypee Institute of information Technology
Noida, Uttar Pradesh, India

Neetigyata Pratap
Department of Biotechnology
Jaypee Institute of Information and
  Technology
Noida, Uttar Pradesh, India

Megha Rathi
Department of Computer Science
Jaypee Institute of Information Technology
Noida, Uttar Pradesh, India

Jatin Shad
Department of Computer Science
Jaypee Institute of Information Technology
Noida, Uttar Pradesh, India

Garima Sharma
Department of Biotechnology
Jaypee Institute of Information and
  Technology
Noida, Uttar Pradesh, India

Shubham Sharma
Department of Computer Science
Jaypee Institute of Information Technology
Noida, Uttar Pradesh, India

Amit Singh
Department of Computer Science
Jaypee Institute of Information Technology
Noida, Uttar Pradesh, India

Deepti Singh
Department of Computer Science
Jaypee Institute of Information Technology
Noida, Uttar Pradesh, India

Ananya Singhal
Department of Computer Science
Jaypee Institute of Information Technology
Noida, Uttar Pradesh, India

Adwitiya Sinha
Department of Computer Science
Jaypee Institute of Information Technology
Noida, Uttar Pradesh, India

Ayush Srivastava
Department of Computer Science
Jaypee Institute of Information Technology
Noida, Uttar Pradesh, India

Mayank Deepak Thar
Department of Computer Science
Jaypee Institute of Information Technology
Noida, Uttar Pradesh, India

Ishant Tyagi
Department of Computer Science
Jaypee Institute of Information Technology
Noida, Uttar Pradesh, India

Ankita Verma
Department of Computer Science
Jaypee Institute of Information Technology
Noida, Uttar Pradesh, India

Ankit Vidyarthi
Department of Computer Science
Jaypee Institute of Information Technology
Noida, Uttar Pradesh, India

Japsehaj Singh Wahi
Department of Computer Science
Jaypee Institute of Information Technology
Noida, Uttar Pradesh, India

1

Big Data Analytics in Healthcare

Priti Bhardwaj
Indira Gandhi Delhi Technical University for Women
Centre for Development of Advanced Computing

Niyati Baliyan
Indira Gandhi Delhi Technical University for Women

CONTENTS

1.1 Introduction: Background and Driving Forces

Today's world experiences big data from every domain. Thus, big data means lots of data or huge amount of data. When we have business problems, big data does not solve technical problems or give us a technical edge; rather, it solves large and complex business problems that cannot be solved with conventional approaches. So, a note can be taken as follows:

Big data: a problem statement arising out of a business situation

As shown in Figure 1.1, various characteristics of big data may be defined as follows:

- Volume: Data is huge and cannot be stored in a single server.
- Velocity: This indicates the speed at which data enters a system.
- Variety: Data captured is not in a single format. It can be log files, images, audios, or sensors.
- Veracity: Veracity indicates truthfulness. Data comes from multiple sources; so before going into the final picture, it should be free from ambiguities.

Healthcare organizations can experience wonderful benefits through big data analytics (BDA). Existing study has not provided enough awareness to the discovery of big business worth of big data. To enlighten the development of BDA abilities and to obtain profits from these abilities in a healthcare firm, a model has been introduced by Wang and Hajli (2017)

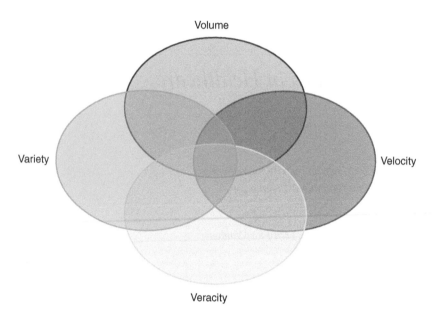

FIGURE 1.1
Characteristics of big data.

using source-based theory and ability structure vision. Sixty-three healthcare bodies were explored to find the underlying associations linking BDA abilities and business value. New visions have to be reflected in healthcare on how to comprise BDA abilities for business revolution and present a practical basis that can motivate a more detailed exploration of BDA execution.

One of the most common neurodegenerative anarchies is Parkinson's disease (PD). To enhance the accomplishment of PD discovery, a source blending procedure containing a combination of gray (GM) and white matter (WM) tissue maps and a decision fusion technique merging all classifiers' output through correlation-based feature selection (CFS) method by mass selection were used (Cigdem & Demirel, 2018).

For all five classification algorithms, CFS gave the maximum outcome for all five diverse feature selection methods, while Support Vector Machine (SVM) provides the best classification performance, where 95% accuracy has been achieved with this fusion technique of GM and WM.

A significant research topic in healthcare is determining an individual's risk of developing a certain disorder. An important step in personalized healthcare is precisely recognizing the level of likeness among patients based on their past reports. We need an efficient way to compute individual similarity on electronic health record (EHR) because EHRs are unevenly distributed and have various individual visit lengths and cannot be used to evaluate patient similarity because of inappropriate representation. In Suo et al. (2018), two new deep parallel learning schemes concurrently discover patient exhibitions and compute match up similarity. Convolutional neural network (CNN) has been used to detain neighboring vital statistics in EHRs. Disease predictions and patient clustering were also carried out in experiments using the similarity information. The outcome was that CNN can enhance representations of longitudinal EHR patterns.

There has to be an assurance of improved elasticity in industries along with group personalization, superior quality, and enhanced output such that organizations can deal with threats of progressively manufacturing more individualized products with a short lead time to market and advanced value. Intellectual production has to play an important role. We can convert resources into intellectual things so that they can respond spontaneously within a well-turned-out environment. For this, intellectual production, Internet of Things (IoT) and cloud manufacturing have been reviewed by Zhong et al. (2017). Similarities and dissimilarities have been discussed corresponding to these topics. Some core technologies such as IoT, cyberphysical systems, cloud computing, BDA, and information and communications technology have also been taken into consideration.

Research has shown that big data and prophetic analytics (BDPA) communicate a different governmental ability, and little is known about their performance effects, in particular contextual conditions (inter alia, national context and culture, and firm size). A trial has been done on 205 Indian manufacturing firms. The effects of BDPA have been investigated by Dubey et al. (2017) on public performance (PP) and ecological performance (EP) using variance-based structural equation modeling. It has been found that BDPA has an important bang on PP/EP.

The growth of information and communication technology is giving us a flow of new and computerized data associated with how nation and organizations work together. To convert this information into facts, considering the primary behavior of social and monetary mediums, organizations and researchers must tackle large amounts of unstructured and assorted data. To obtain success in task data analysis, the process should be carefully planned and organized considering the characteristics of economic and societal analysis and should include a vast multiplicity of heterogeneous sources of data and a strict supremacy strategy. A big data structural design has been constructed by Blazquez and Domenech (2018), which appropriately combines most of the nonconventional information resources and data analysis methods so as to offer a particularly planned structure for predicting public and profitable behaviors, trends, and changes.

As information technology is growing fast, people can shop online as well as provide feedbacks on social websites. The content that is generated by customers on social media is helpful to understand the shopping pattern of customers and to predict the future purchase. Today, customers are visiting the websites and see a lot of recommendations.

In Table 1.1, there are two customers: customer 1 and customer 2, and their buying patterns on a shopping website have been shown. Like Amazon has a lot of products and users, it needs to find the buying pattern of users and the relation between users. Customer 1 and customer 2 are matched, since their buying patterns are matched. So, the recommendation engine will give a choice of iPhone to customer 2.

It is difficult to analyze the customer-generated content on social media. Xu et al. (2017a) examined the characteristics of hotel products and services to observe consumer contentment and disappointment on the basis of online consumer textual feedbacks. Significant attributes motivating contentment and disappointment have been recognized using text mining approach. Latent semantic analysis (LSA) has been applied toward hotel products

TABLE 1.1

Buying Patterns of Customers

Customer 1	Customer 2
Bought items: 1. Titan watch	Bought items: 1. Mac laptop
2. Mac laptop	2. Titan watch
3. iPhone	

and service attributes. Business managers are helped to gain a better understanding of consumer's requests through customer-generated content on websites. We are living in an electronic world, and fresh technologies or implementations are arising with an exponential growth of data. A three-aspect model is proposed by Stylianou and Talias (2017), taking the concern of big data in medical background and to increase the alertness of the considerations that a healthcare person may face in the upcoming time.

Increased higher load on healthcare and the subsequent sprain on funds give rise to the need for ways to increase treatment efficiency. The solution is to use a forecast model to recognize the risk factors for the entire duration of treatment. Execution of a new prediction tool and the first use of an active interpreter in professional therapy practice have been presented by Haraldsson et al. (2017). The tool is rationalized from time to time and enhanced with hereditary upgrading of software. The consequences have shown the consistency and accuracy of predictions for the entire treatment duration. The predictor classified the patients with 100% accuracy and correctness based on formerly hidden records after a learning period of 3 weeks. Professionals are using this predictor to make decisions in complex live systems.

To concentrate on all aspects of care delivery, a standard operating procedure through patient information analysis is medical brainpower. Medical intelligence techniques have been presented through data mining and procedure mining (Giacalone, Cusatelli, & Santarcangelo, 2018). It shows the comparison between these two approaches.

People fitness management (PFM) has been proposed by Wan (2018), and it pays attention on people having risk of chronic disorders who also have the utmost healthcare expenses. People health and PFM have been explained, along with problems in harmonized care. The performance and assessment of People Health Management (PHM) made use of EHRs and other data; and projected PHM practice and exploration.

Cloud computing, BDA, and other rapidly increasing technologies are growing, so the amalgamation of intellectuality and e-commerce systems is required to make a system with improved efficiency, minimized business costs, and groomed information. The expansion of these kinds of systems is still to be achieved (Song et al., 2017). To offer a better understanding of this smart system and assist for upcoming research, Song et al. (2017) explain this type of system in terms of cloud computing, IoT, mobile network, social media, and BDA.

Thus far, we know that big data application functions are the main part of healthcare operations. The study by Van den Broek and van Veenstra (2018) also provided a widespread, detailed, and organized reading of the advanced tools in the big data associated to healthcare uses in five types, including heuristic-based, cloud-based, machine learning, representative-based, and hybrid techniques.

Storing, processing, transporting, mining, and serving the data are big data challenges. The concept of shared computing is being provided by cloud computing. This study by Yang et al. (2017) surveyed the two frontlines—cloud computing and big data. It focuses on the benefits and outcomes of using cloud computing to handle big data in this universe and applicable discipline. This study introduces upcoming revolutions and a research outline that cloud computing will sustain the renovation of the characteristics of big data, that is, volume, velocity, variety, and veracity into morals of big data for local global applications.

The enormous population growth is giving rise to new questions of managing a huge amount of population vital statistics. With the development of digitization, various measures have been presented to tackle big data. The majority of measures deal with a conventional coherent database; therefore, we are unable to utilize big data proficiently and precisely. The well-known platform available is Apache Hadoop to deal with problems of big data. In Bukhari, Park, and Shin (2018), a big data managing structure has been presented beneath Hadoop ecology to resolve the subject of large data scaling of growing population. Sqoop, HBase, and Hive have been considered as main mechanisms. A method is being given to transfer the data from various Relational Database Management Systems (RDBMSs) to Hadoop HBase. Additionally, HBase–Hive amalgamation is a nice structural design to pile up and query data for analyzing the data professionally. This approach will provide expansion in handling big data and will gradually enhance analytics, such as encouraging rational agriculture, prohibiting poverty, and minimizing mortality.

Currently, obesity is posing a grave health concern and thereby causing numerous diseases like diabetes, cancer, and heart ailments. The ways to measure obesity levels are not common enough to be practical in every context (such as an expecting woman or an aged person) and also present precise results. Therefore, Jindal, Baliyan, and Rana (2018) employ the R ensemble prediction model and Python interface and observe that predicted values of obesity are 89.68% accurate. Their work may be expanded to predict other body-illness parameters and recommend rectification based on obesity values.

In this world of information technology, where everyone is busy with their day-to-day activities, we may call it a more digitized world. However, health of an individual is important at the same time. Data is dispersed in the form of statistics, reports, forms, etc. Although a lot of research has already been implemented in several domains, healthcare is providing a broad horizon to utilize previously prepared data and obtain innovative outcomes for humanity. Healthcare generates a large amount of big data in different varieties.

Every human being needs a healthy heart to lead a happy life. If the heart does not work well, many other problems develop in the body. There are chances of loss of human life if the heart becomes nonoperational. If blood flow is not regular, it affects the normal functioning of body. Sometimes it leads to heart attack. Therefore, the heart acts as a significant organ in human body, and thus prediction of heart diseases with accuracy is crucial. The objective is to predict a disease in advance, i.e., diseases should be prevented with early intervention rather than treating the disease after it is diagnosed. We need a system where one will be able to know the details of a disease just by one identity, i.e., fingerprint of the concerned person. Also, we know very well that human fingerprints are the detailed identity of a person. Fingerprints are difficult to change during the lifetime of an individual. Thus, people should be prevented from the risk of diseases.

Data mining and machine learning have been used to get insight about large amounts of medical records that are being generated in healthcare sector. This chapter studies the relationships among various diseases and the machine learning algorithms used for the same. With the enormous accessible data, it is important to bring some perception that can facilitate decision management in actual conditions.

1.2 Related Work

Big data is of no use until and unless it derives some significant information out of the resources in healthcare industry. There are amazing advantages of BDA in healthcare firm from an extent of disease prediction to hospitality. Some of the previous works done in applications of BDA in healthcare are as follows.

In the work of Al Mayahi, Al-Badi, and Tarhini (2018), the objective is to explore the possible benefits of BDA in healthcare to magnify the productivity of healthcare resources.

Naïve Bayesian and J48 algorithms have been used with Weka 3.8 tool on kidney disease dataset from University of California (UCI) website, giving an accuracy of 95% and 100%, respectively, for predictive analysis. Al Mayahi, Al-Badi, and Tarhini proposed evidence-based treatment, predictive analysis, and decision making in healthcare.

Wang, Kung, and Byrd (2018) aimed at understanding the strategic implementations of big data. Twenty-six big data cases from healthcare are collected followed by a three-phase research process: elementary content analysis (i.e., construction, arrangement, summarizing). It recommended data governance, fostering information sharing culture in target healthcare organizations, use of cloud computing for data storage in healthcare industry, and generation of new business ideas.

Rajamhoana et al. (2018) analyze various research works carried out on heart disease prediction and classification and then determine the effective ones. Machine learning and deep learning techniques are applied on the heart disease dataset of 303 records from UCI repository with input, key, and predictable attributes. It was revealed that artificial neural network (ANN) gives better performance.

Saini, Baliyan and Bassi (2017) focus on the treatment of heart disease at the correct time with greater accuracy. Bagging, boosting techniques, and hybrid classifier with weighted voting (HCWV) are applied on a dataset of 76 attributes, and these attributes are compared in SVM, linear Generalized Linear Model (GLM-SVM) bagging, and linear and GLM boosting. Greater accuracy was achieved in heart disease prediction with hybridization of data mining approaches.

Yuvaraj and SriPreethaa (2017) present the use of machine learning algorithms in Hadoop-based clusters for diabetes prediction, and the results show promise for extremely accurate diabetes predictive healthcare systems. For validation of algorithm's working, the dataset used is Pima Indians Diabetes Database from National Institute of Diabetes and Digestive Diseases (2016).

The objective of Maji and Arora (2019) was to predict and prevent heart disease with data mining approaches. Here, decision tree technique C4.5 has been hybridized with ANN technique and applied on 270 × 13 Another RDF Encoding Form (AREF) format dataset in UCI using Weka. The hybrid model gave good results with greater accuracy.

Jain and Singh (2018) aimed at prediction of chronic disease by feature selection and classification system. Filter, wrapper, embedded, and hybrid feature selection has been used, and traditional, adaptive, and parallel classification has been compared. Accuracy, reactivity, specificity, correctness, F-measure, and false positive rate are computed mathematically to measure the performance of classification methods. It proposed that feature selection filter method is more efficient for accurate classification of disease.

The objective of Vlachostergiou et al. (2018) was to improve PD prediction. Multitasking learning (MTL) layer was adopted as a research methodology. Primary task was Dopamine Transporter (DaT) scan, and auxiliary tasks were patient's age and sex. The following features were taken into consideration: Magnetic Resonance Imaging (MRI) of the brain; DaT scans; epidemiological data, age, and gender; time span of a disease; medical information; and clinical data. MTL outperforms the single task learning model, and 83% accuracy was achieved after choosing sex as auxiliary task.

This study was conducted to develop an economic solution for remote consultation by doctors. Patient care monitoring system based on website was developed with a Windows, Apache, MySQL and PHP (WAMP) server and RDBMS. A cost-effective prototype was established to communicate between a patient with sensor application and a remote specialist (Choudhury et al., 2017).

Suo et al. (2017) focused on personalized disease prediction models. The following methods were adopted: measuring patient similarity and preparation of personalized prediction model using K-Nearest Neighbor (KNN), discrimination, and weighted sampling on a dataset of clinical applications of 10,000 patients over 2 years for diabetes, obesity, and chronic obstructive pulmonary disease. It interpreted that there is better vector representation by CNN-based models, and individual disease prediction is a better fit for patients.

Christensen et al. (2018) focused on conversion of dissimilar data sources into significant measures of a person's health. An experiment was conducted on a dataset of 466,715 patients that focused on predicting five high-impact preventable chronic conditions. It interpreted that eXtreme Gradient Boosting (XGBoost) (XGB) is highly interpretable and performs consistently better than long short-term memory (LSTM) (Table 1.2).

1.3 Observations

From the review conducted, it has been observed that big data is impacting the healthcare domain. With the changing business spectra, people face business challenges every day, so we have to find a platform to make this big data beneficial to humanity. Mostly, researchers focused on using data mining and machine learning techniques for disease prediction in healthcare. A new approach of deep learning has been used in some research papers. The research focused on evidence-based treatments, predictive analysis, and decision making in healthcare; importance of ANN in heart disease prediction; and fusion of data mining approaches for analysis of heart problems with greater accuracy. The main thing research emphasized is not to ignore the importance of simple models. Various classification algorithms have been used: generalized linear model, Lasso, Bayesian regularized neural network, SVM, neural network, decision tree, regression tree, multivariate adaptive regression spline, XGB, and LSTM. Accuracy of each algorithm has been computed by examining each algorithm on a training dataset. Bagging and boosting techniques have been employed.

CNN, a technique of deep learning, has been used to show that MTL outperforms the single task learning model. With the help of CNN, a time-fusion framework has been developed to perform the process of individual disease projection. A research work has shown that XGB is a highly interpretable model of disease prediction.

We should look toward hybrid approaches. One approach has been proposed—HCWV. Another was the technique of decision tree, i.e., C4.5 was integrated with ANN and termed as hybrid decision tree.

We can remove the noisy and redundant features by hybrid approaches. Efficient feature selection method can be used for accurate classification of disease.

To improve success rate and reduce the decision-making time for diagnosis of chronic disease, adaptive and parallel classification systems can be used for chronic disease prediction.

Figure 1.2 gives a pictorial representation of various methodologies employed toward BDA in healthcare, particularly disease prediction. It has been found that most researchers have tried to follow hybrid and deep learning approaches (Wang & Hajli, 2017).

TABLE 1.2

Summary of Recent Related Works

Work	Objective	Methodology	Tools/Data	Contributions	Limitations
Al Mayahi, Al-Badi, and Tarhini (2018)	To explore advantages of BDAs in healthcare	Naïve Bayesian and J48 tree algorithms	Weka3.8, kidney disease dataset from UCI website	Naïve Bayesian and J48 gave 95% and 100% accuracy for predictive analysis	Other data mining algorithms may be compared on the given dataset for performance
Wang, Kung, and Byrd (2018)	To address the lack of understanding of strategic implementations of big data	Elementary content analysis (i.e., construction, arrangement, summarizing)	26 big data cases from healthcare industries	Recommendations for fostering information sharing culture and use of cloud computing for data storage in healthcare	Need for efficient unstructured data analytical algorithms and applications
Rajamhoana et al. (2018)	To analyze the various research works on heart disease prediction for effectiveness and accuracy	Machine learning and deep learning	UCI dataset of 303 records with input, key, and predictable attributes	Adjudged better performance of ANN in heart disease prediction	Ensemble methods and hybrid system can be used for improving prediction accuracy
Saini, Baliyan and Bassi (2017)	To prevent heart disease with greater accuracy at the right time	Bagging, boosting, and HCWV	76 attributes compared in SVM, linear GLM-SVM bagging, linear and GLM boosting	Achieved a greater accuracy in heart disease prediction with hybridization of data mining approaches	Majority/weighted voting and other fusion scheme for classifiers need to be explored further
Maji and Arora (2019)	Prediction and prevention of heart disease by data mining	Decision Tree C4.5 hybridized with ANN	270×13 AREF format data in UCI, Weka	Hybrid model with greater accuracy	Need for upscaling datasets and increasing the number of experimental runs
Jain and Singh (2018)	Prediction of chronic disease by feature selection and classification	Filter, wrapper, embedded and hybrid feature selection; traditional, adaptive, and parallel classification	Accuracy, reactivity, specificity, correctness, F-measure, false positive rate computed mathematically	Feature selection filter method is more efficient for accurate classification of disease	Noisy and redundant features can be removed by introducing hybrid approaches
Vlachostergiou et al. (2018)	To improve PD prediction	MTL layer, primary task: DaT scans, auxiliary task: patient's age and sex	Features: MRI of the brain, DaT scans, epidemiological data, age, gender, time span of a disease, medical information, clinical data	MTL outperforms the single task learning model, 83% accuracy achieved after choosing sex as auxiliary task	MRI of the brain, time span of disease, duration of dopaminergic treatment, medical dose can be taken into account for more models

(Continued)

TABLE 1.2 (Continued)

Summary of Recent Related Works

Work	Objective	Methodology	Tools/Data	Contributions	Limitations
Choudhury et al. (2017)	To develop an economic solution for remote consultation by doctors	Patient Care Monitoring System based on website	WAMP server, RDBMS	Cost-effective prototype established to communicate between one patient with sensor application and remote specialist	Different types of sensors to be used to store the data into cloud, and upgradation of disease analysis module with more accurate prediction
Suo et al. (2017)	To focus on personalized disease prediction models	Measuring patient similarity and preparation of personalized prediction model using KNN, discriminate and weighted sampling	Dataset of clinical applications of 10,000 patients over 2 years for diabetes, obesity, chronic obstructive pulmonary disease	Better vector representation by CNN-based models, individual disease prediction is better fit for patients	Deep learning models can be used in other scenarios
Christensen et al. (2018)	Conversion of dissimilar data sources into significant measures of person health	Experiment focuses on predicting five high-impact preventable chronic conditions	Dataset of 466,715 patients	XGB is highly interpretable and consistently the best performer in comparison to LSTM	Could combine the strength of XGB and LSTM to create better classifier
Narayanan, Paul, and Joseph (2017)	To provide some research idea in big data in healthcare	Rough set theory and neural network	Literature survey of 70 papers	Security and neural network are future research areas	Vulnerability of big data has to be taken into account
Johri et al. (2017b)	To address the issue of patient matching records in EHRs	Fuzzy logic BDA	30 individual evidences from 5 different equipment	Improved individual data matching technique for high-volume and high-velocity data	Combined fuzzy algorithms on Hadoop ecology
Johri et al. (2017a)	To focus on the use of large datasets for the end user	Hadoop, Hive, and R	Records of India and China and measure blood pressure	Increase in systolic blood pressure leads to more diabetic patients	More analytic techniques to increase national income
Tse et al. (2018)	To study about the supremacy of big data in healthcare	A qualitative approach of studying research papers	Google scholar	A data ascendancy strategy should be prepared.	Balance between medical data and security concerns
Popovic (2017)	Importance of distributed data networks in healthcare	Machine learning	U.S. Food and Drug Administration	An approach of machine learning for population health analytics	Distributed networks as a data analytical tool

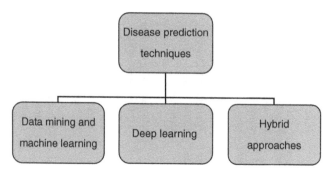

FIGURE 1.2
Disease prediction techniques.

1.4 Open Challenges

Coupled with the advent of big data, the healthcare data is perennially and promptly expanding, with humongous and varied values. There is a broad range of variable data in the form of images, text, video, unprocessed raw sensor data, etc., which are produced and need to be effectively saved, processed, retrieved, indexed, and analyzed. These datasets may serve different purposes while answering different research questions and solving different real-world problems, patient-oriented data such as electronic medical records, public-oriented data such as public health data, and knowledge-oriented data such as drug-to-drug, drug-to-disease, and disease-to-disease interaction repositories. Examples of works on disease-specific big data researches include the following: survival time prediction in breast cancer (Mihaylov, Nisheva, & Vassilev, 2018), a survey to outline the progress in machine learning solutions as applied to cardiac computed tomography as well as to provide clinicians with an understanding of its pros and cons (Singh et al., 2018), a survey of analytical techniques to predict cancer risk that aims to improve patient outcomes and reduce healthcare costs (Richter & Khoshgoftaar, 2018), a practical cardiovascular diseases risk prediction system based on data mining techniques to provide auxiliary medical service (Xu et al., 2017b), mild cognitive impairment prediction method based on an ensemble of one versus all multiclass classifiers which uses the revised Analysis of variance (ANOVA) feature selection method of MRI cortical and subcortical features and analyzes feature dimension reduction via multiclass partial least squares (Ramírez et al., 2018), etc.

Among generic works on leveraging big data technologies coupled with machine learning algorithms, specially ensemble techniques, are works such as prediction of infectious disease using deep learning and big data (Chae, Kwon, & Lee, 2018), using a structural graph-coupled ensemble model for disease risk prediction in a Telehealthcare scenario (Lafta et al., 2018), classification and prediction of disease likelihood using machine learning on multi-GPU cluster MapReduce system (Li, Chen, & Liu, 2017), multilevel incremental influence measure-based classification of medical data for enhanced classification (Ananthajothi & Subramaniam, 2018), etc.

The open issue in aforementioned and related research is that the clinical data must be structured, frequently captured, and clinically relevant. Effective improved modeling methods are lacking in current work. Big data in healthcare brings great challenges but plays an important role in healthcare transformation. The traditional techniques do not compromise end-users' Quality of Service (QoS) in terms of data availability, data response delay, etc. It is urgent to develop software tools and techniques that support rapid query processing, speed up data analytics, and provide awareness and knowledge in real time (Zhang et al., 2018).

We may outline the following research gaps based on our analysis of the limitations of existing works.

- To understand the unstructured data in healthcare, i.e., unspecified patient's information in the form of clinical notes.
- To compare different data mining algorithms to increase the performance.
- To develop significant algorithms and applications to perform analysis of unstructured data.
- To plan multiple learning methods and hybrid systems (combination of artificial intelligence (AI) methods and techniques) for improving the disease prediction rate, thus improving the survival rate of mankind.
- To focus on the hybridization of classification methods to enhance the precision of classifier and optimize computational efficiency of results.
- To ensure the best use of healthcare resources, more parameters are considered such as time span of disease, MRI of the brain, dopaminergic treatment, and medical data.

1.5 Proposed Solutions

As data is growing in the form of big data in healthcare, a cost-effective smart healthcare solution needs to be proposed, which will try to remove the barriers of using big data in healthcare and will assist doctors to make decisions in no time and enhance individual care. Patients having complicated medical stories, distressed from numerous situations will be benefitted with this model. Innovative mechanisms are yet to be projected for the prediction of diseases, for instance, patients who have been predicted with diabetes can be suggested to take a periodical supervision of their weight. Data mining algorithms, multiple learning methods and hybrid systems and deep neural network can be used for improving the prediction rate, thus improving survival rate. Figure 1.3 outlines the proposed framework incorporating the aforementioned aspects. Figure 1.4 gives a pictorial representation of various data analysis techniques.

First, we have to take care of the following challenges of big data.

$$\text{Storing} + \text{processing} + \text{transporting} + \text{mining} + \text{serving the data}$$

And the following perception may be taken.

$$\text{Machine learning models} + \text{Clarifications for the decisions taken} + \text{Medical knowledge}$$

$$= \text{Significant judgment}$$

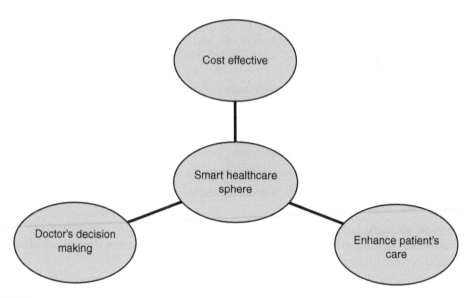

FIGURE 1.3
Proposed solution.

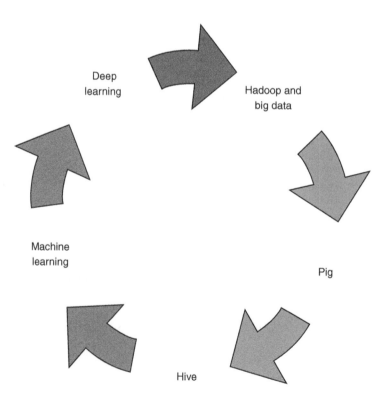

FIGURE 1.4
Data analysis techniques.

1.6 Conclusion

We interpreted that healthcare group accepts BDA's power and abilities and assists them to develop further valuable data analysis techniques. There is a need for integrating big data with healthcare. We have to retain time, strength, and funds for using big data in healthcare to enhance patients' condition, spectacularly, as well as superiority of medical care and contentment; that is, in general, health of the people ought to be enhanced eventually.

References

Al Mayahi, S., Al-Badi, A., & Tarhini, A. (2018, August). Exploring the potential benefits of big data analytics in providing smart healthcare. In *International Conference for Emerging Technologies in Computing* (pp. 247–258). Springer, Cham, London, UK.

Ananthajothi, K., & Subramaniam, M. (2018). Multi level incremental influence measure based classification of medical data for improved classification. *Cluster Computing*, 1–8. doi: 10.1007/s10586-018-2498-z.

Blazquez, D., & Domenech, J. (2018). Big Data sources and methods for social and economic analyses. *Technological Forecasting and Social Change, 130*, 99–113.

Bukhari, S. S., Park, J., & Shin, D. R. (2018, June). Hadoop based demography big data management system. In *19th IEEE/ACIS International Conference on Software Engineering, Artificial Intelligence, Networking and Parallel/Distributed Computing (SNPD), 2018* (pp. 93–98). IEEE, Busan Gwang'yeogsi, South Korea.

Chae, S., Kwon, S., & Lee, D. (2018). Predicting infectious disease using deep learning and big data. *International Journal of Environmental Research and Public Health, 15*(8), 1596.

Cigdem, O., & Demirel, H. (2018). Performance analysis of different classification algorithms using different feature selection methods on Parkinson's disease detection. *Journal of Neuroscience Methods, 309*, 81–90.

Choudhury, A., Krishnan, R., Gupta, A., Swathi, Y., & Supriya, C. (2017, August). Remote patient care monitoring system for rural healthcare. In *International Conference on Energy, Communication, Data Analytics and Soft Computing (ICECDS), 2017* (pp. 2593–2598). IEEE, Chennai, India.

Christensen, T., Frandsen, A., Glazier, S., Humpherys, J., & Kartchner, D. (2018, June). Machine learning methods for disease prediction with claims data. In *IEEE International Conference on Healthcare Informatics (ICHI), 2018* (pp. 467–4674). IEEE, Hilton Metropolitan, NY.

Dubey, R., Gunasekaran, A., Childe, S. J., Papadopoulos, T., Luo, Z., Wamba, S. F., & Roubaud, D. (2017). Can big data and predictive analytics improve social and environmental sustainability? *Technological Forecasting and Social Change*. doi: 10.1016/j.techfore.2017.06.020.

Giacalone, M., Cusatelli, C., & Santarcangelo, V. (2018). Big data compliance for innovative clinical models. *Big Data Research, 12*, 35–40.

Haraldsson, S. O., Brynjolfsdottir, R. D., Woodward, J. R., Siggeirsdottir, K., & Gudnason, V. (2017, July). The use of predictive models in dynamic treatment planning. In *IEEE Symposium on Computers and Communications (ISCC), 2017* (pp. 242–247). IEEE, Heraklion.

Jain, D., & Singh, V. (2018). Feature selection and classification systems for chronic disease prediction: A review. *Egyptian Informatics Journal, 19*(3), 179–189.

Jindal, K., Baliyan, N., & Rana, P. S. (2018). Obesity prediction using ensemble machine learning approaches. In Sa, P., Bakshi, S., Hatzilygeroudis, I., Sahoo, M. (eds.) *Recent Findings in Intelligent Computing Techniques* (pp. 355–362). Springer, Singapore.

Johri, P., Singh, T., Das, S., & Anand, S. (2017a, December). Vitality of big data analytics in healthcare department. In *International Conference on Infocom Technologies and Unmanned Systems (Trends and Future Directions) (ICTUS), 2017* (pp. 669–673). IEEE, Crete.

Johri, P., Singh, T., Yadav, A., & Rajput, A. K. (2017b, December). Advanced patient matching: Recognizable patient view for decision support in healthcare using big data analytics. In *International Conference on Infocom Technologies and Unmanned Systems (Trends and Future Directions)(ICTUS), 2017* (pp. 652–656). IEEE, Amity University Dubai, Dubai International Academic City, Dubai.

Lafta, R., Zhang, J., Tao, X., Li, Y., Diykh, M., & Lin, J. C. W. (2018). A structural graph-coupled advanced machine learning ensemble model for disease risk prediction in a telehealthcare environment. In Roy, S., Samui, P., Deo, R., Ntalampiras, S. (eds) *Big Data in Engineering Applications* (pp. 363–384). Springer, Singapore.

Li, J., Chen, Q., & Liu, B. (2017). Classification and disease probability prediction via machine learning programming based on multi-GPU cluster MapReduce system. *The Journal of Supercomputing*, 73(5), 1782–1809.

Maji, S., & Arora, S. (2019). Decision tree algorithms for prediction of heart disease. In Fong, S., Akashe, S., Mahalle, P. (eds.) *Information and Communication Technology for Competitive Strategies* (pp. 447–454). Springer, Singapore.

Mihaylov, I., Nisheva, M., & Vassilev, D. (2018, September). Machine learning techniques for survival time prediction in breast cancer. In *International Conference on Artificial Intelligence: Methodology, Systems, and Applications* (pp. 186–194). Springer, Cham, Varna, Bulgaria.

Narayanan, U., Paul, V., & Joseph, S. (2017, August). Different analytical techniques for big data analysis: A review. In *International Conference on Energy, Communication, Data Analytics and Soft Computing (ICECDS), 2017* (pp. 372–382). IEEE, Chennai, India.

Pima Indians Diabetes Database (2016), Retrieved from https://www.kaggle.com/uciml/pima-indians-diabetes-database.

Popovic, J. R. (2017). Distributed data networks: A blueprint for Big Data sharing and healthcare analytics. *Annals of the New York Academy of Sciences*, 1387(1), 105–111.

Ramírez, J., Górriz, J. M., Ortiz, A., Martínez-Murcia, F. J., Segovia, F., Salas-Gonzalez, D., Castillo-Barnes, D., Illán, I. A., Puntonet, C. G. & Alzheimer's Disease Neuroimaging Initiative (2018). Ensemble of random forests One vs. Rest classifiers for MCI and AD prediction using ANOVA cortical and subcortical feature selection and partial least squares. *Journal of Neuroscience Methods*, 302, 47–57.

Rajamhoana, S. P., Devi, C. A., Umamaheswari, K., Kiruba, R., Karunya, K., & Deepika, R. (2018, July). Analysis of neural networks based heart disease prediction system. In *11th International Conference on Human System Interaction (HSI), 2018* (pp. 233–239). IEEE, Gdansk, Poland.

Richter, A. N., & Khoshgoftaar, T. M. (2018). A review of statistical and machine learning methods for modeling cancer risk using structured clinical data. *Artificial Intelligence in Medicine*, 90, 1–14.

Saini, M., Baliyan, N., & Bassi, V. (2017, August). Prediction of heart disease severity with hybrid data mining. In *2nd International Conference on Telecommunication and Networks (TEL-NET), 2017* (pp. 1–6). IEEE, Greece.

Singh, G., Al'Aref, S. J., Van Assen, M., Kim, T. S., van Rosendael, A., Kolli, K. K., Dwivedi, A., Maliakal, G., Pandey, M., Wang, J. & Do, V. (2018). Machine learning in cardiac CT: Basic concepts and contemporary data. *Journal of Cardiovascular Computed Tomography*, 12(3), 192–201.

Song, Z., Sun, Y., Wan, J., Huang, L., & Zhu, J. (2017). Smart e-commerce systems: Current status and research challenges. *Electronic Markets*, 1–18. doi: 10.1007/s12525-017-0272-3.

Stylianou, A., & Talias, M. A. (2017). Big data in healthcare: A discussion on the big challenges. *Health and Technology*, 7(1), 97–107.

Suo, Q., Ma, F., Yuan, Y., Huai, M., Zhong, W., Gao, J., & Zhang, A. (2018). Deep patient similarity learning for personalized healthcare. *IEEE Transactions on NanoBioscience*, 17(3), 219–227.

Suo, Q., Ma, F., Yuan, Y., Huai, M., Zhong, W., Zhang, A., & Gao, J. (2017, November). Personalized disease prediction using a cnn-based similarity learning method. In *IEEE International Conference on Bioinformatics and Biomedicine (BIBM), 2017* (pp. 811–816). IEEE, Kansas City, MO.

Tse, D., Chow, C. K., Ly, T. P., Tong, C. Y., & Tam, K. W. (2018, August). The challenges of big data governance in healthcare. In *17th IEEE International Conference on Trust, Security And Privacy In Computing and Communications/12th IEEE International Conference On Big Data Science And Engineering (TrustCom/BigDataSE), 2018* (pp. 1632–1636). IEEE, New York, NY.

Van den Broek, T., & van Veenstra, A. F. (2018). Governance of big data collaborations: How to balance regulatory compliance and disruptive innovation. *Technological Forecasting and Social Change, 129,* 330–338.

Vlachostergiou, A., Tagaris, A., Stafylopatis, A., & Kollias, S. (2018, October). Investigating the best performing task conditions of a multi-tasking learning model in healthcare using convolutional neural networks: Evidence from a Parkinson's disease database. In *25th IEEE International Conference on Image Processing (ICIP), 2018* (pp. 2047–2051). IEEE, Athens, Greece.

Wan, T. T. (2018). Evolving public health from population health to population health management. In Wan, T. T. (ed.) *Population Health Management for Poly Chronic Conditions* (pp. 3–15). Springer, Cham.

Wang, Y., & Hajli, N. (2017). Exploring the path to big data analytics success in healthcare. *Journal of Business Research, 70,* 287–299.

Wang, Y., Kung, L., & Byrd, T. A. (2018). Big data analytics: Understanding its capabilities and potential benefits for healthcare organizations. *Technological Forecasting and Social Change, 126,* 3–13.

Xu, X., Wang, X., Li, Y., & Haghighi, M. (2017a). Business intelligence in online customer textual reviews: Understanding consumer perceptions and influential factors. *International Journal of Information Management, 37*(6), 673–683.

Xu, S., Zhang, Z., Wang, D., Hu, J., Duan, X., & Zhu, T. (2017b, March). Cardiovascular risk prediction method based on CFS subset evaluation and random forest classification framework. In *IEEE 2nd International Conference on Big Data Analysis (ICBDA), 2017* (pp. 228–232). IEEE, Beijing, China.

Yang, C., Huang, Q., Li, Z., Liu, K., & Hu, F. (2017). Big Data and cloud computing: Innovation opportunities and challenges. *International Journal of Digital Earth, 10*(1), 13–53.

Yuvaraj, N., & SriPreethaa, K. R. (2017). Diabetes prediction in healthcare systems using machine learning algorithms on Hadoop cluster. *Cluster Computing,* 1–9. doi: 10.1007/s10586-017-1532-x.

Zhang, Y., Wang, H., Chen, M., Wan, J., & Humar, I. (2018). IEEE access special section editorial: Healthcare big data. *IEEE Access, 6,* 50555–50558.

Zhong, R. Y., Xu, X., Klotz, E., & Newman, S. T. (2017). Intelligent manufacturing in the context of industry 4.0: A review. *Engineering, 3*(5), 616–630.

2

Smart Medical Diagnosis

Raghav Maheshwari, Amit Singh, Siddharth Agrawal, and Adwitiya Sinha
Jaypee Institute of Information Technology

CONTENTS

2.1 Introduction: Background and Driving Forces

Smart Medical Diagnosis was made, keeping in mind, to ease the medical processes of detecting severe diseases and their treatment. Covering major diseases, like heart, diabetes, and cancers in human, we tried to provide an easy, user-friendly, and near-perfect prediction for general people (Agarwal & Sebastian, 2016). Simply through a search via the internet, a user can know if his/her symptoms will lead to anything serious or are just temporary.

We incorporated the datasets of diseases from named online resources like UCI Repository, Kaggle, and other medical servers. The dataset was sanitized initially, and standard machine learning algorithms were used in the disease prediction later on using R programming language. We have provided an amiable website for users to enter their symptoms and medical values to predict their disease. Just by clicking, one will get to know what is wrong with their heart or lungs or diabetes level. Moreover, it is an age-free application, i.e., it could be applicable for people of all age groups (Koh & Tan, 2011). The website is made with the help of a new technology, R Shiny. With the help of Hyper Text Markup Language (HTML), we were able to integrate various diseases under one URL.

Our purpose was to find the best algorithm that could work for all diseases. To do so, we have applied six different machine learning algorithms. These are linear, Bayesian, random forest, extreme gradient boosting, decision trees, and genetic algorithms. At the end, we found that extreme gradient boosting gives the most promising results in all disease datasets. Besides classifications, we have also provided data visualization to show relationship between different attributes for a disease (Bates et al., 2014). We have used various packages of R, like ggplots, pie charts, time analysis, etc., for a better experience.

2.2 Description and Experimentation

Smart Medical Diagnosis majorly covers five diseases: heart diseases, diabetes, Parkinson's disease, kidney diseases, and breast cancer.

The datasets were found from known online resources, such as UCI Repository, Kaggle, and other medical servers (Archenaa & Anita, 2015). The dataset was first cleaned, and only relevant parameters were chosen to which the various models could be applied.

For sanitization of data, we replaced the null values with the mean of the respective column. Rows having null values in more than 50% of its columns were removed completely. Relevant parameters were scaled and normalized as per the needs.

2.2.1 Heart Dataset

The heart dataset had ten attributes that highly affected the outcome of the disease. These attributes included the type of pain in the chest, cholesterol level, blood pressure, pulse rate, and other factors (Palaniappan & Awang, 2008). Though there were around 20 parameters, we narrowed it down to ten as per their importance on the prediction of the disease.

2.2.2 Diabetes Dataset

Not only the fluctuations in the insulin level of the body (Breault et al., 2002) but also many other factors, such as body mass index and age, have impacts on the level of diabetes. After cleaning the data, the correlation matrix was generated to check the relevance of the taken parameters; based on that, nine important factors were chosen.

2.2.3 Breast Cancer Dataset

In the case of breast cancer dataset, parameters like concavity, symmetry, texture, and others paved the way for the prediction of the disease (Reis-Filho & Pusztai, 2011). In total, 11 constraints were found to be the most valuable ones for breast cancer disease prediction.

2.2.4 Parkinson's Dataset

Parkinson's disease had several closely related yet distinct attributes, which increased the size of parameter list to 25. Apart from the average, maximum, and minimum vocal frequency, several measures like variation of fundamental frequency and amplitude, scaling factors, and so on contributed to disease prediction (Hughes et al., 2000).

2.2.5 Kidney Dataset

Parameters like red blood cells, white blood cells, pus cells, amount of urea in the blood, body sugar, blood glucose, and others raised the tally of favorable parameters to 25. The factors were chosen according to their position in the importance matrix and correlation matrix for the prediction of kidney disease.

2.3 Visualization

It is very important to visualize data before actually applying different algorithms. Visualization helps in seeing different kinds of relationship between different attributes of datasets.

2.3.1 Heart Disease

We saw that the attribute "Cp" (pain type of the chest) affects the most in predicting heart diseases, with "Chol" (cholesterol) following it (Figure 2.1). Many other attributes also play a prominent role in predicting heart disease (Soni et al., 2011).

The relationship between "Thalach" (max heart rate) and "Old Peak (OP)" (exercise relative excursion) was also interesting. As we can see, most of the occurrences are between 0.3

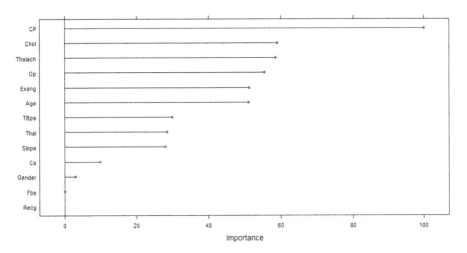

FIGURE 2.1
Relationship graph between attributes of heart and their importance.

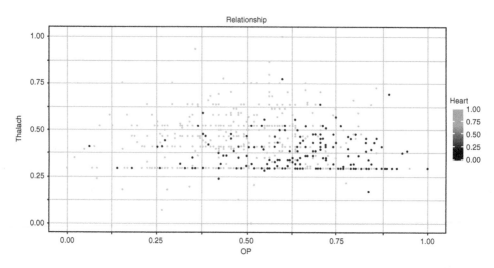

FIGURE 2.2
Comparison graph between Thalach and OP.

and 0.8 of OP and above 0.25 of Thalach, which implies that maximum heart rate is almost above 0.25, as shown in Figure 2.2.

2.3.2 Diabetes

Diabetes could attack anyone, but most importantly, pregnant women risk the chances of catching diabetes. We can clearly see in Figure 2.3 that as the rate of pregnancy increases, the risk of diabetes increases.

The correlation plot gives all 1s in the final boxes, which clearly indicates that all the attributes depend on each other for the correct prediction of diabetes, as shown in Figure 2.4.

Also, in Figure 2.5, the relationship between blood pressure and body mass index shows that they are closely related to each other. Increase in the value of one parameter directly affects the other, which at the end corresponds to diabetes level.

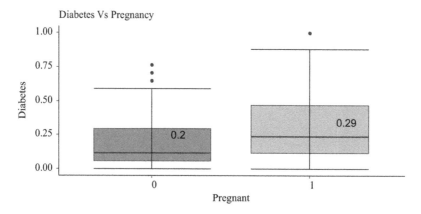

FIGURE 2.3
Graph between the pregnant women versus threat of diabetes.

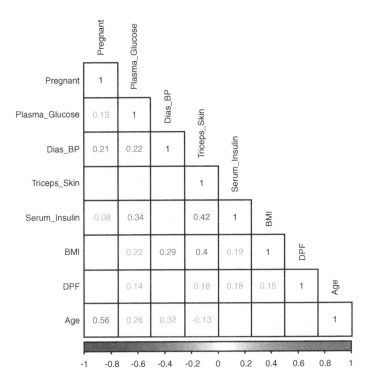

FIGURE 2.4
Correlation plot between the attributes of diabetes.

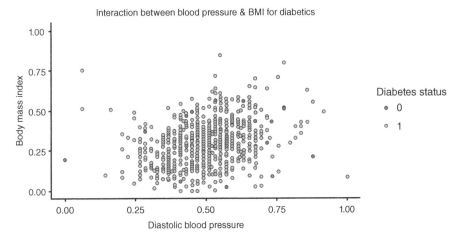

FIGURE 2.5
Relationship between blood pressure and Body Mass Index (BMI).

2.3.3 Breast Cancer

The graph in Figure 2.6 between the perimeter and diagnosis of breast cancer is pretty simple, as women who have a breast perimeter of 100–150, which is normal, have shown no signs of breast cancer, whereas women with perimeters ranging from 50 to 140 have a higher probability of breast cancer.

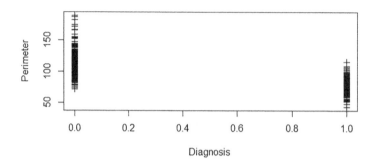

FIGURE 2.6
Distribution of cancer patients' dataset on perimeter versus diagnosis graph.

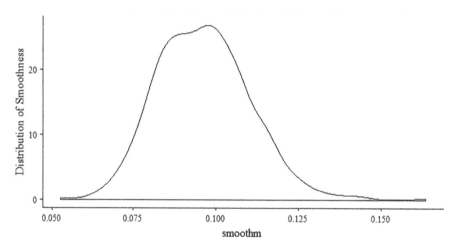

FIGURE 2.7
Distribution of smoothness.

Smoothness of breasts ranging from 0.075 to 0.125 is an indication of having normal breasts, whereas women with extremely low or high smoothness can be an indication of having breast cancer, as in Figure 2.7.

2.3.4 Parkinson's Disease

The decision tree given later predicts the outcome of disease with considerable accuracy (Mahieux et al., 1998). The Pitch Period Entropy (PPE) attribute becomes the root of the tree, followed by Amplitude Perturbation Quotient (APQ) and so on, as shown in Figure 2.8.

We saw, in Figure 2.9, that the attribute "PPE," a nonlinear measure for fundamental frequency measure, affects the most in predicting the Parkinson's disease with "spread1" following it. Other attributes have also played an important role in predicting Parkinson's.

2.3.5 Kidney Disease

The interaction between random blood glucose and blood urea, as in Figure 2.10, is quite interesting, as we can say that people who do not have kidney disease have low levels of urea and glucose when compared with people suffering from kidney disease.

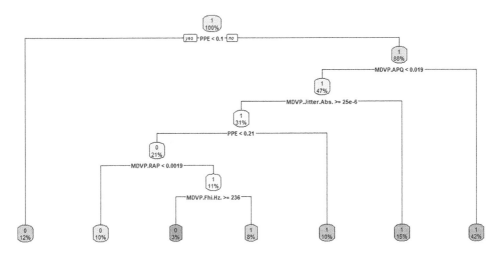

FIGURE 2.8
Decision tree of Parkinson's disease.

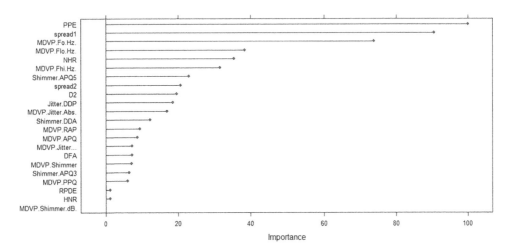

FIGURE 2.9
Relationship graph between attributes of Parkinson's disease and their importance.

Graph of hypertension and threat of chronic kidney disease (CKD), shown in Figure 2.11, implies that people with low hypertension levels have a higher rate of kidney disease, those with moderate levels of hypertension show low rate of CKD, and those with higher levels of hypertension show higher rate of CKD (Levey et al., 2003).

2.4 Classification

Classification is the technique that classifies the whole dataset according to the class variable. To maintain the credibility of prediction, we incorporated seven machine learning algorithms for classifying the dataset.

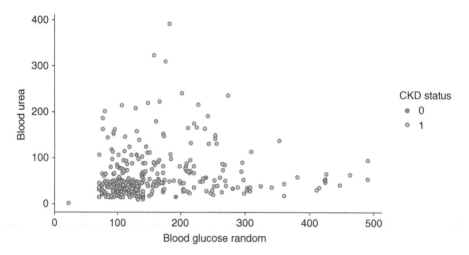

FIGURE 2.10
Plotting of kidney patients on blood glucose and blood urea.

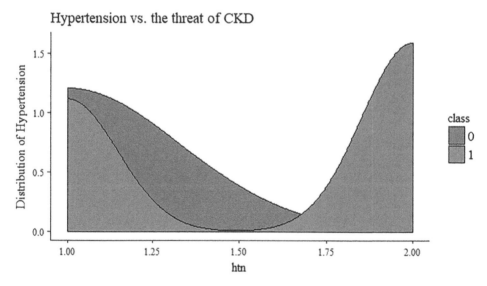

FIGURE 2.11
Graph between hypertension versus threat of CKD.

2.4.1 Logistic Regression

Logistic regression is similar to linear regression, but unlike it, logistic regression is a classification algorithm. In the project, we used the caret module to implement the logistic regression on the given data to predict and classify tests.

Logistic regression simply uses the technique of reducing the error function and hence deducing the equation for the line of predicted values as in linear regression, but it uses a damping function to contain the values between 1 and 0. In general, it proved to be a very accurate algorithm as it gave an accuracy of 75% in all datasets we used. Its average accuracy was 78.3%.

2.4.2 Bayesian Logistic Regression

Bayesian method works on the principle of probability. It is a sophisticated regression model that gives a vivid view of data points, which in turn helps in predicting values more accurately by following a Bayesian approach (Hayes, 2013).

Bayesian logistic regression provides accurate results of around 80%. It is an efficient algorithm, especially in the Parkinson's dataset, which gave an accuracy of 87%.

2.4.3 Decision Trees

Decision trees tend to find the best splits among various parameters to obtain more precise predictive values. It forms a tree-like structure, where nodes contain parameters, while the leaf nodes give us class values. Decision tree is a cataloging practice that is easy to interpret and understand and hence is easy to use (Safavian & Landgrebe, 1991). It can be used in both normal and hard data and is pretty accurate if the data is not overfitting to the classifiers.

2.4.4 Random Forest

Random forest comprises of multiple trees of varied parameters to predict the values. First, the dataset is split into random samples by using bootstrap aggregating algorithm. A new dataset is created by sampling n random cases from original data, leaving about one-third of data (Segal, 2004).

Then the new data obtained is trained using the given model in which very small columns of data are selected at random. At the end, each selected data is allowed to grow fully, and a final prediction is obtained by averaging.

2.4.5 Extreme Gradient Boosting

Gradient boosting is an algorithm that uses weak prediction models to create a final prediction model. At first, data is modeled onto simple models like decision trees to check for error residuals. For further models, we fit the data onto error residuals as target with same input variables (Chen et al., 2015).

The new error residuals with the original ones are added, and the data is fitted onto updated error residuals. Repetition of the steps is done until the sum of residuals become constant. In the end, all predictors are added to predict the outcome.

2.4.6 Genetic Algorithm

Genetic algorithms are search-based algorithms based on natural selection, recombination, and mutation to evolve solutions to a problem. First, we have a pool of different solutions in hand. These solutions undergo recombination and mutation and, in the process, produce new solutions. Each solution is given a fitness score accordingly (García et al., 2009).

Crossover is performed by randomly selecting solutions to produce offspring on the basis of fitness score. The fitter the solutions are, the fitter is their offspring. The process is repeated till a new batch of fitter solutions is created.

2.4.7 Comparison Model

After applying seven algorithms, i.e., linear regression, Bayesian regression, decision tree, random forest, extreme gradient boosting, and genetic algorithm, on all the five datasets and comparing their accuracies, we came to a conclusion that extreme gradient boosting is giving the best accuracy on all datasets. Hence, we have proceeded using extreme gradient boosting algorithm for predicting the outcomes. Other algorithms were giving varying results in different datasets, thus convincing us not to rely on them. Figures 2.12–2.16 show the comparison of all models used on the diseases.

As shown in Figure 2.17, extreme gradient boosting and genetic algorithm, though not giving 100% accuracy, were reliable. It gave considerable results with around 90% accuracy for each disease dataset. We saw that extreme gradient boosting had an upper edge than genetic algorithm; hence, we chose extreme gradient booster as an optimal algorithm for Smart Medical Diagnosis.

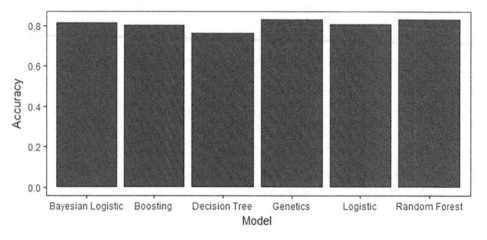

FIGURE 2.12
Accuracy graph among different models of heart disease.

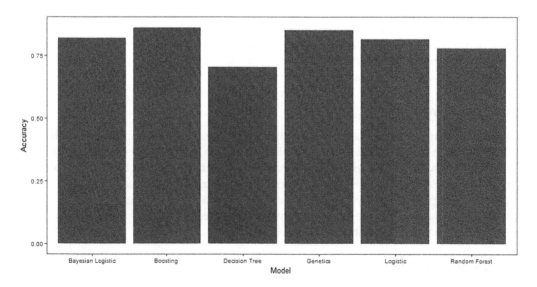

FIGURE 2.13
Accuracy graph among different models of diabetes.

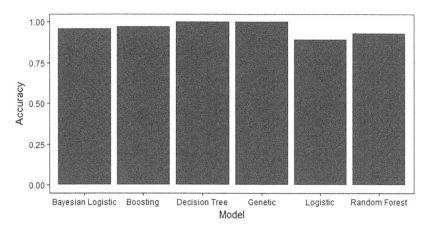

FIGURE 2.14
Accuracy graph among different models of breast cancer.

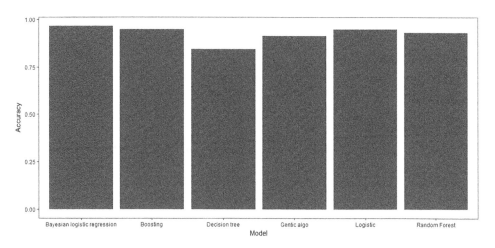

FIGURE 2.15
Accuracy graph among different models of Parkinson's.

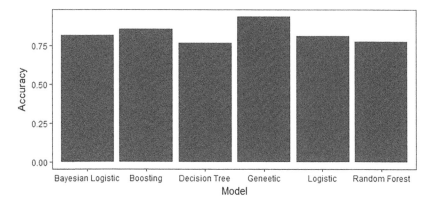

FIGURE 2.16
Accuracy graph among different models of kidney disease.

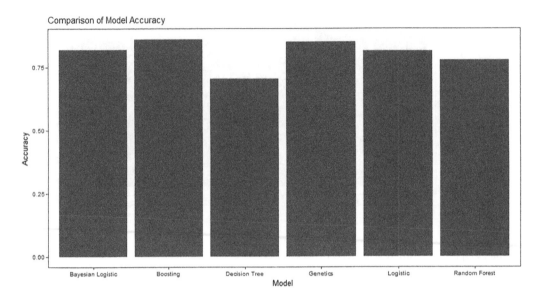

FIGURE 2.17
Combined comparison model of different algorithms used.

2.5 Web Application

We incorporated a responsive web-based frontend for easier and better experience for the users. They could easily enter the values of various parameters and see the output, thus taking steps accordingly. The web-based application was made with R Shiny. The User Interface (UI) is highly responsive, i.e., changing the value of the single parameter will enable the computation to repeat, as shown in Figure 2.18.

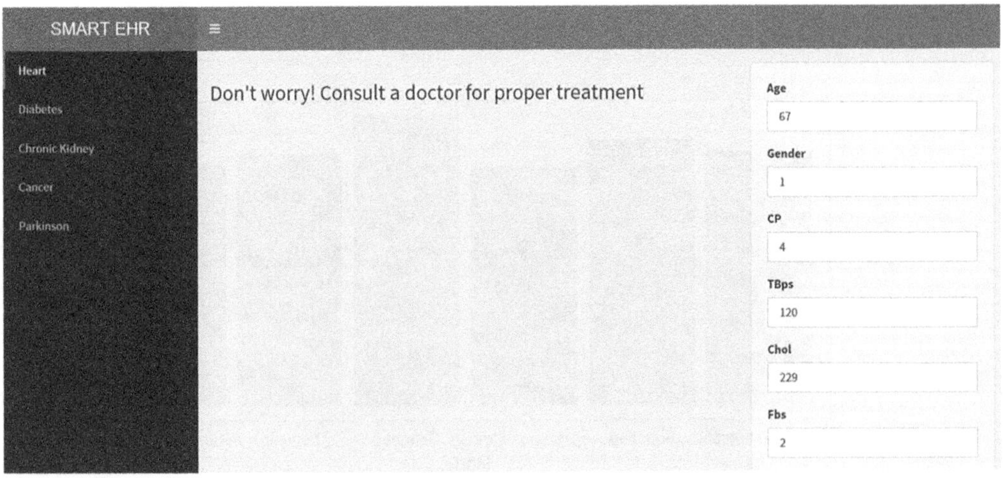

FIGURE 2.18
Screenshot one of the responsive web interface.

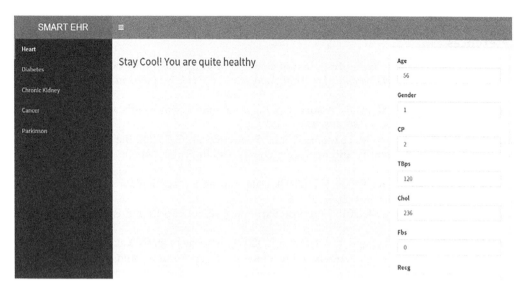

FIGURE 2.19
Screenshot two of the responsive web page.

Users have the choice to test any of the diseases provided: heart disease, diabetes, kidney disease, Parkinson's disease, and cancer. In Figure 2.19, they could easily shuffle through tabs to enter their parameter value, thus giving them a user-friendly web experience.

2.6 Conclusion

Machine learning is a drastically developing field, where it is being used virtually in every aspect related to the digital world. Even in the medical field, as the machines are starting to become a big part of the procedures and monitoring process, the use of machine learning in that aspect is expected. Our project is developed to predict the possibilities of what disease the patient has, based on the monitored vitals of a patient and test results. It uses a range of different algorithms and techniques to ensure high accuracy and more functionality.

For our experimentation, five different datasets were taken, which include kidney disease, heart disease, diabetes, cancer, and Parkinson's disease. There were too many attributes in the dataset, so first we chose the most relevant attributes from them and then preprocessed it using the R's mice package. After visualizing the important graphs of the attributes, we implemented seven algorithms on each dataset for prediction purposes. The gradient boosting tree gave the most accurate result among the applied algorithms, followed by the genetic algorithm as the second best. The web interface enables a user to enter their vitals and predicts whether they might have the disease or not. The designed structure can predict the disease at above 80% accuracy. The project only gives a binary result on whether the user has the disease or not; it does not tell the stage or severity of the disease. That can be included in the future work for people interested in doing so.

References

Agarwal, N., & Sebastian, M. P. (2016). Use of cloud computing and smart devices in healthcare. *International Journal of Computer, Electrical, Automation, Control and Information Engineering, 10*(1), 1–4.

Archenaa, J., & Anita, E. M. (2015). A survey of big data analytics in healthcare and government. *Procedia Computer Science, 50,* 408–413.

Bates, D. W., Saria, S., Ohno-Machado, L., Shah, A., & Escobar, G. (2014). Big data in health care: using analytics to identify and manage high-risk and high-cost patients. *Health Affairs, 33*(7), 1123–1131.

Breault, J. L., Goodall, C. R., & Fos, P. J. (2002). Data mining a diabetic data warehouse. *Artificial Intelligence in Medicine, 26*(1–2), 37–54.

Chen, T., He, T., & Benesty, M. (2015). Xgboost: Extreme gradient boosting. *R Package Version, 0*(4-2), 1–4.

García, S., Fernández, A., Luengo, J., & Herrera, F. (2009). A study of statistical techniques and performance measures for genetics-based machine learning: Accuracy and interpretability. *Soft Computing, 13*(10), 959.

Hayes, A. F. (2013). *Introduction to Mediation, Moderation, and Conditional Process Analysis: A Regression-Based Approach.* New York: The Guilford Press. In: Bolin, J. H. (Ed.), (2014). *Journal of Educational Measurement, 51*(3), 335–337.

Hughes, T. A., Ross, H. F., Musa, S., Bhattacherjee, S., Nathan, R. N., Mindham, R. H. S., & Spokes, E. G. S. (2000). A 10-year study of the incidence of and factors predicting dementia in Parkinson's disease. *Neurology, 54*(8), 1596–1603.

Koh, H. C., & Tan, G. (2011). Data mining applications in healthcare. *Journal of Healthcare Information Management, 19*(2), 65.

Levey, A. S., Coresh, J., Balk, E., Kausz, A. T., Levin, A., Steffes, M. W., ... Eknoyan, G. (2003). National Kidney Foundation practice guidelines for chronic kidney disease: Evaluation, classification, and stratification. *Annals of Internal Medicine, 139*(2), 137–147.

Mahieux, F., Fénelon, G., Flahault, A., Manifacier, M. J., Michelet, D., & Boller, F. (1998). Neuropsychological prediction of dementia in Parkinson's disease. *Journal of Neurology, Neurosurgery & Psychiatry, 64*(2), 178–183.

Palaniappan, S., & Awang, R. (2008, March). Intelligent heart disease prediction system using data mining techniques. In *AICCSA 2008. IEEE/ACS International Conference on Computer Systems and Applications, 2008* (pp. 108–115). IEEE, Malaysia.

Reis-Filho, J. S., & Pusztai, L. (2011). Gene expression profiling in breast cancer: Classification, prognostication, and prediction. *The Lancet, 378*(9805), 1812–1823.

Safavian, S. R., & Landgrebe, D. (1991). A survey of decision tree classifier methodology. *IEEE Transactions on Systems, Man, and Cybernetics, 21*(3), 660–674.

Segal, M. R. (2004). Machine Learning Benchmarks and Random Forest Regression. UCSF: Center for Bioinformatics and Molecular Biostatistics. Publication Date: 2004-04-14.

Soni, J., Ansari, U., Sharma, D., & Soni, S. (2011). Predictive data mining for medical diagnosis: An overview of heart disease prediction. *International Journal of Computer Applications, 17*(8), 43–48.

3

Lifestyle Application for Visually Impaired

Megha Rathi and Ananya Singhal

Jaypee Institute of Information Technology

CONTENTS

3.1 Introduction

Applications have made life simpler for a number of individuals with blindness or those diagnosed with visual impairment. The estimated number of visually impaired people in the world is 285 million. A standout among the most well-known issues that numerous visually impaired individuals encounter is their day-to-day challenges in adapting to their weakness. It is uncommon to find someone not glued to their smartphones nowadays, but with the reliance on technology, many have found independence for themselves. Various equipment, such as Braille, reading glass, or a walking stick, are only a portion of a couple of things that assist such individuals in their lives. With the advancement of technology, a common android smartphone equipped with specific applications can aid the visually impaired and blind to carry out their tasks.

Need to know how far you've walked in a day? There's an application present. Need to find your keys or a TV remote? There's an app for that too. Every basic activity is now implemented via an application. But what if one needs exact directions, because they can't visually identify the landmarks or the map of the city they are currently in? Or you can't tell if that is a bottle of tomato sauce or mustard sauce until you open it? Or you feel incompetent at work because you can't identify people in a meeting, thus disturbing the decorum? Well, for those with blindness, thankfully there's an app for that too.

Having the ability to peruse things that are just in visual print, choosing a cloth of specific color or texting someone are some of the tasks that require a handicapped person to seek the help of another (Wang et al., 2012). Be that as it may, applications when combined with the rapid advancements in technology provide such individuals with new and better approaches of reading things and doing anything in different but easier ways: they learn to read with their voices. Voice-over features available on smartphones are of a distinct advantage, conceding the same access to the digital world of visually impaired users just like everyone else.

The definition of "to look" is now being redefined. Numerous applications are helping people to level the playing field and be more confident and independent, and the main focus of this project "Lifestyle App for the Visually Impaired" involves reading printed documents, identifying objects or people or colors that come across, i.e., in real time, connecting them with sighted volunteers for visual assistance, and texting using a Braille keyboard—all operating with touch gestures and presenting the result in audio form (Neumann & Matas, 2012).

It applies algorithms used in the framework of modern-day technologies like optical character recognition (OCR), principal component analysis (PCA) for face recognition, and deep convolutional neural network (CNN) used in Tensorflow with some modifications for object detection and recognition. It is further extended to detect color and product information and description using a barcode reader. The application developed also captures images of people and saves the images as a training set into a database. Then, it uses the saved images as a training set to train the system to recognize a particular person in real time whenever he/she comes in front of the camera. For object detection, an already trained dataset has been used for around 1,000 classes of objects, while text recognition is done using Tesseract library with OpenCV. Also, it provides the blind users to sign up for a community, where they can ask for help from volunteers in real time—via video calling features enabled in the application and can text with a modified design of keyboard that operates over Braille language. This new system has additional advantages that include easy to setup and install, high portability, and low start-up costs.

3.2 Related Work

There has been a rapid advancement in the area of recognition and detection systems over the years and yet the development growth in this field is not slowing down at all. However, there are still many lingering issues that need to be resolved.

Bonner et al. (2010) proposed a type of keyboard for blind people. For that, they divided the mobile screen into eight segments, where each segment represents the letters in the alphabetic series. This keyboard works using two-finger interaction. When the user touches a segment, the device pronounces the letters of that segment and the user will use the next finger for selecting the letters from the list of letters that are alphabetically displayed on the screen. While face recognition using PCA method (Paul & Al Sumam, 2012) worked on the principle of preparing a set of a linear combinations of weighted eigenvectors called eigenfaces, performing the recognition process by anticipating a test picture onto the subspace spreads over the eigenfaces, after which the classification is finished by estimating the least Euclidean separation, real-time face recognition (Haji & Varol 2016) focuses on developing a face recognition system for its use in the field of biometrics. In Haji & Varol (2016), the authors first stored 5–10 pictures of a person in different angles and calculated the Euclidean distance using the weights sent from the client and the weights at the server, and the closest match will be found out and the image identification will be successfully completed.

Coates et al. (2011) partition the project into two stages: (i) text location and (ii) text recognition. They took the help from International Conference on Document Analysis and Recognition, wherein one utilizes a paired classifier that aims to recognize 32-by-32 windows for the text location part and implemented the same. They utilized the word-bounding box obtained for perceiving the content in those particular area using recognition libraries. Vezhnevets et al. (2003) used pixel-based techniques and then compared the results of each technique for skin color detection. The technique was based on an RGB format, in which they collected the red, green, and blue content of each pixel and then normalized the stored RGB values, after which they calculated the hue, saturation, value and R/B ratio for showing skin tone. The study of Kutiyanawala & Kulyukin (2010) focus on helping visually impaired users in shopping. So for getting the details of products in supermarket, they used barcode localization and decoding modules. For barcode localization, they worked on a homogeneous area consisting of interchange high-contrast lines consolidated in a little area, where each line can be decoded as a bit specifier: black line denoted by 1 and white line denoted by 0.

Ohtsuka et al. (2010) focused on making a communication device for deaf and blind people. Using this, a blind–deaf person is able to recognize any known person standing nearby. Hearing impaired and visually impaired individuals can use this communication device, which contains two small-scale vibrators for body Braille, switches for Braille information input, infrared information/yield gadgets, and a controller. Nonhandicapped individuals will carry a little gadget that tells them that a blind person needs help. Using mobile assistive technologies, Hakobyan et al. (2013) conducted a survey for the visually impaired, where they focused on the visually impaired users and how they use their mobile phone in daily life to ease out their tasks. So, they researched about the existing developments in the field of portable assistive innovations implemented till now for helping the visually disabled ones to lead more autonomous lives. In conclusion, the authors mentioned that usually a blind person does not believe in using his/her mobile phones that much and would rather prefer a person who can help him/her in every problem to solve his/her query.

Mednis et al. (2011) focus on object detection and recognition and its implementation on android devices using CNN models. CNN is yet another alternative approach to deep neural network (DNN). The main aim of the convolutional layer is to simply extract the basic information at high resolution from among the input data and then transform it to more complex representations at much unrefined resolutions. It is achieved by applying filters to extract out the local data followed by min or max pooling of the layers that cause them to be invariant to translations as a form of dimensionality reduction. Lastly, DNN is applied to complete the classification process.

The network used in Mednis et al. (2011) is SqueezeDet, which implements a fully yet low-power CNN for object detection, which uses convolutional layers not only to extract

feature maps but also as an output layer to compute bounding boxes and class probabilities. Smith (2007) gave a review of the method behind the Tesseract OCR Engine used for
the acknowledgment of content from images. The algorithm used starts off with a prees-
sential of the high-resolution picture being captured and further handling it for line finding for deskewing the picture, baseline fitting, chopping of individual letters from words,
thus enhancing it. However, the recognition of characters from the image is extracted out
from a well-trained classifier.

The project Lifestyle App for the Visually Impaired is hence an additional combination
to both the areas, since it not only gives a supplementary experience on these subjects
but also presents some foundations to develop applications based on them for android
devices, choosing the best proposed algorithm from the researches already applied in a
scalable manner.

3.3 Methodology

The proposed framework aims at making the visually impaired self-sufficient by providing them various features and to overcome the problems faced by them in their day-
to-day life. The problem is solved in various steps by keeping in mind that the whole
application is accessed via voice commands or touch gestures, thereby guiding them
at every step. Images captured from the camera are first preprocessed using OpenCV
library in an android. Then, the images are converted to gray scale, noise is removed, and
then skew detection and correction are implemented. Although a lot of work has been
done in this area, none of it focuses on effective implementation for users not having iOS
devices. While face detection and recognition are implemented using a PCA algorithm
that builds its dataset of feature extraction and trains the dataset using machine learning,
information of a product is extracted using a barcode reader and searched over an UPC
database. We propose to add object recognition and color recognition for the help and
ease of users (Figure 3.1).

Object is detected using a modified CNN, while color is detected by specifying a range
of colors and extracting an individual pixel's information. Daily-used objects are identified
in real time in minimal amount of time, and identified objects are spoken aloud in the app
for it to be heard by the visually impaired.

The application intends to help them in carrying out the daily life activities more easily
and efficiently with reference to recognizing objects, their brands, and people, providing
them with a community of volunteers to help them cross hurdles via web real-time proto-
cols (RTPs). Given later is the description of core modules of this framework.

3.3.1 Text Recognition

For text recognition, the first step is to get a clean image of the document one wants to
make it editable.

For this, a high-resolution camera is used to capture the image, which is then processed
using OpenCV library functions like skew detection, luminance enhancement, etc. to
extract out the best results from it before segmentation is applied. The next step is to pass
the processed image through a trainer to separate the words out after detecting separate

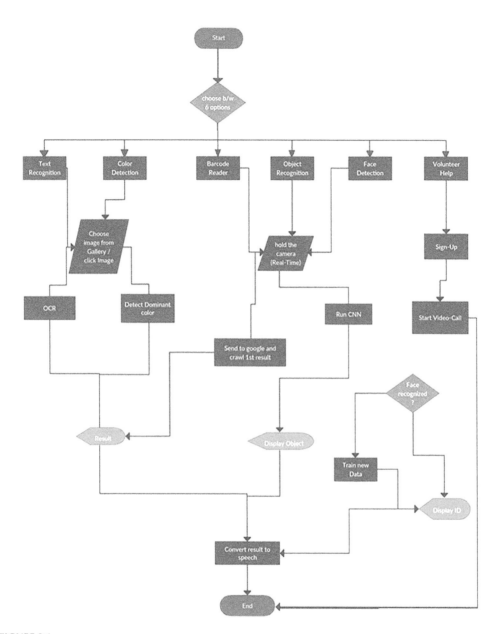

FIGURE 3.1
Control flow diagram for the application.

lines from the image. Character recognition is the last step in the OCR technology, which is then shown to the user on the screen via a text-to-speech tool (Figures 3.2 and 3.3).

3.3.2 Color Recognition

This module required the user to extract the most dominant color in the image provided by the user (Lenneberg, 1961). For this, we first defined a set of around 150 colors based on the assumption that a particular range of colors will fall in the defined dominant color

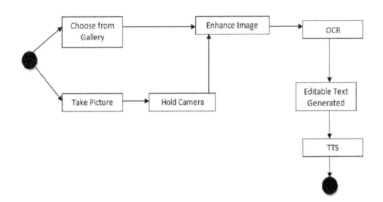

FIGURE 3.2
Text recognition.

```
if (rgbBytes == null) {
  rgbBytes = new int[previewWidth * previewHeight];
}
try {
  final Image image = reader.acquireLatestImage();

  if (image == null) {
    return;
  }

  if (isProcessingFrame) {
    image.close();
    return;
  }
  isProcessingFrame = true;
  Trace.beginSection("imageAvailable");
  final Plane[] planes = image.getPlanes();
  fillBytes(planes, yuvBytes);
  yRowStride = planes[0].getRowStride();
  final int uvRowStride = planes[1].getRowStride();
  final int uvPixelStride = planes[1].getPixelStride();

  imageConverter =
      (Runnable) () -> {
          ImageUtils.convertYUV420ToARGB8888(
              yuvBytes[0],
              yuvBytes[1],
              yuvBytes[2],
              previewWidth,
              previewHeight,
```

FIGURE 3.3
Text recognition model using OCR.

category (Berwick & Lee, 1998). When an image is passed, it is divided into a grid of $N \times N$ pixels. For each pixel, the dominant color is found out via conversion from HSV to RGB color panel. The R, G, B count of every pixel is noted down, which is further passed for shade comparison, and the deviation from it is calculated to get a more detailed color. Also, the brightness of every pixel is considered for a further change in the shade of the color. The hexadecimal value further obtained is changed to an RGB panel and displayed (Figures 3.4 and 3.5).

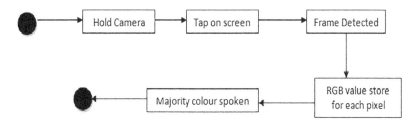

FIGURE 3.4
Color recognition.

```
@Override
protected void processImage() {
    rgbFrameBitmap.setPixels(getRgbBytes(), 0, previewWidth, 0, 0, previewWidth, previewHeight);
    final Canvas canvas = new Canvas(croppedBitmap);
    canvas.drawBitmap(rgbFrameBitmap, frameToCropTransform, null);

    // For examining the actual TF input.
    if (SAVE_PREVIEW_BITMAP) {
        ImageUtils.saveBitmap(croppedBitmap);
    }
    runInBackground(
        () → {
            final long startTime = SystemClock.uptimeMillis();
            final List<Classifier.Recognition> results = classifier.recognizeImage(croppedBitmap);
            lastProcessingTimeMs = SystemClock.uptimeMillis() - startTime;
            LOGGER.i("Detect: %s", results);
            cropCopyBitmap = Bitmap.createBitmap(croppedBitmap);
            if (resultsView == null) {
                resultsView = (ResultsView) findViewById(R.id.results);
            }
            resultsView.setResults(results);
            requestRender();
            readyForNextImage();
```

FIGURE 3.5
Color recognition model.

3.3.3 Face Recognition

A colored face image is converted to a grayscale image, as they are easier for applying computational techniques in image processing (Graham & Allinson, 1998). A grayscale face image is scaled for a particular pixel size as 250×250, because many input images can be of different sizes whenever we take an input face for recognition. Different expressions of a single person are captured under different conditions, because size variations, illumination, etc. can lead to a significant change in output. A test image for recognition is tested by comparing the stored dataset. Mean face is obtained by

$$\psi = (1/M) \sum M\mu_i \quad i = 1 \tag{3.1}$$

where $\mu_1, \mu_2, \ldots \mu_n$ are training set images, and the mean centered images are evaluated by

$$\xi = \mu_i \psi \tag{3.2}$$

for further computations. The eigenvectors corresponding to the covariance matrix define the eigenface that has a ghostly appearing face-like appearance, and a match is found if a new face is close to these images (Turk & Pentland, 1991) (Figures 3.6 and 3.7).

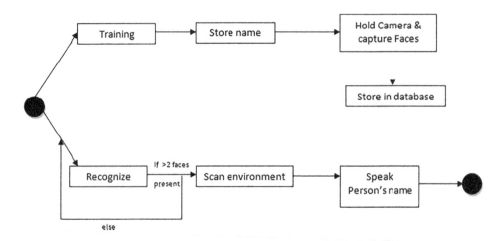

FIGURE 3.6
Face recognition.

```
String line;
while ((line = br.readLine()) != null) {
  LOGGER.w(line);
  d.labels.add(line);
}
br.close();


d.inferenceInterface = new TensorFlowInferenceInterface(assetManager, modelFilename);

final Graph g = d.inferenceInterface.graph();

d.inputName = "image_tensor";

final Operation inputOp = g.operation(d.inputName);
if (inputOp == null) {
  throw new RuntimeException("Failed to find input Node '" + d.inputName + "'");
}
d.inputSize = inputSize;
// The outputScoresName node has a shape of [N, NumLocations], where N
// is the batch size.
final Operation outputOp1 = g.operation("detection_scores");
if (outputOp1 == null) {
  throw new RuntimeException("Failed to find output Node 'detection_scores'");
}
final Operation outputOp2 = g.operation("detection_boxes");
if (outputOp2 == null) {
  throw new RuntimeException("Failed to find output Node 'detection_boxes'");
}
final Operation outputOp3 = g.operation("detection_classes");
if (outputOp3 == null) {
  throw new RuntimeException("Failed to find output Node 'detection_classes'");
}
```

FIGURE 3.7
Face recognition model.

3.3.4 Braille Touch Keyboard

The main thought behind this module is just not simply tapping on the Braille keys but associated with the required specks together to get the genuine letter as they are displayed in Braille dialect using fingers (Litschel, 1997). We have created this keyboard for helping blinds. This keyboard contains six dots. Using these dots, a user can type any letter using Braille. The letter thus recognized is stored in a fixed size array list. We have used the speech feature that tells the user the whole word and tells the position of keyboard and supports talk back and every other application (Figure 3.8).

3.3.5 Help from Volunteers

A web RTP tool is required to connect the community of blind to the community of volunteers that register on the sign-up page and enter which category they lie in before using the app. The contact details of every person are kept anonymous for a safer environment. In this, the blind person can send the call notification, and whoever wants to volunteer can connect to him on the video chat for help.

```
final int backgroundColor = Color.argb(100, 0, 0, 0);
canvas.drawColor(backgroundColor);

final Matrix matrix = new Matrix();
final float scaleFactor = 2;
matrix.postScale(scaleFactor, scaleFactor);
matrix.postTranslate(
    canvas.getWidth() - copy.getWidth() * scaleFactor,
    canvas.getHeight() - copy.getHeight() * scaleFactor);
canvas.drawBitmap(copy, matrix, new Paint());

final Vector<String> lines = new Vector<~>();
if (detector != null) {
  final String statString = detector.getStatString();
  final String[] statLines = statString.split("\n");
  for (final String line : statLines) {
    lines.add(line);
  }
}
lines.add("");

lines.add("Frame: " + previewWidth + "x" + previewHeight);
lines.add("Crop: " + copy.getWidth() + "x" + copy.getHeight());
lines.add("View: " + canvas.getWidth() + "x" + canvas.getHeight());
lines.add("Rotation: " + sensorOrientation);
lines.add("Inference time: " + lastProcessingTimeMs + "ms");

borderedText.drawLines(canvas, 10, canvas.getHeight() - 10, lines);
});
```

FIGURE 3.8
Braille touch implementation code.

3.3.6 Object Recognition

In this module, the entry point is the object recognition process in real time (Prokop & Reeves, 1992). In this, one can detect several objects that come across the screen using mobile camera with the help of object tracking and multibox detector class provided by Tensorflow along with image processing functions to enhance every frame captured per 5 s to pick out the best frame for further recognition. A trained dataset in Python using Tensorflow library is converted to .pb extension to be used in android, which is then fed to the convolutional network models for further process by applying filters and calculating a score for every set of pixels and building a graph to get the confidence score for feature matching (Figures 3.9 and 3.10).

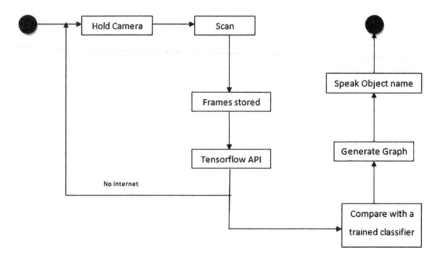

FIGURE 3.9
Object recognition.

```
/deprecation/
private void onSelectFromGalleryResult(Intent data) {
    Bitmap bm=null;
    if (data != null) {
        try {
            bm = MediaStore.Images.Media.getBitmap(getApplicationContext().getContentResolver(), data.getData());
        } catch (IOException e) {
            e.printStackTrace();
        }
    }
    processImage(bm);
}

private void onCaptureImageResult(Intent data) {
    Bitmap thumbnail = (Bitmap) data.getExtras().get("data");
    ByteArrayOutputStream bytes = new ByteArrayOutputStream();
    thumbnail.compress(Bitmap.CompressFormat.JPEG,  quality: 90, bytes);
    File destination = new File(Environment.getExternalStorageDirectory(),
                child: System.currentTimeMillis() + ".jpg");
    FileOutputStream fo;
    try {
        destination.createNewFile();
        fo = new FileOutputStream(destination);
        fo.write(bytes.toByteArray());
        fo.close();
    } catch (FileNotFoundException e) {
        e.printStackTrace();
    } catch (IOException e) {
```

FIGURE 3.10
Object recognition module.

3.3.7 Barcode to Product Description

The barcode of the various products helps to identify the product as well as its brand. Its implementation requires the use of an autofocus tool that can enhance the brightness, pixel density, and reduce the noise on the real-time image frame captured. When the barcode is decoded, the 12-digit number captured helps to extract the product information. The first digit specifies the product category, while the next five digits determine the manufacturer's name. The set of next five digits tells about the specific type of product, and the last digit is a testing number used by scanners to verify whether scanning is done correctly. The number extracted out is searched accordingly in the UPC database, and the detailed information is displayed to the user (Figures 3.11 and 3.12).

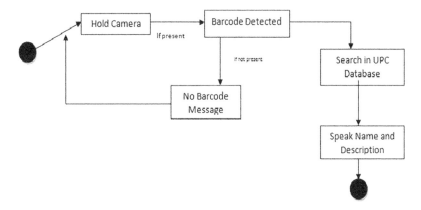

FIGURE 3.11
Barcode recognition.

```
public class SinchService extends Service {
    private static final String APP_KEY = "d2d52a0f-21ca-4275-b99e-b07632fa45b0";
    private static final String APP_SECRET = "xgJl/TmTi0+QrMIZQtHmpw==";
    private static final String ENVIRONMENT = "clientapi.sinch.com";

    public static final String CALL_ID = "CALL_ID";
    static final String TAG = SinchService.class.getSimpleName();

    private SinchServiceInterface mSinchServiceInterface = new SinchServiceInterface();
    private SinchClient mSinchClient;
    private String mUserId;

    private StartFailedListener mListener;

    @Override
    public void onCreate() { super.onCreate(); }

    @Override
    public void onDestroy() {
        if (mSinchClient != null && mSinchClient.isStarted()) {
            mSinchClient.terminate();
        }
        super.onDestroy();
    }

    private void start(String userName) {
        if (mSinchClient == null) {
            mUserId = userName;
            mSinchClient = Sinch.getSinchClientBuilder().context(getApplicationContext()).userId(userName)
                    .applicationKey(APP_KEY)
```

FIGURE 3.12
Barcode recognition module.

3.4 Algorithms Used

A detailed description of all techniques and algorithms used in the study is presented in this section. Object recognition, text recognition, face recognition, Braille touch implementation, and barcode to product recognition are the main modules of the developed lifestyle android app for visually impaired persons. This section provides a brief summary of all the techniques deployed in the proposed work.

3.4.1 Tesseract Algorithm

Blobs are organized into text lines, and the lines and regions are analyzed for proportional text. Piece of writing is torn into words divergently according to the type of character spacing. Confirmed piece of writing is drastically reduced immediately by character cells. Identification then advanced as a two-step process. In the initial step, a trail is made to identify each word in rotation. Each phrase that is reasonable is progressed to a compatible classifier as training data (Mithe et al., 2013). The standard classifier then gets the opportunity to more precisely identify text bottom down the page. Since the standard classifier may have gained useful knowledge slowly to make a contribution close to the top of the page, another pass is run over the page, in which the words that were not identified well enough are identified once more (Smith, 2013).

3.4.2 Scalable Object Detection (Deep Neural Network)

Deep neural network has achieved a remarkable performance upgradation for achieving the task of object recognition. Scalable objects are detected by forecasting a group of closed boxes that constitute a group of principal objects. In this research work, we have utilized CNN, which produces a stagnant count of closed boxes. In deep-learning network, each layer of node trains on a well-defined unique set of attributes established on the antecedent layer's response (Marosi, 2007). More extreme you proceed into the neural net, the advanced and extreme complex the features your nodes can identify, since they integrate and put together again all the attributes from the previous layer. Initially, we elucidate object identification as a regression problem to the geometric points of several closed boxes. In inclusion, for each forecasted box, the net response is a confidence score of how likely this box contains that object (Deng & Yu, 2014).

3.4.3 Single Shot Multibox Detector

Single shot multibox detector (SSD) works by finding out the discrete value of response space of bounding boxes into a group of default boxes over divergent facet ratios and scales per feature map position (Liu et al., 2016). For the purpose of prediction, the closed net foster scores for the existence of each object class in each default box and foster adjustments to the box to superiorly match the object shape. SSD model is simple when compared with the techniques that need object proposals, because it perfectly abolishes proposition generation and the ensuing pixel or feature resampling phase that encloses all computation in a single network (Zhang et al., 2017). Training of this algorithm is quiet easy and can be integrated with other tools and techniques for further use.

3.4.4 Principle Component Analysis

PCA is a dimensionality reduction algorithm that is actually fruitful with a redundant dataset. PCA works by reducing the count of variables or dimensions into a smaller set of variables, and these variables are known as principal components, which is actually responsible for most of the discrepancies in the observed variables (Jolliffe, 2011). Emphasis of PCA is to lessen the dimensionality of the dataset by keeping maximum possible variations in the original dataset. On the contrary, dimensionality reduction leads to an indirect data loss. Best principal components are discovered by preeminent low-dimensional space. The utmost advantage of PCA is using it in eigenface approach, which aids in decreasing the size of the database for identification of test images (Abdi & Williams, 2010). The images are stored as their feature vectors in the database, which is retrieved by predicting each and every trained image to the set of eigenfaces obtained. PCA is applied on eigenface approach to lessen the dimension or size of a large dataset.

3.5 Results and Findings

Use of external assistive devices is common nowadays for visually impaired people. However, not every individual is able to afford them. But one can find a mobile phone almost with everyone. While surveying for its development, we found out that almost every other blind person knows Braille language. Although external keyboards operating over this language are available, no one has yet developed a mobile application based on touch gestures corresponding to Braille dot alphabets. Also, the efficiency of Tesseract engine is highly increased once processed images are fed to the classifier.

Real-time tracking creates a lag and consumes time, but simpler yet efficient algorithms can be implemented to compensate for the same.

Software development kit (SDK) version greater than 21 along with 3 GB RAM is required for the application to work properly. Also, some issues listed are as follows:

Tables and symbols are not recognized using the algorithm.

1. Images with background color and images are difficult to process.
2. Slow connection leads to noisy videoconferencing.
3. Face detection requires stillness to face/frame capture.
4. Objects that look the same as cup and kettle are categorized as cup only.
5. Objects like pen or fan are difficult to train, since feature extraction for such objects becomes hard.

However, the application developed is the best possible solution to the models stated that could be available for free. Figures 3.13–3.20 unfold the results of running a lifestyle app for visually impaired patients.

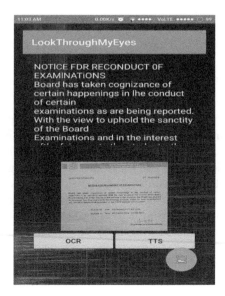

FIGURE 3.13
Output of text recognition module.

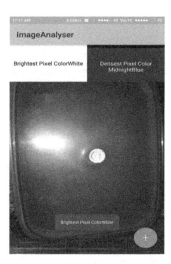

FIGURE 3.14
Output of color recognition module.

3.6 Conclusion and Future Work

Using this project, visually impaired people will be able to do their daily life work independently with the help of different types of detection and recognition modules, namely face detection, object detection, text recognition, barcode detection, and color detection, using algorithms that are both simple and efficient. Visually impaired individuals do not believe in assistive devices and always seek help from others thus becoming dependent. So, the

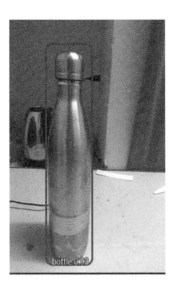

FIGURE 3.15
Output of object recognition.

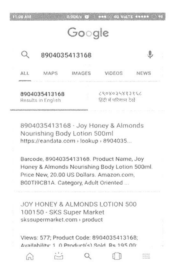

FIGURE 3.16
Output of barcode to product recognition. (Google and the Google logo are registered trademarks of Google LLC, used with permission.)

application will provide volunteers help, wherein the nondisabled ones can also contribute to this application by connecting via videoconferencing. Thus, the user will be able to perform most of the tasks himself using the application that will guide them through every step using voice output and touch input gestures.

Camera usage becomes an important part when dealing with visually impaired users. Since every mobile consists of different camera quality, thus providing with different efficiencies in modules implemented, it becomes important that the quality issue be totally eliminated by the use of Internet of Things (IoT) devices. The application can be further

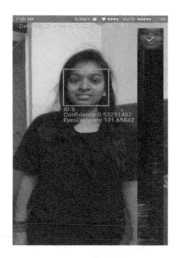

FIGURE 3.17
Output of face detection.

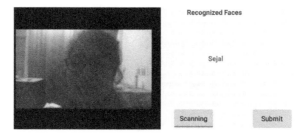

FIGURE 3.18
Output of face detection.

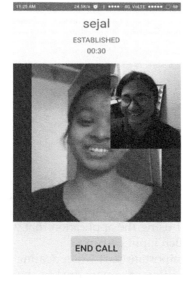

FIGURE 3.19
Videoconferencing required for communication.

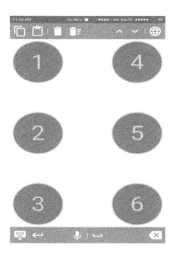

FIGURE 3.20
Braille keyboard.

extended to denomination recognition, wherein the user will be able to detect the denomination of any currency that comes under the camera. Efficiency of object and face recognition can be further enhanced using better and complex algorithms. Also, the text-to-speech conversion in every module in this application will be further improvised to speak in the native language of the user and not just English.

References

Abdi, H., & Williams, L. J. (2010). Principal component analysis. *Wiley Interdisciplinary Reviews: Computational Statistics*, 2(4), 433–459.

Berwick, D., & Lee, S. W., (1998, January). A chromaticity space for specularity, illumination color- and illumination pose-invariant 3-D object recognition. In *6th International Conference on Computer Vision (IEEE Cat. No. 98CH36271)* (pp. 165–170). IEEE, Mumbai, India.

Bonner, M. N., Brudvik, J. T., Abowd, G. D., & Edwards, W. K. (2010, May). No-look notes: Accessible eyes-free multi-touch text entry. In *International Conference on Pervasive Computing* (pp. 409–426). Springer, Berlin, Heidelberg.

Coates, A., Carpenter, B., Case, C., Satheesh, S., Suresh, B., Wang, T., ... Ng, A. Y. (2011, September). Text detection and character recognition in scene images with unsupervised feature learning. In *International Conference on Document Analysis and Recognition (ICDAR), 2011* (pp. 440–445). IEEE, Beijing, China.

Deng, L., & Yu, D. (2014). Deep learning: Methods and applications. *Foundations and Trends® in Signal Processing*, 7(3–4), 197–387.

Graham, D. B., & Allinson, N. M. (1998). Characterising virtual eigensignatures for general purpose face recognition. In Wechsler, H., Phillips, P. J., Bruce, V., Soulié, F. F., Huang, T. S. (eds.) *Face Recognition* (pp. 446–456). Springer, Berlin, Heidelberg.

Haji, S., & Varol, A. (2016, April). Real time face recognition system (RTFRS). In *4th International Symposium on Digital Forensic and Security (ISDFS), 2016* (pp. 107–111). IEEE, Barcelos, Portugal.

Hakobyan, L., Lumsden, J., O'Sullivan, D., & Bartlett, H. (2013). Mobile assistive technologies for the visually impaired. *Survey of Ophthalmology*, 58(6), 513–528.

Jolliffe, I. (2011). Principal component analysis. In Lovric, M. (ed.) *International Encyclopedia of Statistical Science* (pp. 1094–1096). Springer, Berlin, Heidelberg.

Kutiyanawala, A., & Kulyukin, V. (2010). Eyes-free barcode localization and decoding for visually impaired mobile phone users. In *International Conference on Image Processing, Computer Vision and Pattern Recognition, 2010* (Vol. 1, pp. 130–135), Las Vegas, Nevada, USA.

Lenneberg, E. H. (1961). Color naming, color recognition, color discrimination: A re-appraisal. *Perceptual and Motor Skills*, 12(3), 375–382.

Litschel, D. (1997). U.S. Patent No. 5,627,566. Washington, DC: U.S. Patent and Trademark Office.

Liu, W., Anguelov, D., Erhan, D., Szegedy, C., Reed, S., Fu, C. Y., & Berg, A. C. (2016, October). Ssd: Single shot multibox detector. In *European Conference on Computer Vision* (pp. 21–37). Springer, Cham, Munich, Germany.

Marosi, I. (2007, January). Industrial OCR approaches: Architecture, algorithms, and adaptation techniques. In *Proceedings on SPIE 6500, Document Recognition and Retrieval XIV* (Vol. 6500, p. 650002). International Society for Optics and Photonics, Bellingham.

Mednis, A., Strazdins, G., Zviedris, R., Kanonirs, G., & Selavo, L. (2011, June). Real time pothole detection using android smartphones with accelerometers. In *International Conference on Distributed Computing in Sensor Systems and Workshops (DCOSS), 2011* (pp. 1–6). IEEE, Santorini Island, Greece.

Mithe, R., Indalkar, S., & Divekar, N. (2013). Optical character recognition. *International Journal of Recent Technology and Engineering (IJRTE)*, 2(1), 72–75.

Neumann, L., & Matas, J. (2012, June). Real-time scene text localization and recognition. In *IEEE Conference on Computer Vision and Pattern Recognition (CVPR), 2012* (pp. 3538–3545). IEEE, Rhode Island, USA.

Ohtsuka, S., Hasegawa, S., Sasaki, N., & Harakawa, T. (2010, January). Communication system between deaf-blind people and non-disabled people using body-braille and infrared communication. In *7th IEEE Conference on Consumer Communications and Networking Conference (CCNC), 2010* (pp. 1–2). IEEE, Las Vegas, Nevada, USA.

Paul, L. C., & Al Sumam, A. (2012). Face recognition using principal component analysis method. *International Journal of Advanced Research in Computer Engineering & Technology (IJARCET)*, 1(9), 135.

Prokop, R. J., & Reeves, A. P. (1992). A survey of moment-based techniques for unoccluded object representation and recognition. *CVGIP: Graphical Models and Image Processing*, 54(5), 438–460.

Smith, R. (2007, September). An overview of the Tesseract OCR engine. In *ICDAR 2007, 9th International Conference on Document Analysis and Recognition, 2007* (Vol. 2, pp. 629–633). IEEE, Sydney, Australia.

Smith, R. W. (2013, February). History of the Tesseract OCR engine: What worked and what didn't. In *Proceedings on SPIE 8658, Document Recognition and Retrieval XX* (Vol. 8658, p. 865802). International Society for Optics and Photonics, Bellingham.

Turk, M. A., & Pentland, A. P. (1991, June). Face recognition using eigenfaces. In *Proceedings on CVPR'91, IEEE Computer Society Conference on Computer Vision and Pattern Recognition, 1991* (pp. 586–591). IEEE, Lahaina, Maui, Hawaii.

Vezhnevets, V., Sazonov, V., & Andreeva, A. (2003, September). A survey on pixel-based skin color detection techniques. In *Proceedings on Graphicon* (Vol. 3, pp. 85–92).

Wang, T., Wu, D. J., Coates, A., & Ng, A. Y. (2012, November). End-to-end text recognition with convolutional neural networks. In *21st International Conference on Pattern Recognition (ICPR), 2012* (pp. 3304–3308). IEEE, Tsukuba Science City, Japan.

Zhang, S., Zhu, X., Lei, Z., Shi, H., Wang, X., & Li, S. Z. (2017, October). S^ 3FD: Single shot scale-invariant face detector. In *IEEE International Conference on Computer Vision (ICCV), 2017* (pp. 192–201). IEEE, Venice, Italy.

4

Classification of Genetic Mutations

Megha Rathi, Ishant Tyagi, Jatin Shad, Shubham Sharma, and Siddharth Gaur
Jaypee Institute of Information Technology

CONTENTS

4.1 Introduction

Mutations can be defined as permanent changes that may occur in a genetic sequence. The word mutation basically refers to changes affecting nucleic acid. They are the reason why every organism is different (Davies et al., 2002). These changes can have different consequences for different organisms as they occur at distinct levels. Some of these changes only affect the organism carrying them, while some others affect the descendants of the organism as well. These rates of mutation can differ between genomes and also within a genome. Mutations are a common occurrence. They may benefit us, harm us, or do nothing to us. This depends on the location where gene change occurs. Mutations that are non-neutral are dangerous. Generally, base pairs are affected by mutations, where the effect of mutation is greater and the probability of mutation to be hazardous is more (Nigro et al., 1989). A single mutation is unlikely to be responsible for cancer. Multiple mutations throughout our life can cause cancer. This is the reason behind the fact that older people are more susceptible to cancer than younger people, as they have more chances for those mutations to add up. Many types of genes may contribute toward the development of cancer. The gene that is mutated most commonly of all is TP53 (Omoto et al., 2004), which leads to the production of a protein that hinders the growth of tumors. Le-Fraumeni syndrome, a rare inherited disorder leading to higher risk of developing cancer, is caused by a germ line mutation in the gene. BRCA1 and BRCA2 (Brooker, 2009) genes are two inherited mutations linked with breast and ovarian cancer syndrome, a disorder marked by an enhanced lifelong danger of these two cancers (breast and ovarian) in women. Other types of cancers have been linked with this particular syndrome, like prostate and pancreatic cancers and breast cancer in males. PTEN (Omoto et al., 2004) is another protein producer gene that suppresses tumor growth. Mutation in these genes increases the risk of breast, thyroid, and endometrial cancer. These genes are actually protective genes. But when these genes mutate, cells grow without any control and a tumor may form.

4.2 Related Work

Significant research has been carried out in the field of gene classification and prediction. In a recent research, authors have presented each and every letter in a gene sequence by a layer image (Abdelwahab & Abdelrahman, 2017). The last four layers are combined with 2-Dimensional Principle Component Analysis (2DPCA) to build an algorithm for predicting lung cancer. They have used 2DPCA for reflecting four layers of gene into eigenspace. The selection of dominant eigenvectors is done using the prevalent or dominant eigenvalues. The feature matrix for the layers is made by projecting the layer on the dominant or prevalent eigenvectors. While testing, the dominating eigenvector was used to find the feature matrices of tested genes. The database was from the Catalog of Somatic Mutations in Cancer, and sequences of normal or nonmutated candidate genes were extracted from the National Center for Biotechnological Information (NCBI). They attained an accuracy of 98.55% in predicting the mutation and 88.18% in substitution type identification.

In another research, a priori algorithm and decision tree algorithms are used to match the DNA sequence of mutations that may lead to adenocarcinoma, i.e. Epidermal growth factor (EGFR), Anaplastic lymphoma kinase (ALK), Vascular endothelial growth factor (VEGF), and Echinoderm microtubule-associated protein-like 4 (EML4) (Ham et al., 2015). In a priori algorithm, due to the difference in length of four sequences, classes 2, 3, and 4 were amplified to match class 1. They used excel to classify the results and remove frequency less than 0.8. In decision tree, they blocked every sequence into 17, 9, and 13 windows. In window 13, each gave result as 13 of L proteins, in window 17, EGFR gave the result as 16, but the other two gave the result as 17, whereas in windows 9, all of ALK, EGFR, and EML gave an outcome as 9 L of proteins. Sequence of S in ALK, EGFR, and EML4 (0, 1, and 2 each in the order) also exhibited the same tendency.

A study conducted by Abdelrahman and Abdelwahab (2018) identified the class of genes responsible for lung cancer. For gene representation, a novel new technique has been proposed, i.e., AGLI, also known as accumulated gray level image method. It is used with 2DPCA for building an algorithm that eventually classifies genetic mutations. Proposed algorithm has been applied on the most prevalent ten genes in lung cancer, and they managed to achieve an accuracy of 99.27%. Also, authors optimize the proposed algorithm, as they were able to reduce their classification time and dimensionality as well.

Another contribution highlighted that frequent pattern (FP) mining is applied to build the relationship between characteristics of patient and response of tumor in advanced nonsmall cell lung cancer (Kureshi et al., 2016). They also did univariate analysis to deduce that smoking condition, EGFR mutation, histology, and drug (targeted) are the highly linked factors with response to targeted therapy. Four classification algorithms are applied to predict the result or outcome variable, i.e., treatment from EGFR tyrosine kinase inhibitors. They recorded their highest accuracy at 76.57% using decision tree. The combination of attributes used by decision tree was the associated factors. Also, authors concluded that decision tree and support vector machines (SVMs) were the promising algorithms for their prediction of the outcome variable.

In another novel work, authors utilized advanced data mining algorithm to diagnose breast cancer (Khan & Chouhan, 2015). Breast cancer affects a lot of people, and early diagnosis is crucial for saving many lives. Accurate classification leads to early diagnosis. They have applied genetic programming, which is excelling these days in the field of classification. Under genetic programming, they applied mutation method and knowledgeable crossover. This method is the fusion of conventional method and hill climbing approach, which was enforced on both mutation and recombination. The dataset they used was from University of California, Irvine (UCI) archive and comprised nine attributes and two classes. After tenfold cross-validation method, they recorded their highest accuracy at 99.6%.

A research was conducted over the classification of mutations by deploying hidden Markov models (Liu et al., 2014). These classifications were done by functional effect types like loss of function, switch of function, and gain of function. This research work utilizes K-means clustering to group the arrangement into distinct subgroups. So, they eventually concluded that a pipeline is suitable to determine mutations of various distinct types. Also, gains of function mutations are often variants that are activating, and the losses of function mutations are often destructive variants. Their condensed prediction on the mutations' outcome was dependent on only two cutoff values, 2 and 1. So, they have used hidden Markov models only.

Researchers have used mutation data from ovarian cancers to find the informative genes for cancer (Ma et al., 2014). Gene mutation profile of patient is used, and gene–gene interactions network and gene expression data are used to construct a graphical depiction of patients and genes and build Markov processes for patients and mutations distinctly. Led by the Cancer Genome Atlas, the data for experiment was taken from the study of Integrated Genomic Analyses of Ovarian Carcinoma. They have set $\alpha = 0.75$. For the additive model (RW–AM), they have set $\gamma = 0.4$, $\alpha = 0.3$, and $\beta = 0.3$. Higher occurrences of mutation assist higher rank for a frequency-based model. They have calculated gene rank vector after performing random walk on gene correlation network and patient mutation network individually.

An integrated classification decision tree on micro RNAs, genes and their proteins is carried out by Dass et al. (2014). They further applied cross-validation technique to increase the accuracy of J48 Algorithm in Weka. The datasets were obtained by a vast survey of literature from a PubMed module of NCBI. They were a combination of genomic, micro RNAs, and proteomic markers collectively. This classification technique affirms a way for arithmetical analysis of cancers based on learning of varying or unregulated biomolecules.

Furthermore, Bhardwaj et al. (2014) used Genetically Optimized Neural Network (GONN) algorithm to solve the problem of division into classes. To hone its construction for division, they genetically trained a neural network. They introduced new mutation operations and crossover that differs from an ordinary genetic programming life cycle to shorten the damaging type of these procedures. To segregate breast cancer tumors as mild or lethal, they use the GONN algorithm. Their accuracy was found to be 98.52%. Although their attributes do not contain any genetic mutation history, their classification is primarily based on physical form factors of cancer cells.

4.3 Dataset Collection

The dataset used here was taken from kaggle (Kaggle Dataset, 2017) and made available by Memorial Kettering Cancer Center (MSKCC). MSKCC made available a database anno-tated by experts, where oncologists and researchers around the globe have annotated thousands of mutations manually. The genetic mutations have to be classified automati-cally using this knowledge base as a baseline.

The detailed description of contents of the dataset is

- training_variants: File having the explanation of genetic mutations. Attributes are ID (unique ID for each row), gene (the gene where genetic mutation is tak-ing place), variation (the amino acid change occurring in the mutation), and class (class of the genetic mutation).
- training_text: File containing the medical proof (text) is used to distinguish genetic mutations using double pipe (||) delimiter. Columns are ID (unique ID for each row) and text (the clinical proof of the genetic mutation).

Figures 4.1–4.3 present the pictorial representation of dataset used in the study. Figure 4.1 presents the list of top occurring genes in the dataset, Figure 4.2 presents classes, and Figure 4.3 outlines the uppermost existing genes in a specific class of genetic mutation.

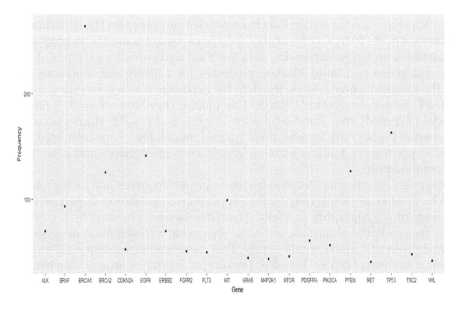

FIGURE 4.1
Top occurring genes in the dataset.

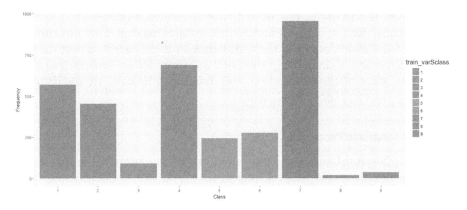

FIGURE 4.2
Most occurring classes in the dataset.

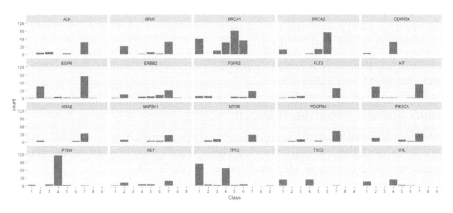

FIGURE 4.3
Top occurring genes in a specific class of genetic mutation.

4.4 Methodology

A detailed description of all techniques and algorithms for gene classification is presented in this section. First step is the assemblage of genes data, after that data preprocessing techniques are applied to make it suitable for the execution of machine learning algorithm for the purpose of gene classification. Various machine learning techniques have been used to find out the best optimal algorithm in the domain of genes. A web-based user interface is created for making prediction regarding genes and its associated class values.

4.4.1 Data Preprocessing

Data preprocessing is one of the essential steps of data-oriented process. It involves transmuting data from raw state to a more interpreting state. Data collected from various sources is inconsistent, erroneous, and incomplete and contain many more anomalies (García et al., 2015). Data preprocessing techniques are applied to remove such anomalies from the real-world dataset. It actually works out with data for further processing. Quality results depend upon quality data, so it is essential to utilize data that contributes in enhancing the classification results. Raw data goes through various progressions during the process of preprocessing. Cleaning of data, integration of data from various sources into a single file format, data alteration, attribute selection, and data discretization are the different steps involved in preprocessing (Zhao et al., 2018).

4.4.1.1 Natural Language Processing

The main use of Natural Language Processing (NLP) is to analyze the text data. In text data, all words become a column of a dataset (i.e., predictor variables), and their count in each instance will be the value for that particular column and row (Silge & Robinson, 2017). So, cleaning the text data becomes very important here. Also remember that not all words are important for the analysis, so removing some unnecessary words become a very important task, as it will also reduce the size of the dataset (Aggarwal & Zhai, 2012).

Some basic preprocessing applied are as follows:

- First of all, convert every word to lowercase, as it is not advisable to have two same words in the dataset with different cases.
- Sometimes, numbers in the text data are also not important, so it becomes important to remove those numbers.
- It is also important to remove punctuations from the text data like full stop, comma, brackets, colon, semicolon, etc.
- Removing irrelevant words is an important task. Some irrelevant words are as follows: for, a, and, the, etc. So, removing these words may largely reduce the size of dataset and improve model fitting (Kao & Poteet, 2007).
- Stemming the text data is also very beneficial. Stemming means getting the root for each word. For example, work, worked, will work, working, all are derived from work. Keeping only one word for all the earlier words is called stemming (Figure 4.4) (Prather et al., 1997).

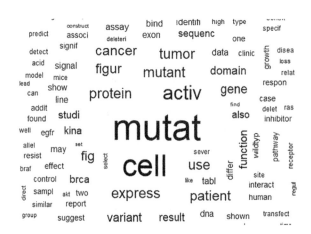

FIGURE 4.4
Word cloud for most occurring words.

This word cloud is made after applying NLP. For example, "mutating" word that was appearing in textual reports is being shown as "mutat"; that is, "ing" is removed from the original word due to stemming.

4.5 Machine Learning Algorithms

Machine learning is one the specialized fields of artificial intelligence that proffer system with the capability to learn from the past experiences and improve the technical ability from those experiences without being directly programmed (Kotsiantis et al., 2007). Main emphasis of machine learning is on the enlargement of software programs that can explore past data and further utilize it for attaining perfection without human intervention. Learning process starts with exploring data, surveying the data, or finding some hidden pattern from the given dataset for providing effective decisions on future test datasets (Callahan & Shah, 2018). Random forest, decision tree, SVM, ANN, extreme gradient boosting (XGBoost), and naïve Bayes are some machine learning techniques that are applied in this study for classification and future prediction (Witten et al., 2016).

4.5.1 Decision Tree

In this algorithm, information gain is first calculated for all the attributes, which is done in accordance with its entropy value (Lantz, 2013). A single decision tree is then created based on the attribute that has the highest entropy value. Now, the process is repeated on the remaining values. So, it basically divides the data on the basis of the attribute having the highest information gain value (Safavian & Landgrebe, 1991). The approach followed is top-down greedy, also called as recursive binary splitting. The process runs until the user-defined criteria (meant for stopping the algorithm) is met (Freund & Mason, 1999). For example, the algorithm can terminate if the number of observations per node is less than 40, as decided by the user.

4.5.2 Random Forest

This algorithm is based on several decision trees instead of just a single one. It does the job of adding randomness to the decision trees that have been generated. The attributes and training data are randomly selected from the given sets, and the decision trees are based on these selected inputs. The output of this algorithm is based on the votes by individual trees (Lantz, 2013). Let's suppose that the numbers of input variables are K, a number $k < K$ is stated in a way that at each and every node, k variables are chosen out of the total K. To split the node, the best split on this "k" is used. Aggregation of the prediction of trees (i.e., majority votes for classification, average for regression) is used for predicting new data (Liaw & Wiener, 2002).

4.5.3 XGBoost

In XGBoost, by a combination of prediction of each weak learner using methods like weighted average, weak learners are converted to strong learners (Chen & Guestrin, 2016). To find the weak rules, base learning (Machine Learning (ML)) algorithms are applied with a different distribution (Lantz, 2013). A weak prediction rule is made every time a machine learning algorithm is applied. This is a single round of the process or iteration. After many rounds or iterations, this algorithm does the combination of weak rules into a single yet strong rule for prediction. It is more efficient when compared with gradient boosting. It has tree learning algorithms as well as a linear model solver (Torlay et al., 2017).

4.5.4 Artificial Neural Networks

Artificial neural network (ANN) exactly works like a human brain. So, the first challenge is to recreate a neuron (Yegnanarayana, 2009). The most important thing about neurons is that they work together. In ANN, a neuron is nothing but a node. Weights are given to each node. Weights are how neural networks learn (Abraham, 2005). By weights, it learns which signal or value is important, which is not, or to what extent a signal is passed along. Now, inside the neuron, two steps take place:

Step 1. Compute

$$\sum (w_i x_i) \tag{4.1}$$

Step 2. Apply activation function on the earlier weighted sum, as in Equation (4.1).

$$\Phi\left(\sum (w_i x_i)\right) \tag{4.2}$$

Based on these steps, neuron passes this signal or value to the next neuron and so on (Hopfield, 1988). Activation function used is rectifier function. Rectifier function is basically

$$\Phi(x) = \max(x, 0) \tag{4.3}$$

i.e., if $x > 0$, then x is returned, else 0 is returned by the rectifier function. ANN contains an input layer, hidden layer, and output layer. There may be many hidden layers. In the hidden layer, there are many neurons. Activation function is applied in the hidden layer. This follows the working of ANNs. Suppose y_i is the actual value and $\hat{y}$ is the predicted value. Then, the cost function becomes

$$c = \sum (\tfrac{1}{2})\left(\hat{y}_i - y_i\right)^2 \tag{4.4}$$

It tells us the error that we have in our prediction. Our goal is to minimize this error. To minimize the cost function, weights given to each node or neuron are updated. This whole process of updating the weights are done by a method called gradient descent. In gradient descent, the slope of the line at a given point in the graph between c (y-axis) and $\hat{y}$ (x-axis) is tried to be made 0. But the problem with gradient descent is that it requires the cost function to be convex. However, the cost function cannot be convex in two ways:

- Choose a cost function, $c \neq \sum (\tfrac{1}{2})\left(\hat{y}_i - y_i\right)^2$
- If there are multiple minima in a cost function, then it is necessary to select a global minima.

So, stochastic gradient descent comes into play, which does not require a cost function to be convex. In stochastic gradient descent, one row is taken at a time, the cost function is calculated, and then the weights are updated to minimize the cost function. Then, the next row is taken and so on, and the procedure continues for all the rows. So, here the weights are updated for each row rather than taking all the rows at once and then updating the weights (He & Xu, 2010). Updating or adjusting the weights is known as backpropagation.

4.5.5 Support Vector Machine

It is a supervised machine learning algorithm that works on support vectors. Support vectors are basically vectors to the extreme boundary points that are useful for the classification. So basically, those extreme points support the algorithm. A line or a plane is drawn, which makes a good partition in the data for the classification (Steinwart & Christmann, 2008). This line is called maximum margin linear hyperplane. However, this method is good for linear data only, and in the case of nonlinear data, there may be a situation where the boundary line may not be found. In that case, kernel SVM is used.

In kernel SVM, Gaussian kernel is used, which becomes

$$K(x,l) = \frac{e^{\left(|x-l|\right)^2}}{2\sigma^2} \qquad (4.5)$$

In the earlier formula, $|x-l|^2$ is the distance and σ is a constant which determines the circumference, i.e., the area around the landmark which is the value of K. If distance is very large, then K is small. So here, K value is used to build the boundary for classification (Shmilovici, 2009). There can be two or more kernel functions depending on the data.

4.5.6 Naïve Bayes

Naïve Bayes is a probabilistic model. It works according to Bayes theorem (Pawlak, 2002), which is formulated as in Equation (4.6):

$$P(A/B) = \frac{P(B/A)P(A)}{P(B)} \qquad (4.6)$$

Here, B denotes attributes or predictor variables and A denotes the outcome variable. For each class of A, the earlier probability is calculated, and for whichever class the probability value comes highest, that class is predicted (Rish, 2001).

Bayes theorem requires each predictor variable to be independent of other predictor variables, but still we use it even when there is some correlation among the predictor variables, so it is called naïve Bayes.

4.6 System Architecture

After building the machine learning models, a web-based application is developed using R software through a *shiny* interface. Any shiny application consists of two files:

- ui.r: This is used for creating the user interface. Here, one can give the input and display the output.

- server.r: This is used for processing the input so as to convert it into the desired output. This is the file where algorithms are applied and analysis is done.

In our application, the user is first prompted to upload the text-based report through ui.r. The data of the file is received in server.r, and prediction regarding the gene and class value is done for that specific report. Also, the word cloud regarding the report is made. All these are transferred back to ui.r, where they are displayed.

4.7 Block Diagram of Proposed Model

Figure 4.5 presents the overall design of the proposed machine learning model for finding out the gene alteration of DNA sequence. A web-based user interface is created for easy accessibility. A user can enter the medical reports for finding out the corresponding outcome for a given input file. For the same, we have created a "ui.r" interface that can take input and generate output. After the input of medical data, the proposed model starts its function, first data preprocessing is applied, and for the same proposed model, it uses text-preprocessing using NLP to make clinical data appropriate for further application

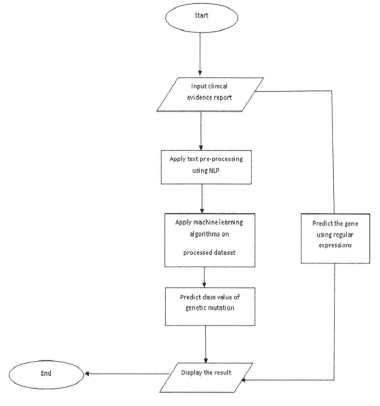

FIGURE 4.5
Overall architecture of a proposed gene classification model.

of machine learning models. "Server.r" interface is developed, which is used for the process of classification. All machine learning models are applied on the clinical report for the prediction of class value of genetic mutation, and response is sent back to "ui.r" for displaying final reports to the user. Regular expressions are used for searching the gene mutation patterns. R language is used to implement the proposed gene classification model (Team, 2013).

4.8 Evaluation Methods

To calculate the accuracy, precision, and recall of our model, the following formulae (Han et al., 2011) were used.

Accuracy can be defined as the ratio of correct predictions to the total predictions (both correct and incorrect).

$$\text{Accuracy} = \frac{TP + TN}{TP + TN + FP + FN} \tag{4.7}$$

Precision can be defined as the ratio of positive observations that are correctly predicted to the sum of total predicted positive observations.

$$\text{Precision} = \frac{TP}{TP + FP} \tag{4.8}$$

Recall is the ratio of positive observations that are correctly predicted to the total observations in actual class.

$$\text{Recall} = \frac{TP}{TP + FN} \tag{4.9}$$

where TP is the number of cases that were positive and predicted positive, TN is the number of cases that were negative and predicted negative, FP is the number of cases that were negative but predicted positive, and FN is the number of cases that were positive but predicted negative.

For finding various genetic mutations, the pattern ([A-Z0-9]{3,10}[ ][m|M][u][t][a][t][i][o][n] ([s]?)) was used as the regular expression (Li et al., 2008).

4.9 Experimental Result

We applied six machine learning algorithms on the dataset, and nine types of class variables were predicted using machine learning algorithms (Figures 4.6–4.12). After applying ML algorithms on our original dataset, we obtained the following accuracies (Table 4.1).

```
Confusion Matrix and Statistics

            Reference
Prediction   1   2   3   4   5   6   7   8   9
         1  42  12   2  22   4   8  18   1   6
         2   0   8   0   2   0   0   0   0   0
         3   0   0   0   0   0   0   0   0   0
         4  51  19   6 113  13   8  32   1   2
         5  21   0   1   7  26   5   0   0   0
         6   5   0   0   0   2  28   0   0   0
         7  23  74  13  27  15  19 188   2   1
         8   0   0   0   0   0   0   0   0   0
         9   0   0   0   0   0   0   0   0   0

Overall Statistics

               Accuracy : 0.4897
                 95% CI : (0.4551, 0.5244)
    No Information Rate : 0.2878
    P-Value [Acc > NIR] : < 2.2e-16

                  Kappa : 0.3445
 Mcnemar's Test P-Value : NA

Statistics by Class:

                     Class: 1 Class: 2 Class: 3 Class: 4 Class: 5 Class: 6 Class: 7 Class: 8 Class: 9
Sensitivity           0.29577 0.070796   0.0000   0.6608  0.43333  0.41176   0.7899 0.000000  0.00000
Specificity           0.89343 0.997199   1.0000   0.7988  0.95567  0.99078   0.7046 1.000000  1.00000
Pos Pred Value         0.36522 0.800000      NaN   0.4612  0.43333  0.80000   0.5193      NaN      NaN
Neg Pred Value         0.85955 0.871481   0.9734   0.9003  0.95567  0.94949   0.8925 0.995163  0.98912
Prevalence            0.17170 0.136638   0.0266   0.2068  0.07255  0.08222   0.2878 0.004837  0.01088
Detection Rate        0.05079 0.009674   0.0000   0.1366  0.03144  0.03386   0.2273 0.000000  0.00000
Detection Prevalence  0.13906 0.012092   0.0000   0.2963  0.07255  0.04232   0.4377 0.000000  0.00000
Balanced Accuracy     0.59460 0.533998   0.5000   0.7298  0.69450  0.70127   0.7473 0.500000  0.50000
```

FIGURE 4.6
Confusion matrix for a decision tree.

```
Confusion Matrix and Statistics

            Reference
Prediction   1   2   3   4   5   6   7   8   9
         1  79   4   3  21  14   4  10   1   2
         2   7  58   0   8   3   0  47   1   0
         3   2   2   6   4   1   1   4   0   0
         4  27   2   3 115   7   4   5   0   2
         5  10   2   4   5  29   6   7   0   0
         6  14   8   0  13   2  49   9   1   0
         7   3  37   6   5   4   4 156   0   0
         8   0   0   0   0   0   0   0   1   1
         9   0   0   0   0   0   0   0   0   4

Overall Statistics

               Accuracy : 0.601
                 95% CI : (0.5667, 0.6345)
    No Information Rate : 0.2878
    P-Value [Acc > NIR] : < 2.2e-16

                  Kappa : 0.5128
 Mcnemar's Test P-Value : NA

Statistics by Class:

                     Class: 1 Class: 2 Class: 3 Class: 4 Class: 5 Class: 6 Class: 7 Class: 8 Class: 9
Sensitivity           0.55634 0.51327 0.272727   0.6725  0.48333  0.72059   0.6555 0.250000 0.444444
Specificity           0.91387 0.90756 0.982609   0.9238  0.95567  0.93808   0.8998 0.998785 1.000000
Pos Pred Value         0.57246 0.46774 0.300000   0.6970  0.46032  0.51042   0.7256 0.500000 1.000000
Neg Pred Value         0.90856 0.92176 0.980173   0.9154  0.95942  0.97401   0.8660 0.996364 0.993925
Prevalence            0.17170 0.13664 0.026602   0.2068  0.07255  0.08222   0.2878 0.004837 0.010883
Detection Rate        0.09553 0.07013 0.007255   0.1391  0.03507  0.05925   0.1886 0.001209 0.004837
Detection Prevalence  0.16687 0.14994 0.024184   0.1995  0.07618  0.11608   0.2600 0.002418 0.004837
Balanced Accuracy     0.73510 0.71042 0.627668   0.7981  0.71950  0.82933   0.7776 0.624392 0.722222
```

FIGURE 4.7
Confusion matrix for an SVM (linear).

```
Confusion Matrix and Statistics

          Reference
Prediction   1    2    3    4    5    6    7    8    9
         1  67    4    1   12   13    8    0    0    1
         2   2   28    0    0    1    0    5    0    0
         3   1    1    3    0    0    1    1    0    0
         4  23    2    5  126    6    5    4    1    2
         5   9    0    2    9   22    2    2    0    0
         6   6    4    0    0    2   41    0    0    0
         7  34   74   11   24   16   11  226    2    3
         8   0    0    0    0    0    0    0    1    0
         9   0    0    0    0    0    0    0    0    3

Overall Statistics

               Accuracy : 0.6252
                 95% CI : (0.5912, 0.6583)
    No Information Rate : 0.2878
    P-Value [Acc > NIR] : < 2.2e-16

                  Kappa : 0.5191
 Mcnemar's Test P-Value : NA

Statistics by Class:

                     Class: 1 Class: 2 Class: 3 Class: 4 Class: 5 Class: 6 Class: 7 Class: 8
Sensitivity           0.47183 0.24779 0.136364   0.7368  0.36667  0.60294   0.9496 0.250000
Specificity           0.94307 0.98880 0.995031   0.9268  0.96871  0.98419   0.7029 1.000000
Pos Pred Value        0.63208 0.77778 0.428571   0.7241  0.47826  0.77358   0.5636 1.000000
Neg Pred Value        0.89598 0.89254 0.976829   0.9311  0.95134  0.96512   0.9718 0.996368
Prevalence            0.17170 0.13664 0.026602   0.2068  0.07255  0.08222   0.2878 0.004837
Detection Rate        0.08102 0.03386 0.003628   0.1524  0.02660  0.04958   0.2733 0.001209
Detection Prevalence  0.12817 0.04353 0.008464   0.2104  0.05562  0.06409   0.4849 0.001209
Balanced Accuracy     0.70745 0.61829 0.565697   0.8318  0.66769  0.79357   0.8262 0.625000
                     Class: 9
Sensitivity          0.333333
Specificity          1.000000
```

FIGURE 4.8
Confusion matrix for an SVM (radial).

```
Confusion Matrix and Statistics

          Reference
Prediction   1    2    3    4    5    6    7    8    9
         1  84    3    4   22   21    7    0    2    1
         2   3   44    0    1    1    0   17    0    1
         3   1    0    5    0    1    0    2    0    0
         4  26    3    3  128    4    3    4    1    2
         5   6    1    4    6   26    7    8    0    0
         6  10    5    0    1    0   46    1    0    0
         7  12   57    6   13    7    5  205    1    2
         8   0    0    0    0    0    0    0    0    0
         9   0    0    0    0    0    0    1    0    3

Overall Statistics

               Accuracy : 0.6542
                 95% CI : (0.6206, 0.6866)
    No Information Rate : 0.2878
    P-Value [Acc > NIR] : < 2.2e-16

                  Kappa : 0.5659
 Mcnemar's Test P-Value : NA

Statistics by Class:

                     Class: 1 Class: 2 Class: 3 Class: 4 Class: 5 Class: 6 Class: 7 Class: 8 Class: 9
Sensitivity           0.5915 0.38938 0.227273   0.7485  0.43333  0.67647   0.8613 0.000000 0.333333
Specificity           0.9124 0.96779 0.995031   0.9299  0.95828  0.97760   0.8251 1.000000 0.998778
Pos Pred Value        0.5833 0.65672 0.555556   0.7356  0.44828  0.73016   0.6656      NaN 0.750000
Neg Pred Value        0.9151 0.90921 0.979218   0.9342  0.95579  0.97120   0.9364 0.995163 0.992710
Prevalence            0.1717 0.13664 0.026602   0.2068  0.07255  0.08222   0.2878 0.004837 0.010883
Detection Rate        0.1016 0.05320 0.006046   0.1548  0.03144  0.05562   0.2479 0.000000 0.003628
Detection Prevalence  0.1741 0.08102 0.010883   0.2104  0.07013  0.07618   0.3724 0.000000 0.004837
Balanced Accuracy     0.7520 0.67858 0.611152   0.8392  0.69581  0.82704   0.8432 0.500000 0.666055
```

FIGURE 4.9
Confusion matrix for a random forest.

```
Confusion Matrix and Statistics

          Reference
Prediction  1  2  3   4  5  6   7  8  9 mutation
    1      76  6  2  34  7  8   5  0  0    4
    2       1 55  0   1  2  7  44  0  0    3
    3       4  0  8   2  2  0   6  0  0    0
    4      15  2  3 128  6  3   9  0  0    5
    5      17  2  3   2 29  0   5  0  0    2
    6       5  0  0   3  8 48   2  0  0    2
    7       3 43  4   4  7  2 164  0  1   10
    8       0  1  0   1  0  0   1  1  0    0
    9       1  1  0   1  0  0   0  1  5    0
 mutation   0  0  0   0  0  0   0  0  0    0

Overall Statistics

            Accuracy : 0.6215
              95% CI : (0.5875, 0.6547)
 No Information Rate : 0.2854
 P-Value [Acc > NIR] : < 2.2e-16

               Kappa : 0.537
 Mcnemar's Test P-Value : NA

Statistics by Class:
```

	Class: 1	Class: 2	Class: 3	Class: 4	Class: 5	Class: 6	Class: 7	Class: 8	Class: 9	Class: mutation
Sensitivity	0.6230	0.50000	0.400000	0.7273	0.47541	0.70588	0.6949	0.500000	0.833333	0.00000
Specificity	0.9064	0.91911	0.982652	0.9339	0.95953	0.97365	0.8748	0.996364	0.995128	1.00000
Pos Pred Value	0.5352	0.48673	0.363636	0.7485	0.48333	0.70588	0.6891	0.250000	0.555556	NaN
Neg Pred Value	0.9328	0.92297	0.985093	0.9268	0.95828	0.97365	0.8778	0.998785	0.998778	0.96856
Prevalence	0.1475	0.13301	0.024184	0.2128	0.07376	0.08222	0.2854	0.002418	0.007255	0.03144
Detection Rate	0.0919	0.06651	0.009674	0.1548	0.03507	0.05804	0.1983	0.001209	0.006046	0.00000
Detection Prevalence	0.1717	0.13664	0.026602	0.2068	0.07255	0.08222	0.2878	0.004837	0.010883	0.00000
Balanced Accuracy	0.7647	0.70955	0.691326	0.8306	0.71747	0.83977	0.7849	0.748182	0.914231	0.50000

FIGURE 4.10
Confusion matrix for ANN.

```
Confusion Matrix and Statistics

          Reference
Prediction  1   2  3   4  5  6   7  8  9
    1      81   5  1  30  6 11   8  0  0
    2       8  43  0   5  0  4  53  0  0
    3       4   0  7   2  3  0   6  0  0
    4      22   3  1 128  2  0  15  0  0
    5      20   1  0   6 23  0  10  0  0
    6       9   0  1   3  6 43   6  0  0
    7       2  18  1   3  7  2 205  0  0
    8       1   0  0   2  0  0   1  0  0
    9       1   1  0   1  0  0   1  1  4

Overall Statistics

            Accuracy : 0.6457
              95% CI : (0.612, 0.6783)
 No Information Rate : 0.3688
 P-Value [Acc > NIR] : < 2.2e-16

               Kappa : 0.5549
 Mcnemar's Test P-Value : NA

Statistics by Class:
```

	Class: 1	Class: 2	Class: 3	Class: 4	Class: 5	Class: 6	Class: 7	Class: 8	Class: 9
Sensitivity	0.54730	0.60563	0.636364	0.7111	0.48936	0.71667	0.6721	0.000000	1.000000
Specificity	0.91016	0.90741	0.981618	0.9335	0.95256	0.96741	0.9368	0.995157	0.993925
Pos Pred Value	0.57042	0.38053	0.318182	0.7485	0.38333	0.63235	0.8613	0.000000	0.444444
Neg Pred Value	0.90219	0.96078	0.995031	0.9207	0.96871	0.97760	0.8302	0.998785	1.000000
Prevalence	0.17896	0.08585	0.013301	0.2177	0.05683	0.07255	0.3688	0.001209	0.004837
Detection Rate	0.09794	0.05200	0.008464	0.1548	0.02781	0.05200	0.2479	0.000000	0.004837
Detection Prevalence	0.17170	0.13664	0.026602	0.2068	0.07255	0.08222	0.2878	0.004837	0.010883
Balanced Accuracy	0.72873	0.75652	0.808991	0.8223	0.72096	0.84204	0.8045	0.497579	0.996962

FIGURE 4.11
Confusion matrix for XGBoost.

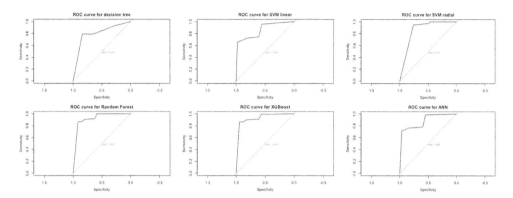

FIGURE 4.12
Receiver operating characteristic curve for the implemented models.

TABLE 4.1

Accuracies of Implemented Models

Algorithm	Accuracy (%)
Decision tree	48.97
SVM (linear)	60.10
SVM (radial)	62.52
Random forest	65.42
ANN	62.15
XGBoost	64.57

Area under the curve (AUC) (Fawcett, 2006) is given later for all the algorithms we applied, and the following outcome is received:

- AUC for decision tree is 0.801
- AUC for SVM linear is 0. 860
- AUC for SVM radial is 0. 863
- AUC for random forest is 0.921
- AUC for XGBoost is 0.926
- AUC for ANN is 0.881

Low accuracy and low AUC of ANN than random forest and XGBoost show that the data is linear, and we know the fact that neural networks work better when data is nonlinear. Here are a few screenshots of the running shiny application. Figure 13.15 shown below presents few snapshots of working of the proposed web-based tool for predicting gene mutation. In Figure 4.13, we can see that once a user uploads the text report on the webpage, the result regarding the webpage will be printed. In the screenshot in Figure 4.13, the gene predicted is CBL, and the class predicted is 4. As we can see, the word cloud regarding the text reported is also printed, and it shows the words that have occurred most of the times (Figure 4.14).

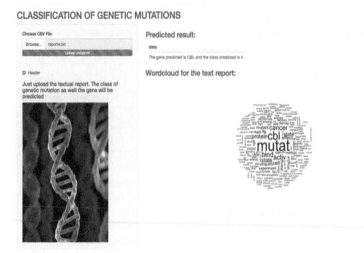

FIGURE 4.13
Gene class prediction.

In this case, the gene predicted was EGFR, and the class predicted was 7. The word cloud shows mutat and egfr as the two dominant words (Figure 4.15).

Similarly, the gene in this report was CBL, and the class was 2. Mutat and ccbl were the two most occurring words in this report.

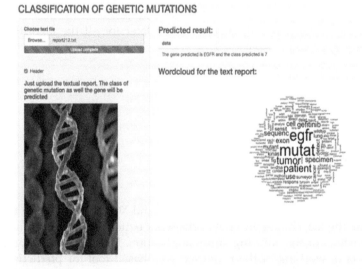

FIGURE 4.14
Word cloud along with gene class prediction.

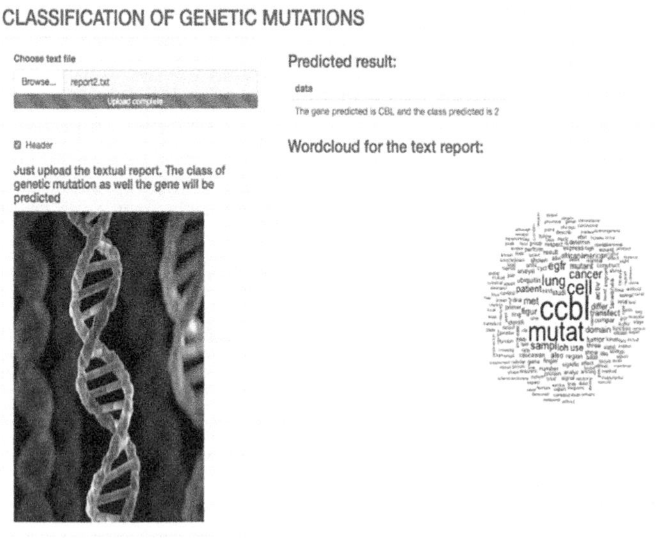
CLASSIFICATION OF GENETIC MUTATIONS
Choose text file
Browse...
report2.txt
Upload complete
Header
Just upload the textual report. The class of genetic mutation as well the gene will be predicted
Predicted result:
data
The gene predicted is CBL and the class predicted is 2
Wordcloud for the text report:
egfr
cancer
lung
cell
patient
met
ccbl
mutat
domain
sampl
use

FIGURE 4.15
Prediction model.

4.10 Conclusion

Cancer is one of the leading causes of death worldwide. Early diagnosis is essential for improving the survivability of cancer patients. Classification of cancerous genes is significant in personalizing cancer treatment. The proposed work plays a significant role in the classification of gene mutation. Cancer genes are the growth of unwanted cells from genetic alterations that outperform other normal cells and stop normal cells from functioning. Advanced machine learning techniques are extensively used for the identification of mutated genes. ML techniques are experimented in gene analysis for finding out the hidden gene pattern that can ultimately lead to abnormal genes that contribute to life-threatening disease like cancer. Classifying genetic mutations is crucial, as not all mutations cause cancer. So, if the manual work of doctors is saved, they can spend that extra time for curing the never ending line of patients. The proposed system imposes on searching the mutated genes so that one can diagnose severe diseases at an early stage. The proposed machine learning model for gene mutation classification is able to classify mutated genes, and for the same, we have experimented six different machine learning techniques (random forest, decision tree, SVM, ANN, XGBoost, Naïve Bayes) to find out more accurate results. Experimental analysis shows that random forest and XGBoost surpass other classification techniques in the classification of gene mutation. This classification of mutations can be instrumental in redefining cancer treatment. In future, we would like to increase the accuracy of our predictions that can further enhance cancer treatment.

References

Abdelrahman, S. A., & Abdelwahab, M. M. (2018). Accumulated grey-level image representation for classification of lung cancer genetic mutations employing 2D principle component analysis. *Electronics Letters*, 54(4), 194–196.

Abdelwahab, M. M., & Abdelrahman, S. A. (2017, August). Four layers image representation for prediction of lung cancer genetic mutations based on 2DPCA. In *IEEE 60th International Midwest Symposium on Circuits and Systems (MWSCAS), 2017* (pp. 599–602). IEEE, USA.

Abraham, A. (2005). Artificial neural networks. *Handbook of Measuring System Design*. doi: 10.1002/0471497398.mm421.

Aggarwal, C. C., & Zhai, C. (Eds.) (2012). *Mining Text Data*. Springer Science & Business Media, Berlin.

Bhardwaj, A., Tiwari, A., Chandarana, D., & Babel, D. (2014, October). A genetically optimized neural network for classification of breast cancer disease. In *7th International Conference on Biomedical Engineering and Informatics (BMEI), 2014* (pp. 693–698). IEEE, China.

Brooker, R. J. (2009). *Genetics: Analysis and Principles*.

Callahan, A., & Shah, N. H. (2018). Machine learning in healthcare. In *Key Advances in Clinical Informatics* (pp. 279–291), Academic Press.

Chen, T., & Guestrin, C. (2016, August). Xgboost: A scalable tree boosting system. In *Proceedings of the 22nd ACM SIGKDD International Conference on Knowledge Discovery and Data Mining* (pp. 785–794). ACM, Sydney, Australia.

Dass, M. V., Rasheed, M. A., & Ali, M. M. (2014, January). Classification of lung cancer subtypes by data mining technique. In *International Conference on Control, Instrumentation, Energy and Communication (CIEC), 2014* (pp. 558–562). IEEE, Kolkata, India.

Davies, H., Bignell, G. R., Cox, C., Stephens, P., Edkins, S., Clegg, S., … Davis, N. (2002). Mutations of the BRAF gene in human cancer. *Nature*, 417(6892), 949.

Fawcett, T. (2006). An introduction to ROC analysis. *Pattern Recognition Letters*, 27(8), 861–874.

Freund, Y., & Mason, L. (1999, June). The alternating decision tree learning algorithm. In ICML (Vol. 99, pp. 124–133).

García, S., Luengo, J., & Herrera, F. (2015). *Data Preprocessing in Data Mining* (pp. 195–243). Springer International Publishing, Switzerland.

Ham, C., Kim, J., Ahn, S., Kim, Y., Kim, S., & Yoon, T. (2015, August). Analysis of gene mutation that cause lung cancer by using data miningand study of common remedy. In *IEEE Conference on Computational Intelligence in Bioinformatics and Computational Biology (CIBCB), 2015* (pp. 1–5). IEEE, Siena - Tuscany, Italy.

Han, J., Pei, J., & Kamber, M. (2011). *Data Mining: Concepts and Techniques*. Elsevier, USA.

He, X., & Xu, S. (2010). *Artificial Neural Networks. Process Neural Networks: Theory and Applications*, Springer-Verlag, Berlin Heidelberg, pp. 20–42.

Hopfield, J. J. (1988). Artificial neural networks. *IEEE Circuits and Devices Magazine*, 4(5), 3–10.

Kaggle Dataset (2017). Personalized Medicine: Redefining Cancer Treatment. https://www.kaggle.com/c/msk-redefining-cancer-treatment/data

Kao, A., & Poteet, S. R. (Eds.) (2007). *Natural Language Processing and Text Mining*. Springer Science & Business Media, Berlin.

Khan, A., & Chouhan, M. (2015, December). Intelligent crossover and mutation technique to control bloat for breast cancer diagnosis. In *International Conference on Computational Intelligence and Communication Networks (CICN), 2015* (pp. 387–391). IEEE, Honolulu Hawaii, USA.

Kotsiantis, S. B., Zaharakis, I., & Pintelas, P. (2007). Supervised machine learning: A review of classification techniques. *Emerging Artificial Intelligence Applications in Computer Engineering*, 160, 3–24.

Kureshi, N., Abidi, S. S. R., & Blouin, C. (2016). A predictive model for personalized therapeutic interventions in non-small cell lung cancer. *IEEE Journal Biomedical and Health Informatics*, 20(1), 424–431.

Lantz, B. (2013). Machine learning with R. Packt Publishing Ltd.

Li, Y., Krishnamurthy, R., Raghavan, S., Vaithyanathan, S., & Jagadish, H. V. (2008, October). Regular expression learning for information extraction. In *Proceedings of the Conference on Empirical Methods in Natural Language Processing* (pp. 21–30). Association for Computational Linguistics, Honolulu, Hawaii, USA.

Liaw, A., & Wiener, M. (2002). Classification and regression by random forest. *R News*, 2(3), 18–22.

Liu, M., Watson, L. T., & Zhang, L. (2014, June). Classification of mutations by functional impact type: Gain of function, loss of function, and switch of function. In *International Symposium on Bioinformatics Research and Applications* (pp. 236–242). Springer, Cham, Beijing, China.

Ma, C., Chen, Y., & Wilkins, D. (2014, November). Ranking of cancer genes in Markov chain model through integration of heterogeneous sources of data. In *IEEE International Conference on Bioinformatics and Biomedicine (BIBM), 2014* (pp. 248–253). IEEE, San Diego, USA.

Nigro, J. M., Baker, S. J., Preisinger, A. C., Jessup, J. M., Hosteller, R., Cleary, K., … Glover, T. (1989). Mutations in the p53 gene occur in diverse human tumour types. *Nature*, 342(6250), 705.

Omoto, C. K., Lurquin, P. F., & Lurquin, P. (2004). *Genes and DNA: A Beginner's Guide to Genetics and Its Applications*. Columbia University Press, New York.

Pawlak, Z. (2002). Rough sets, decision algorithms and Bayes' theorem. *European Journal of Operational Research*, 136(1), 181–189.

Prather, J. C., Lobach, D. F., Goodwin, L. K., Hales, J. W., Hage, M. L., & Hammond, W. E. (1997). Medical data mining: knowledge discovery in a clinical data warehouse. In *Proceedings of the AMIA Annual Fall Symposium* (p. 101). American Medical Informatics Association.

Rish, I. (2001, August). An empirical study of the naive Bayes classifier. In *IJCAI 2001 Workshop on Empirical Methods in Artificial Intelligence* (Vol. 3, No. 22, pp. 41–46). IBM, New York.

Safavian, S. R., & Landgrebe, D. (1991). A survey of decision tree classifier methodology. *IEEE Transactions on Systems, Man, and Cybernetics*, 21(3), 660–674.

Shmilovici, A. (2009). Support vector machines. In Maimon, O., Rokach, L. (eds.) *Data Mining and Knowledge Discovery Handbook* (pp. 231–247). Springer, Boston, MA.

Silge, J., & Robinson, D. (2017). *Text Mining with R: A Tidy Approach*. O'Reilly Media, Inc., Sebastopol, California.

Steinwart, I., & Christmann, A. (2008). *Support Vector Machines*. Springer Science & Business Media, Berlin.

Team, R. C. (2013). *R: A Language and Environment for Statistical Computing*. R Foundation for Statistical Computing, Vienna, Austria.

Torlay, L., Perrone-Bertolotti, M., Thomas, E., & Baciu, M. (2017). Machine learning–XGBoost analysis of language networks to classify patients with epilepsy. *Brain Informatics*, 4(3), 159.

Witten, I. H., Frank, E., Hall, M. A., & Pal, C. J. (2016). *Data Mining: Practical Machine Learning Tools and Techniques*. Morgan Kaufmann, Burlington, MA.

Yegnanarayana, B. (2009). *Artificial Neural Networks*. PHI Learning Pvt. Ltd, New Delhi, India.

Zhao, J., Wang, W., & Sheng, C. (2018). Data preprocessing techniques. In *Data-Driven Prediction for Industrial Processes and Their Applications* (pp. 13–52). Springer, Cham, Beijing, China.

5

m-Health: Community-Based Android Application for Medical Services

Mahima Narang, Charu Nigam, and Nisha Chaurasia

Jaypee Institute of Information Technology

CONTENTS

5.1 Motivation

Everyone is currently experiencing a world where mobile utilization is developing exponentially. Innovation has empowered us greatly, where one looks for information at any place and time.

Versatile medicinal services applications offer astounding chances to enhance one's well-being, security, and in some sense, readiness to common illnesses. Because of their moderateness, accessibility, and conveyance of smart devices, well-being applications have prominent chances (Gupta, 2017).

The unique characteristics of m-health apps are as follows:

1. Simple: Apps are expected to be easy to use, and with just a single touch, one can get the desired search results instantly.

2. Context: Apps are customizable according to user's circumstances, and accordingly, services can be offered.

3. Immediacy: m-health apps provide instant results to its users.

There are a lot of cases of accidental situations like fire, road accidents, or natural calamities such as earthquakes. Such situations can cause major loss of life and mishappenings of disabilities due to untimely or delayed attention and treatment given to the victims. It becomes obvious that a person might panic and become helpless at such situations, and it is where such app comes into the picture. The proposed app assists the users to find nearby hospitals, at the same time getting the best ones according to the availability of resources and ratings provided to it. In addition, it fetches nearby available pharmacies and blood banks.

The app is designed to be a community-based application that allows users to access it anywhere even without any logging-in to provide quick access to the required data. It allows people to update information about the availability of resources and share/get guidance from peers (ET Rise, n.d.). Also, in case of emergency, notifications are sent to nearby users about the urgency so that immediate help can be provided.

This aforementioned characteristics of m-health apps inspired the authors to implement medical services on the mobile platform, for which the authors have used Android. It is incorporated with other technologies such as Google Application Program Interfaces (APIs), Geofire, Firebase, and machine learning techniques.

This chapter focuses on making advantageous use of Android and machine learning to provide an integrated platform to deliver health-related information on major healthcare units, such as hospitals, pharmacies, and blood banks. These facilities are provided through a developed app in which, according to the user's location and their specialized needs, data is customized on factors such as distance, availability of required resources, and ratings according to the general and offered specialized services of health units. Firebase is used as the platform approached to store and retrieve data that is dynamically updated for accurate results. In cases of natural disasters or accidents, an emergency button is added for immediate alert to nearby users along with a quick and efficient solution.

5.2 Background

In the ever-increasing rat race of ease-of-access, where people are facing such a highly competitive world, one can easily fall victim to health issues and accidents. According to Moushumi (2017), every hour there is news about 17 deaths due to road accidents. Also, it is to be noted that only 3.7% of total gross domestic product (GDP) is spent on health. The incidents like breaking of fire or occurrence of any natural calamity also lead to health issues. The earlier factors have motivated researchers to make apps using Android to ease health-related issues and assist people in case of emergencies. One such health application is "FinDoctor–Interactive Android Clinic Geographical Information System Using Firebase and Google Maps API" researched by Anisa Rahmi, NyomanPiarsa, and Putu WiraBuana (Rahmi et al., 2017), in which doctors and patients login the application. The firebase authenticates patient's details, and accordingly, the prescriptions are stored using Firebase, which acts as a real-time database. After logging in, the patient gets an availability of all doctors that are available near to his/her location. The patient then sends the request to the doctor that is stored in the firebase database, from where the doctor receives the request. The doctor can either accept or decline the request. In case the doctor accepts the request, the data of patient and doctor are added to the user's database, which is connected to the doctor's database.

There is another app, called "Red Panic Button," that is used in case of an emergency. It has a red button, pressing on which sends an emergency message along with the location of the user to registered email and contact numbers. It is a Global Positioning System (GPS)-based application. There has been the development of similar apps like Life360, First Aid for American Red Cross, etc., which tackles health-related issues. Taking motivation and information from the earlier described prebuilt applications and knowing about technology in which it works, an app that is better and more efficient is implemented and contains all facilities in one; that is, it not only finds the nearest hospital but also can look for a nearest pharmacy as well as blood bank. Also with the implementation of Firebase, one can dynamically update availability of resources in these units with the provision of emergency buttons like "Red Panic button" app to send notification about alert to all nearest users of the detected location using Firebase Cloud Messaging (FCM) and Hypertext Preprocessor (PHP) script.

The two main factors of the project that need to be kept in mind are

1. to help users to search for appropriate health units during emergency
2. to allow people to update information about the availability of resources, health units, and share/get guidance from peers

The aforementioned factors make it a community-based app.

5.3 m-Health App: Description

With billions of users across the globe, Android is an open-source widely available easy-to-use ground for developing and implementing applications for smartphone users today.

5.3.1 Android as a platform

In the world of digital technology, everything is desired to be accessible through one handset. Thus, to provide immediate and efficient healthcare, it is an effective platform for customers or patients to access healthcare providing services at the convenience of a touch.

There are various advantages of using Android:

- Multitasking
- Easy to notify
- Easy access to a huge number of people through Google Playstore
- Phone options are diverse
- Can install a modified read only memory (ROM)
- Widgets

5.3.2 Real-Time Database: Firebase

To maintain the frequently changing database that stores the information about the token IDs (generated by Firebase as the app is installed on the device) and health units, it is important to maintain a real-time database called Firebase. The advantages of using Firebase in the proposed work are as follows:

a. Latency: To overcome latency and get an optimized result for providing the best health unit in a fast and efficient manner, Firebase is used. It is a real-time database that follows the concept of NoSQL that does not hold database and tables like Structured Query Language (SQL); instead, it stores data in key/value pairs. The data is stored in the form of JavaScript Object Notation (JSON) (Firebase Realtime Database, n.d.). In contrast to the relational database framework, for example SQL, NoSQL does not have relationships between tables, which engage in frequent change in values (Leavitt, 2010). The data can be synced with all the end users in realtime, and the data remains stored and its functions work even if there is no internet connection (Alsalemi et al., 2017). This attribute permits agile development of the database as the location of the user can be changed from time to time, accordingly his/her nearby health units are changed. All this need quick data modification, deletion, insertion, and quick information retrieval for the best results.

b. *Compatibility:* Firebase database, owned by Google, can support various platforms and devices, such as Android, iOS, Linux, and Arduino firmware (Su et al., 2011), which adds another factor to use Firebase.

Figures 5.1–5.4 show the database as seen in Firebase Console.

5.3.3 Firebase Cloud Messaging

FCM, earlier known as Google Cloud Messaging, is a utility provided by Firebase, a subsidiary of Google. FCM is a cross-platform cloud-based solution to send messages and display notifications for iOS, Android, and other web-based applications, which can be utilized without any expenses (Wikipedia, 2019).

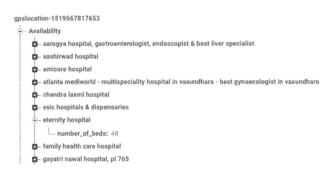

FIGURE 5.1
Nearby hospitals.

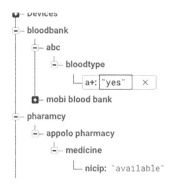

FIGURE 5.2
Nearby blood banks and pharmacies.

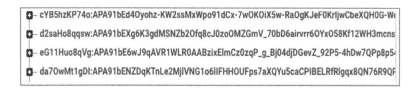

FIGURE 5.3
Tokens generated for different users.

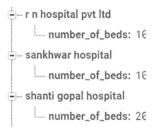

FIGURE 5.4
Total beds available in hospital (generated using Firebase).

1. One of the important parts of the application is to notify the users within a specified radius (determined by Geofire) about the emergency situation that is implemented with the help of FCM technology that sends push notifications whenever necessary. The application notifies all the users within the vicinity of the user that presses the emergency button (on the main page of the app). Whenever the user presses the notification that triggers on his/her device, he/she will be thereafter directed to a page where three options will be available, viz. hospital, blood banks, and pharmacy. Users can choose any one of the options according to their requirement from where they will be directed to Google maps with a marker on it displaying (hospital/pharmacy/blood bank) the optimized result calculated using the algorithm. By clicking the marker on the maps, the best route and estimated time from your location to the marked location on the map are shown. The Firebase, used as the database tool along with Geofire, is connected to the Android application using PHP scripts (Dhivya et al., 2015). One can host the PHP file either

through Firebase or through an online free web hosting service such as the one provided by 000webhost.com. Here, Server Side (PHP) retrieves the token IDs of nearby users from the database, while the Client Side (ANDROID) pushes notification with the emergency message triggered on the user's device.

5.3.4 GeoFire

It is an open-source library that enables users to store and enquire a set of keys depending on their geographic area. It simply stores locations with string keys. It provides the plausibility of recovering only those keys within a given geographic zone—all in real-time (Wenger, 2014).

In the project, GeoFire is integrated with the Firebase Realtime Database for storing the information about user's token IDs, his/her nearby hospitals, pharmacies, and blood banks within a specified radius. Geofire permits results of the query to be upgraded in realtime as they alter. It loads the information selectively for only certain nearby locations, making the application well responsive and lighter, even for extremely large datasets (Wenger, 2014).

To keep things basic, GeoFire stores information in its own format and location within the Firebase database. This permits the existing data format and security rules to remain unaltered while still providing the user with an easy solution for geoqueries. GeoFire client is also available for Objective-C and Java.

5.3.4.1 Example Usage

In the app, an emergency button is displayed, such that if a user presses it, then all the app users within the specified radius of that user's location will receive a notification signaling about the emergency situation and the immediate reaction they should take. To search for users' vicinity within the specified radius, GeoFire comes into play. You can store the location for each user using GeoFire, using the token IDs (user IDs) as GeoFire keys. GeoFire then grants one to easily query which keys (user IDs) are nearby.

5.3.5 Star Rating Prediction

The users can also choose their preference based on the ratings of the health unit calculated by the reviews provided for the hospital. For predicting the rating of responses for queries fired by users, TF-IDF vectorization is used. TF-IDF stands for term frequency–inverse document frequency. First, calculate IDF for each word in the document by performing the logarithmic ratio of the total number of documents to the number of documents in which that word is present. The obtained IDF is multiplied by the total number of that word present in the entire document, which is termed as term frequency. The obtained result is known as TF-IDF vector (Using TF-IDF to Determine Word Relevance in Document Queries). Following includes an example for calculating TF-IDF (Diana, 2016). Our experiment takes into account a collection of four documents given later:

s1:"service very good"

s2:"service very bad"

s3:"doctor quite good"

s4:"doctor very bad"

There are some terms appearing twice, while others appear once. Say N be the total documents present, i.e. $N = 4$. So, the IDF values for the words (terms) are

$$\text{quite} \log 2(4/1) = 2$$

$$\text{doctor } \log 2(4/2) = 1$$

$$\text{service} \log 2(4/2) = 1$$

$$\text{bad} \log 2(4/2) = 1$$

$$\text{good} \log 2(4/2) = 1$$

$$\text{very} \log 2(4/3) = 0.415$$

	Quite	Doctor	Service	Bad	Good	Very
s1	0	0	1	0	1	1
s2	0	0	1	1	0	1
s3	1	1	0	0	1	0
s4	0	1	0	1	0	1

On multiplying the TF scores by the IDF values of each term, the results are obtained in the form of matrix for each term in the document as follows:

	Quite	Doctor	Service	Bad	Good	Very
s1	0	0	1	0	1	0.415
s2	0	0	1	1	0	0.415
s3	2	1	0	0	1	0
s4	0	1	0	1	0	0.415

For a given query: "doctor good good," compute the TF-IDF of the query given, and then it can be compared with the TF-IDF score of all documents present in the group using cosine similarity. Arranging the similarity values in the decreasing order provides a final sequence in which the documents are presented as result to the query.

In the project, each document represents the reviews of a hospital, blood banks, or pharmacies. Since the surveys are composed of clients, obviously, there will be errors or certain words and punctuation marks that won't be required to classify the data using multinomial naive Bayes (MNB) theorem. Thus, tokenization of the documents will be required (Reddy et al., 2017).

Thus, the steps followed are as follows:

1. Removal of punctuations
2. Removing stopwords
3. Tokenize
4. Stemming

Wordnet Lemmatizer can be used for stemming purpose.

5.3.5.1 Feature Vector Generation

Once the tokenization is done, the words are transformed into feature vectors, that is a unigram model of text, that keep records of the frequency(TF-IDF vector) of each word that is used as features to generate the classification of reviews.

5.3.5.2 Training and Rating Prediction

Automatic text classification or text categorization is becoming progressively essential with the consistently developing measure of literary data put away in an electronic frame.

5.3.5.3 Multinomial Naive Bayes Approach

MNB is a supervised learning technique, in which a new document is classified by allocating one or more class labels from a fixed set of predefined classes (Kibriya et al., 2004).

Naive Bayes is an algorithm that is often utilized to tackle text classification problems. It is easy to implement and is efficient in computations.

For the objective of predicting the ratings of hospitals, pharmacies, or blood banks, MNB (Reddy et al., 2017) has been used to train the datasets that are further used to generate ratings based on the review text.

MNB considers that distributions of words are done by applying a specific parametric model, and the parameters can be estimated through a training data. The following equation represents the MNB model (Su et al., 2011):

$$P(c \mid d) = \frac{P(c) \prod_{i=1}^{n} P(w_i \mid c)^{f_i}}{P(d)}$$

where $P(c)$ is the probability that a document with class c may happen in the document collections, n is the number of unique words in document d, $P(w_i \mid c)$ is the conditional probability that a word w_i may occur in a document d given the class value c, f_i shows the count of occurrences of a word w_i in document d.

Figure 5.5 shows Flow diagram for prediction of ratings from reviews.

5.3.6 Flask

Once the ratings are generated using machine learning, one needs to connect it with Android, which is done using Flask. "Flask is a very famous web framework which provides simplicity and flexibility by implementing a bare-minimum web server"

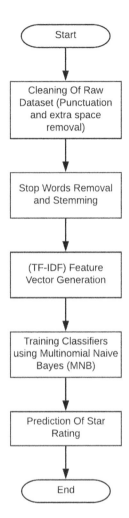

FIGURE 5.5
Flow diagram for prediction of ratings from reviews.

(Vogel et al., 2017), and it creates a local host that sends the generated result from Python to Android in JSON form, from where data is extracted and displayed on the user interface. It contains a proper procedure for implementation, and among it the most important line is app.run ("0.0.0.0," "8010"). The first part tells Flask to serve files on the developer's local Internet Protocol (IP) address (which is always kept as 0.0.0.0, even though if it is not the IP address). The second part tells the port number that can be changed if user wants (Coburn, n.d.).

5.4 Implementation Results

By implementing the above-stated technologies in a developed app sequentially, the app will provide the desired output as shown in Figure 5.6a and b.

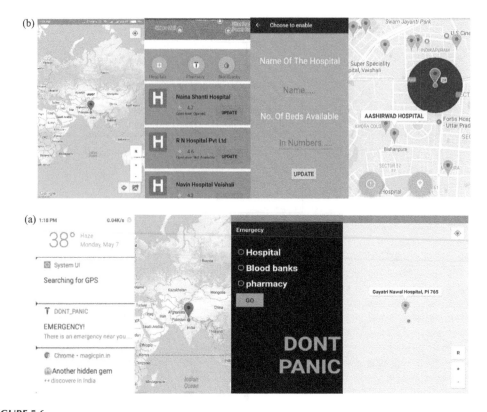

FIGURE 5.6
API screen for (a) locating hospital and (b) emergency service. (Google and the Google logo are registered trademarks of Google LLC, used with permission.)

After clicking on the emergency notification, the user displays the emergency screen. If the user clicks on a hospital, it displays the optimized solution for the best hospital, filtered by relevance.

5.4.1 Process for Results

The user can look for the information of nearby required health unit based on the preferences such as relevance that produces the results based on factors such as distance, availability of resources (beds/medicines/blood bags), and ratings or primarily on the basis of distance or availability or ratings alone.

Figure 5.7a and b shows the algorithm/approach used to obtain the results for the queries to find hospitals, pharmacies, or blood banks, with filtering based on relevance.

5.5 Conclusion

The uniqueness of the app lies in the fact that it gives an effective solution based on three factors such as distance, availability, and ratings of health units. The procedure is as follows: first, generate the token for each user who installs the app, then detect the location of user using Google Maps API that finds the nearby hospitals, and then optimize it even further by showing the nearby health units within the specified radius of the user using "GEOFIRE." The second filtration of data is based on the availability of resources for which data is stored in "FIREBASE," through which data can be updated dynamically, following the concept of community-based app, and the user can himself/herself update the availability of these resources. The third filtration mechanism is to sort according to ratings of these units generated using MNB theorem. There is a provision of the Emergency button to notify nearby users about emergencies implemented using FCM and PHP script.

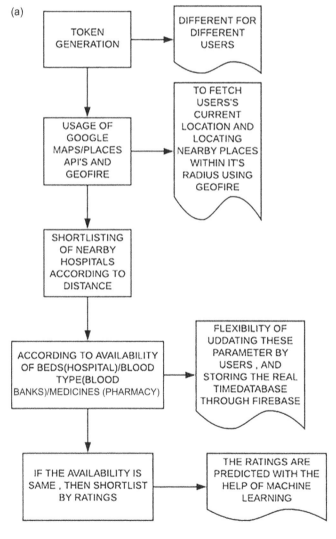

FIGURE 5.7
(a) Android approach and (b) Machine learning approach.

(*Continued*)

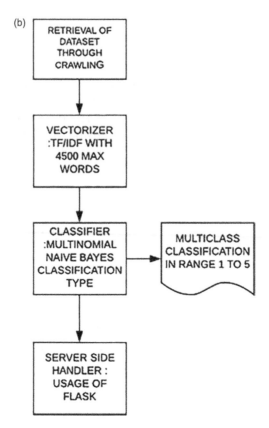

FIGURE 5.7 (CONTINUED)
(a) Android approach and (b) Machine learning approach.

5.6 Future Scope

The authors desire to extend this work by expanding the database of hospitals with the information of doctors in their respective specialized services and then predicting the ratings for the same, thus showing the optimized results after the combination of distance and reviews. For updating the resources by users, the new information regarding the availability of beds/blood group/medicine shall be first authenticated by the concerned health unit (hospitals, pharmacy, etc.) before displaying the changes on the application for correct information.

References

Alsalemi, A., Homsi, Y. A., Al Disi, M., Ahmed, I., Bensaali, F., Amira, A., Alinier, G. (2017). Real-time communication network using firebase cloud IoT platform for ECMO simulation. *IEEE International Conference on Internet of Things (iThings) and IEEE Green Computing and Communications (GreenCom) and IEEE Cyber, Physical and Social Computing (CPSCom) and IEEE Smart Data (SmartData), Exeter* (pp. 21–23). UK: IEEE.

Coburn, J. (n.d.). How to Get Python and JavaScript to Communicate Using JSON. Retrieved from https://www.makeuseof.com/tag/python-javascript-communicate-json/.

Diana, I. (2016). Information retrieval and the Internet. *Presented at University of Ottawa*. Retrieved from syllabus week 2: http://www.site.uottawa.ca/~diana/csi4107/cosine_tf_idf_example.pdf.

Dhivya, B., Lakshmiprabha, G., Nivethitha, P., Kala, K. (2015). Cloud messaging for android is a push. *International Journal of Emerging Technology and Innovative Engineering*, 1(3), 189–194.

ET Rise. (n.d.). GoDaddy Launches Community-Based App for Entrepreneurs Called Flare. Retrieved from https://economictimes.indiatimes.com/small-biz/startups/godaddy-launches-communitybased-app-for-entrepreneurs-called-flare/articleshow/54556972.cms.

Firebase Realtime Database. (n.d.). Retrieved from Firebase: https://firebase.google.com/docs/database/.

Gupta, R. (2017). The Importance of Healthcare Apps within Healthcare. Tech Jini.

Kibriya, A.M., Frank, E., Pfahringer, B., Holmes, G. (2004). Multinomial Naive Bayes for text categorization revisited. In Webb, G.I., Yu, X. (eds.) *Lecture Notes in Computer Science, Advances in Artificial Intelligence*. Springer, Berlin, Heidelberg.

Leavitt, N. (2010). Will NoSQL databases live up to their promise? *Computer*, 43(2), 12–14.

Moushumi, D.G. (2017). Road accidents killed 17 people every hour in India in 2016, Delhi most unsafe. *Hindustan Times*. Retrieved from: https://www.hindustantimes.com/india-news/road-accidents-claimed-nearly-400-lives-every-day-in-india-in-2016/story-7DlmtdnvMYLLZVGxXKOaJN.html.

Rahmi, A., Piarsa, I. N., Buana, P. W. (2017). FinDoctor–interactive android clinic geographical information system using firebase and google maps API. *International Journal of New Technology and Research (IJNTR)*, 3(7), 8–12.

Reddy, C. S. C., Uday Kumar, K., Dheeraj Keshav, J., Prasad, B. R., Agarwal, S. (2017). Prediction of star ratings from online reviews. *IEEE Region 10 Conference (TENCON)* (pp. 1857–1861). Malaysia: IEEE.

Su, J., Shirab, J. S., Matwin, S. (2011). Large scale text classification using semi-supervised multinomial Naive Bayes. *28th International Conference on Machine Learning*. Bellevue, WA.

Vogel, P., Klooster, T., Andrikopoulos, V., Lungu, M. (2017). A Low-Effort Analytics Platform for Visualizing Evolving Flask-Based Python Web Services. *2017 IEEE Working Conference on Software Visualization (VISSOFT)*. Shanghai, China: IEEE.

Wenger, J. (2014). GeoFire 2.0.Firebase. Retrieved from: https://firebase.googleblog.com/2014/06/geofire-20.html.

Wikipedia. (2019). Firebase Cloud Messaging. Retrieved from https://en.wikipedia.org/wiki/Firebase_Cloud_Messaging. Last modified June 10, 2019.

6

Nanoemulsions: Status in Antimicrobial Therapy

Atinderpal Kaur, Rakhi Bansal, Sonal Gupta, Reema Gabrani, and Shweta Dang
Jaypee Institute of Information Technology

CONTENTS

6.1 Introduction

Traditional therapies involve high doses of antimicrobial agents that lead to various side effects and development of drug resistance leading to ineffective therapy. High lipophilicity, low absorption, poor aqueous solubility, and hence, low bioavailability are some of the reasons behind the usage of large doses of conventional antibiotics (Chesa-Jiménez, Peris, Torres-Molina, & Granero, 1994; Padovan, Ralić, Letfus, Milić, & Mihaljević, 2012). From the last few years, the infectious diseases are prevalent due to the development of resistant bacteria. The rise is primarily attributed to poor patient compliance (Kallen et al., 2010). The resistance of antibiotics is developed due to various mechanisms, as bacteria with very short reproductive cycle are responsible for their large population. Due to this, when these come in contact with the antibiotic environment, these easily develop resistance against antibiotics (Seil & Webster, 2012). The primary mechanisms associated with the development of resistance are alteration in the structure of antibiotic drugs by the bacteria. The bacteria have the ability to change their metabolic pathway to ignore the antibiotic disruptive effects or to alter the target sites where the antibiotics are supposed to attach. These also enhance the clearance of drugs from the cells to avoid antibiotic accumulation in the cells (Tenover, 2006; Blair, Webber, Baylay, Ogbolu, & Piddock, 2015). Therefore, new approaches are much needed, which not only decreases the bacterial activities but also enhances the antibiotic activities without development of resistance. Nanotechnology is being utilized for medical applications and is able to kill or reduce the activity of numerous microorganisms. Some of the examples of pharmaceuticals developed on the basis of nanotechnology are nanoemulsions (NEs) (Pangeni, Sharma, Mustafa, Ali, & Baboota, 2014), nanosuspensions (Xu et al., 2012), nanospheres, nanotubes, nanoshells, nanocapsules, lipid nanoparticles, and dendrimers (Wojnarowicz et al., 2016; Zhang, Liu, & Yan, 2012). It suggests the use of NEs, nanoparticles, and dendrimers being used as antimicrobial agents.

6.1.1 NEs as Novel Delivery Systems for Drugs

NEs are formulations made of various dispersed particles of nanorange, used for pharmaceutical applications and could act as a new era of future therapeutics. NEs increase the dissolution rates and bioavailability of partially water-soluble antibiotics (Zhao et al., 2013; Vatsraj, Chauhan, & Pathak, 2014). Due to greater free energy (ΔG) of NEs than zero, these are thermodynamically unstable and kinetically stable systems (Anton, Benoit, & Saulnier, 2008). NEs are nanometric size emulsions with the size of droplets in the range of 20–200 nm (Solans et al., 2003). These are homogenous and polydispersed mixtures of oil and water. The surfactants and cosurfactants are used to make them stabilized (Shah, Bhalodia, & Shelat, 2010). Based on their composition, they could be fabricated as follows: o/w (oil in water), w/o (water in oil), and multiple emulsions (o/w/o (oil in water in oil) and w/o/w (water in oil in water)) (Solans, Izquierdo, Nolla, Azemar, & Garcia-Celma, 2005). Emulsions are developed by applying many internal and external forces on these to make the emulsions stable in nature for longer periods of time. vander Waals interactions and electrostatic interactions maintain the stability of an emulsion. Electrostatic forces are the repulsive forces arising from the similar charge on the surface of particles rendering emulsion stable, whereas vander Waals forces are attractive forces between particles, leading to aggregation and making emulsion unstable (Tadros, Izquierdo, Esquena, & Solans, 2004). As the vander Waals forces are relatively weaker in an NE than electrostatic repulsion, NEs are rendered highly stable, as greater the repulsion between the particles lesser is the particle aggregation, flocculation, and coalescence. Steric stabilization is another reason for the high stability of NE, which occurs due the interfacial layer on the particles of NE formed due the presence of surfactants. As the particles come together, the space between them decreases restricting the movement of particles with decreased entropy, leading to repulsion between particles (Tadros, 2009). In addition, the fine droplet size and surface area of particles of NE make them physically stable against creaming, flocculation, coalescence, and aggregation (Lovelyn & Attama, 2011).

However, Oswald ripening is found to be the most important cause for the instability of NE (Koroleva & Yurtov, 2012). Ostwald ripening directly induces droplet size growth. It occurs due to the particle size difference. The internal phase droplet grows largely due to the diffusion of small droplets with each other (Taylor, 2003). This can be attributed to an increase in chemical potential of components upon the decrease in size. The chemical potential difference in the droplet of formulation causes instability and emulsion breakdown (Lifshitz & Slyozov, 1961). Lifshitz–Slezov–Wagner (LSW) theory was proposed to explain Ostwald ripening (ω), where r is the radius of the particles, t is the time, $C_{(\infty)}$ is the bulk phase solubility, γ is the interfacial tension, V_m is the molar volume of the dispersed phase, D is the diffusion coefficient of the dispersed droplets in the continuous phase, ρ is the density of the oil, R is the gas constant, and T is the absolute temperature, as shown in Equation (6.1) (Wagner, 1961).

$$\omega = \frac{dr^3}{dt} = \frac{8}{9} \frac{C_{(\infty)}}{\rho RT} \gamma V_m D \tag{6.1}$$

Li and Chiang (2012) developed an NE of d-limonene using ultrasonication method and checked its stability studies. Ostwald ripening was the reason behind the instability of NE. The LSW equation, Ostwald ripening, and effect on temperature were studied on the diameter of droplets of NEs. According to the LSW equation, there is a linear relationship between droplet radius (r^3) and time of storage of formulation (t). It was reported that r^3 was in good linear relationship with time when plotted together, suggesting that the main reason for instability of NE is Ostwald ripening (Liu, Sun, Li, Liu, & Xu, 2006; Forgiarini, Esquena, González, & Solans, 2001). LSW equation relates Ostwald ripening with temperature, in which it is inversely proportional to temperature. Ostwald ripening rates calculated were found to be lower at 25°C ($0.39\,\text{m}^3/\text{s} \times 10^{29}$) than at 4°C ($1.44\,\text{m}^3/\text{s} \times 10^{29}$), suggesting LSW theory to be sufficient to explain Ostwald ripening. Thus, Ostwald ripening appeared to be the main reason for NE instability (Li & Chiang, 2012).

Ostwald ripening can be reduced using various methods. For instance, use of compounds less soluble in dispersion media than the internal phase; for example, hydrocarbons with less solubility in water while preparing o/w NE reduces Ostwald ripening. Use of binary internal phase decreases the rate of Ostwald ripening. The second compound with much lower solubility in the dispersion phase is transferred less to the dispersion media and has much higher concentration in small droplets than larger droplets. This becomes the rate limiting step resulting in kinetically stabilized NE (Higuchi & Misra, 1962).

The enzymatic and chemical degradation of drugs can be protected by encapsulating these inside NEs. Moreover, NEs also enhance the bioavailability and decrease the therapeutic dosage requirement of drugs (Han et al., 2009; Nicolaos, Crauste-Manciet, Farinotti, & Brossard, 2003). NEs are easy to prepare at laboratory scale and can be easily exploited for industrial-scale production (Abismail, Canselier, Wilhelm, Delmas, & Gourdon, 1999). NEs are more effective and safe drug delivery systems than the commercial drugs and also enhance the patient compliance (Halnor, Pande, Borawake, & Nagare, 2018). NE can be used for the delivery of drugs at target sites due to their large interfacial tension, which enhances the transport of drugs (Goldberg & Higuchi, 1969) (Table 6.1).

6.1.2 Methods of Preparation of NEs

The methods of preparation of NEs are differentiated on the basis of energy input while preparing NEs (Figure 6.1). Further, the low-energy method is categorized into phase inversion temperature (PIT) method, emulsion inversion point (EIP) method, and spontaneous nanoemulsification. Phase inversions are produced either by maintaining a constant temperature and composition or by changing the composition and temperature (Anton et al., 2008).

TABLE 6.1

List of oils, surfactants and co-surfactants used for nanoemulsion preparation

1	HLB Value	Surfactant	HLB Value
Oleic Acid	2	Tween 20	16.7
Soybean Oil	7	Tween 80	15
Coconut Oil	8	Tween 85	11
Sesame Oil	7	Span 20	8.6
Corn Oil	10	Span 40	6.7
Olive Oil	7	Span 80	4.3
Castor Oil	14	Igepal	13
Jajoba Oil	6	Kolliphor	15
Peanut Oil	6	Cetyl Pyridinium Chloride	26
Mineral Oil	10	Gylceryl Monostearate	3.8
Lauroglycol	4–5	Brij O20	15
Labrafac	2	Myrj 49	15

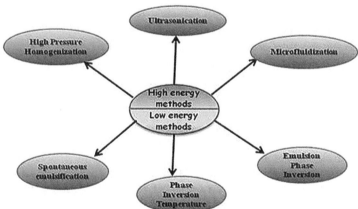

FIGURE 6.1
Various low energy and high energy methods used for the preparation of nanoemulsion.

6.1.2.1 Low-Energy Methods

6.1.2.1.1 PIT Method

This method depends upon the property of the surfactant to change affinity for oil and water upon change in temperature. This property is primarily shown by non-ionic surfactants having ethoxylated groups. At lower temperature, the polar groups are hydrated by increasing its affinity toward the hydrophilic phase. With the increase in temperature, the ethoxylated groups become oil loving in nature and bend toward the oil phase. The surface area becomes larger for the hydrocarbon chains than the polar group, resulting in w/o nanoemulsion (Heurtault, Saulnier, Pech, Proust, & Benoit, 2002). The most widely used method in industries is phase inversion method for the production of NEs. It is the best-suited method that is highly responsible for the development of formulations exhibiting lower size of particles and polydispersity index (PDI) (Jintapattanakit, 2017).

6.1.2.1.2 EIP Method

In this process, an aqueous phase is added slowly with continuous shaking in the mixture containing oil phase and surfactant. The system undergoes phase transitions upon addition of water. At first step, a w/o emulsion is formed, which converts to o/w/o with mixing and finally to o/w emulsion. The value of critical water concentration, emulsion type, and droplet size depend upon the parameters such as surfactant concentration, speed of the stirrer, and percentage of water added. Surfactants other than ethoxylated surfactants can be used, and less dependency on temperature makes EIP a better method than PIT method (Salager et al., 2004).

Borrin, Georges, Moraes, and Pinho (2016) produced curcumin-loaded NE using emulsification inversion point method by optimizing some parameters. The NE contained soybean oil (20%), Tween 80 (10%), and glycerol (20%) and was developed using an impeller system consisting of anchor blade at revolutions of 300 rpm. The prepared NE showed 0.07% encapsulation of curcumin. The formulation was kept on stability, and it was observed that 70% of curcumin still remained in the formulation even after a time period of 60 days. It was a good indication of stability of the formulation compared with other lipid-based encapsulation systems.

Ševčíková, Kašpárková, Vltavská, and Krejčí (2012) prepared NE by phase inversion method using surfactant mixtures of required hydrophile-lipophile balance (HLB) values. The required HLB was obtained by blending pairs of nonionic surfactants (igepals and brij). The low HLB surfactants were added to oil and high HLB to water. At 1,050 rpm and 25°C, water was added dropwise to oil phase, and various oil-to-water ratios (5/95, 10/90, 15/85, 20/80, 25/75, and 30/70) were used. Surfactants of 3 and 5 wt% concentration and HLB values of 9.5, 10, 10.5, 11, and 11.5 were used. The results indicated that the increased oil concentration in the formulation increases the size of particles. The particle size was influenced by the type of surfactant, as igepal showed higher average particle sizes (100–500 nm) than brij (50–300 nm). An oil-to-water ratio of 5/95 and a surfactant HLB of 10.5–11.5 resulted in most transparent NEs (Ševčíková et al., 2012).

6.1.2.1.3 Spontaneous Nanoemulsification

Spontaneous nanoemulsification occurs via the mechanism of rapid diffusion of the solvent at the interface due to the instability originated by decreased interfacial tension (Vitale & Katz, 2003). In this method, there is no need of sophisticated equipment as in the case of high-energy methods or change in temperature or emulsion composition as in the case of PIT and EIP (Komaiko & McClements, 2015).

Kelmann, Kuminek, Teixeira, and Koester (2007) developed an NE loaded with carbamazepine for parenteral use by using spontaneous emulsification process. In this study, 2^2 full factorial design was used to explore the effect of emulsifier and oil on the size of particles, PDI, zeta potential, viscosity of formulation, drug content, and drug association. Drug was mixed in oil (castor oil) to prepare an oily phase. The emulsifier (soybean lecithin) was dissolved in organic solvent (acetone: ethanol) and mixed with the oil phase. To prepare an aqueous phase, water was mixed with hydrophilic emulsifier (polysorbate 80). The oily phase was then added slowly with continuous stirring in an aqueous phase to obtain NE. The developed NEs were found to be more stable with a particle size of 150–212 nm, zeta potential of –35 mV, and low PDI of 0.25. The oil used had no effect on the dispersity of particles and zeta potential, whereas particle size was found to decrease in the NE prepared by using a mixture of castor oil and medium chain triglyceride (MCT) oil (1:1) (Kelmann et al., 2007).

6.1.2.2 High-Energy Methods

6.1.2.2.1 Ultrasonication

In ultrasonication method, ultrasonic waves are used to achieve nanometric size particle, which is based on the mechanism of "cavitation bubble" formation (Tadros, Izquierdo, Esquena, & Solans, 2004). The interrupted compressions and expansions are generated by ultrasound waves. During the expansion phase, bubbles on the interface are filled with vapor or gas. These bubbles grow to a limited size and then collapse. Approximately, the collapsing bubble, high shear fields, and microjets of high liquid velocity are generated (Tal-Figiel, 2007).

Kolmogorov theory of turbulent droplet breakdown is used to predict the size of NE, which can be further used for designing an ultrasonicator (Bechtel, Gilbert, & Wagner, 1999), as shown in Equation (6.2).

$$\eta = \left(v^3/\varepsilon\right)^{\frac{1}{4}}$$

(6.2)

where η is the Kolmogorov length scale, v is the viscosity of media, and ε is the rate of energy dissipation. A typical ultrasonicator works at 20–24 kHz at an amplitude of 20%–100%, consisting of a sonoprobe with a horn of variable diameters depending on the volume of the media. It consists of a transducer that converts the electrical energy into mechanical energy (Hielscher, 2005).

When used to a certain limit, ultrasonic power generates a smaller droplet size. Tang, Manickam, Wei, and Nashiru (2012) studied various ultrasonication parameters such as the effect of amplitude and sonication time on the size of particles and PDI of the NE of aspirin, a highly lipophilic drug. It was found that both the applied amplitude and time of sonication significantly affected the droplet size. The applied amplitude and time of sonication were varied from 20% to 40% and 30 to 70 s, respectively. It was found that with an increase in the applied amplitude and time of sonication, the droplet size is increased. This effect was attributed to the mechanism of overprocessing and excessive heat generation, which may lead to coalescence of droplets. In addition, high processing times may lead to high-energy inputs, which may ultimately lead to exclusion of emulsifier from the surface of oil droplets. At low processing conditions such as 20% amplitude and 70 s sonication time, NE was developed with a particle size of 246 nm and a PDI of 0.35.

Similarly, Li and Chiang (2012) prepared the NE of d-limonene via ultrasonication method and developed a stable NE with a minimum size of particles when the ultrasonic processing conditions were kept at low level. A high power greater than 18 W and a sonication time greater than 140 s resulted in NEs with larger droplet size. The NE prepared using low processing parameter of 18 W power and 120 s sonication time was stable with a particle size of 31.2 nm.

Abbas, Bashari, Akhtar, Li, and Zhang (2014) prepared an NE of curcumin using octenyl succinic anhydride modified starch as stabilizer and a high-intensity sonicator of 20 kHz frequency and 1,200 W power. The power range of 10%, 20%, 30%, 40%, 50%, 60%, and 70% (120, 240, 360, 480, 600, 720, and 840 W, respectively) was applied and a sonication time range of 1, 3, 5, 7, 9, 11, and 13 min was used. It was found that the use of power beyond 40% was unnecessary and insignificant. Similarly, sonication time beyond 7 min did not affect the particle size but only led to a consumption of high energy, which was uneconomical. Optimum conditions of 40% amplitude and 7 min sonication time were found to be suitable for the preparation of NE.

Sugumar, Ghosh, Nirmala, Mukherjee, and Chandrasekaran (2014) prepared an eucalyptus oil formulation using a 20 kHz ultrasonic processor (Sonics, USA) with a maximum power output of 750 W. The applied amplitude was fixed at 40%, and the sonication time was increased from 5 to 30 min. In contrast, a transparent and stable NE with a particle size of 3.8 nm was obtained at a sonication time of 30 min. It was found that the obtained NE could allow active component penetration due to its small particle size and larger surface area of particles.

Kaur et al. (2017)prepared an NE loaded with polyphenon 60 and curcumin using ultrasonication technique at 40% amplitude for 150 s. The developed NE was more stable with a particle size of 167 nm and a PDI of 0.311. The ultrasonication energy decreased the size of particles and enhanced the penetration at the site of action.

However, there is a basic but crucial limitation to the use of ultrasonication in the formulation of NEs. Emulsification occurs due to the nearness of ultrasonic waves requiring constant mixing for larger volume samples. As a result, poor-quality product produced due to the use of high amplitudes leads to product degradation by excessive shear or thermal degradation. Therefore, ultrasonication has only been found to be effective at lab scale level for the production of small batches of NE (Peshkovsky, Peshkovsky, & Bystryak, 2013). A basic setup of ultrasonicator is shown in Figure 6.2.

6.1.2.2.2 Microfluidizers

Microfluidizers are prepared by the collision of two immiscible liquids in a microchannel under high pressure (Zheng, Tice, & Ismagilov, 2004). This was first patented by Cook and Lagace (1985) and was reported in a scientific publication by Washington (1987). A microfluidizer consisted of an air-driven intensifier pump, which produces a high pressure to

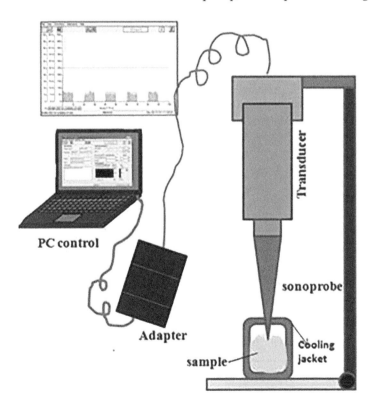

FIGURE 6.2
Basic set-up of ultrasonication.

push the emulsion into the chamber of microfluidizer. The two streams of crude emulsion entered in the chamber get accelerated with a very high velocity. This causes collision between two emulsions at a high velocity under high pressure, generating a tremendous shearing action by producing a final emulsion. High turbulence, shear force, and cavitations result in fine droplets (Olson, White, & Richter, 2004) (Figure 6.3).

Based on the direction of flow streams, microfluidizers can be divided into three types: co-directional, opposite directional, and T-shaped. Codirectional microfluidizers produce monodispersed emulsion, whereas opposite directional and T-shaped microfluidizers efficiently produce smaller size droplets with a narrow range (Koroleva & Yurtov, 2012).

Salvia-Trujillo, Rojas-Graü, Soliva-Fortuny, and Martín-Belloso (2013) studied the effect of processing parameters of microfluidizer (pressure and cycles) on the droplet size stability and viscosity of lemongrass oil NE. The NE was subjected to variable pressures of 50, 100, or 150 MPa and cycles of 1, 2, 3, 4, 5, and 10. It was found that the microfluidizer processing parameters significantly influenced the average size and dispersion of particles. The size of particles is decreased with an increase in pressure and cycle of microfluidizer. The size was reduced from 1,410 ± 366 to 23 ± 2 nm after passing through a microfluidizer at 100 or 150 MPa for 1 cycle and to 7.35 ± 1.67 nm at 150 passing through a microfluidizer. However, change in processing parameters significantly showed no effect on zeta potential. The viscosity decreased from 35.65 ± 2.33 to 16.85 ± 0.21 MPa s when subjected to microfluidization.

It has been shown that microfluidization is sometimes not feasible, as high pressure and high emulsification times lead to overprocessing, degradation of actives, and unstable emulsions (Lobo & Svereika, 2003). Some of the models of microfluidizers available include the following: Model M-110Y (Microfluidics, USA) and M110P (Microfluidics, USA). A typical microfluidizer is shown in Figure 6.3.

6.1.2.2.3 High-Pressure Homogenizer

High-pressure homogenizer (HPH) is used for low- and medium-viscosity liquids. It basically works by putting high pressure on the liquid passing through an orifice (Figure 6.4). Homogenizers work in a wide pressure range from 10 to 350 MPa. The slit width between the plunger and the outlet nozzle is 10–100 mm, resulting in a high velocity greater than 100 m/s (Bałdyga, Orciuch, Makowski, Malski-Brodzicki, & Malik, 2007).

In HPH, the emulsion undergoes a size reduction brought simultaneously by shear forces, turbulence, and cavitations. Droplet size of an emulsion depends upon fluid flow,

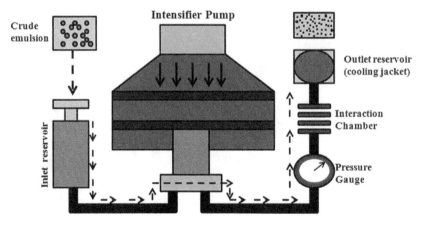

FIGURE 6.3
Basic setup of microfluidizer.

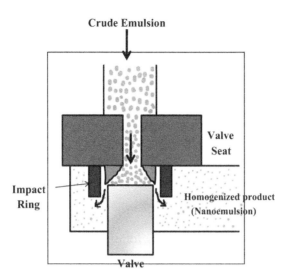

FIGURE 6.4
Basic set up of high pressure homogenization.

fluid viscosity, and applied pressure. HPH is used for lab scale and industrial production of NEs (Floury, Desrumaux, Axelos, & Legrand, 2003). Depending on the direction of flow of media, homogenizers are divided into three types: radial diffusers, capillary jet dispersers, and nozzle devices. In radial diffusers, the direction of flow deviates 90° from the starting point. Mobile valve controls the flow rate and the applied pressure, whereas capillary jet dispersers are based on the collision of two or more flows moving with high velocity. In nozzle devices, two or more liquids flow in the same direction or on the different axes without the use of a moving valve (Mohr, 1987; Huppertz, 2011).

Yuan, Gao, Mao, and Zhao (2008a) checked the effect of HPH processing parameters on the particle size and stability of beta carotene NE. The effect of pressure of homogenization and temperature of HPH was evaluated. The pressure was varied from 79.1 to 140.0 MPa, and temperature was varied from 34.5°C to 65.5°C. The increased pressure of homogenizer decreases the average particle size of formulation. The effect of homogenization temperatures was found to have no significant effect on the particle size.

Yuan, Gao, Zhao, and Mao (2008b) further studied beta carotene NE stability prepared by HPH. The NE was found to be of average particle size in the range of 132–184 nm. It was found that the NE prepared had smallest size of particles prepared by using tween 20 as surfactant. The number of cycles and homogenization pressure affected the average particle with most stable NE prepared at 3 cycles and 100 MPa. The emulsion was found to be more stable at 4°C than 25°C. Twenty-five percent of beta carotene was degraded at 25°C.

Donsì, Annunziata, Vincensi, and Ferrari (2012) encapsulated three essential oils: carcavol, limonene, and cinnamaldehyde in sunflower oil NE were developed by high-pressure homogenization. HPH was carried at 300 MPa for 5 cycles. The prepared NE was in the range of 100–200 nm, and PDI was in the range of 0.1–0.2 with a narrow size distribution. HPH was successfully used for the preparation of NE.

A basic setup of HPH is shown in Figure 6.4. Multiple designs of homogenizers are available commercially. These include Stansted homogenizer, Micron Lab 40 HPH (Microfluidics Corp), "Nanojet" device, Nano DeBEE Electric Bench-Top (BEE International, USA), and Sonic Corp.

6.1.3 Comparison between the Methods

Tang, Shridharan, and Sivakumar (2013) compared the two methods of ultrasonication and microfluidization for the preparation of NE of aspirin. NE was produced by benchtop microfluidizer. Microfluidization was performed at pressures of 200, 400, and 600 bars for 1–10 passes. Ultrasonicator was used at a power amplitude of 50%, 60%, and 70% for 10–100 s. Results showed that ultrasonication and microfluidization produces NEs with approximately similar particle sizes. An ultrasonicator with high shear stress could produce NEs with smaller sizes when compared with a microfluidizer but with a relatively broader peak. NE prepared by a microfluidizer showed better stability when compared with ultrasonication. However, microfluidization was found to be more inconvenient and often lead to overprocessing at longer run times.

Ostertag, Weiss, and McClements (2012) studied the emulsion phase inversion (EPI) method fitness for the preparation of food-grade NE. The low-energy method (EPI) was compared with the high-energy method (microfluidization). The system composition and preparation conditions behavior were evaluated for the preparation of edible NE, and it was found that EPI method was suitable for preparing NEs of a smaller droplet size of 0.16 µm but at a higher concentration of (surfactant oil ratio of 0.7). EPI was found to be feasible for the preparation of nanoparticles requiring less sophisticated methods, less cost, and equipment, whereas microfluidization method could be used for the preparation of NE with low surfactant concentration, resulting in benefits like low ingredient cost, less foaming, and better patient compliance due to reduction of bitter taste caused by surfactants.

Lee and Norton (2013) produced a food-grade NE to examine the difference between high-pressure valve homogenizer and microfluidizer methods for their effect on droplet breakdown. Different parameters, such as oil to aqueous phase viscosity ratio, type of emulsifier, pressure, and number of passes from the chamber, were to analyze the effects on particle size of NE. It was found that when NE was subjected to the same pressure for five passes, a similar particle size was obtained; however, after a single pass, HPH produced larger particle sizes with a broad range than microfluidizer. Oil:aqueous viscosity ratios (0.1–80) had no effect in case of both HPH and microfluidizer. However, emulsifier type (sodium dodecyl sulfate (SDS), Tween 20, and sodium caseinate) affected the droplet size in HPH as the particle size reached a limiting value after two passes with SDS, while with Tween 20 and sodium caseinate, a minimum particle size could be obtained after five passes.

6.2 Characterization of NEs

NEs are unstable in nature and are characterized on the basis of used methods for preparation. There are various methods used for the characterization and optimization of NEs and their ingredients (surfactant, oil phase, and aqueous phase). This study is necessary when the formulation is made by PIT method and self-emulsification method to determine the dispersibility. For this, different ingredients of NEs were placed in varying concentrations in glass vials and homogenized for a certain period of time at a particular temperature to obtain equilibrium. Anisotropic phase can be identified by polarized light (Cazabat & Langevin, 1981). The particle size and distribution should be determined to know the nature of NE. This is done using dynamic light scattering

(DLS) methods for the measurement of particles and further particle size distribution. To check the uniformity among nanodroplets of NE, PDI should be determined via DLS, based on the principal of Brownian motion of scattered droplets in the continuous phase (Candau, Hirsch, Zana, Safran, & Clark, 1987). The surface properties of particles to be assessed is checked by measuring the zeta potential of NE by using mini electrode. Moreover, viscosity should be determined to know the flow of formulation for its better delivery inside the body.

6.3 Advantages of NEs as Antimicrobial Agents

Due to nanodroplet size, NEs have a large surface area that allows rapid penetration, thereby enhancing the dissemination of encapsulated actives and helping in the treatment of infections (Gupta, Gabrani, Ali, & Dang, 2011). Presence of surfactants on the interface of dispersed and continuous phase in the NE system causes increased solubilization of actives, thereby increasing the dose loading capacity when compared with any other drug dosage form. High drug solubilization also results in increased bioavailability of encapsulated actives. Since NEs are biphasic systems, i.e., composed of oil phase as well as aqueous phase, they could be used to encapsulate both lipophilic and hydrophilic drugs at the same time in a single NE system. Various polymers can be used to modify the NEs in a manner that improves the drug residence time and could therefore prolong the release of actives at a particular target site. Nanometric size range results in a large reduction of gravity force, and the Brownian motion of the dispersed phase is sufficient to overcome gravity, thereby surmounting the problem of creaming, flocculation, or sedimentation. In addition, at the interface, the surfactant film (at a particular concentration) prevents disruption of dispersed droplets by a continuous phase (Attwood, Mallon, Ktistis, & Taylor, 1992). The formulation of NEs involves the use of surfactants that are approved for animal and human use (generally regarded as safe). Besides, NEs are effective at relatively lower concentrations and are sufficient to kill/inhibit microorganisms; therefore, NE-based drug delivery systems could be reliably used with minimum side effects. Since these structures are not developed by evolution and there are no indigenous detoxifying genes for these synthetic NEs, they can be considered as supramolecular antibiotics that could not give an unfortunate rise to resistant microorganisms (Karthikeyan, Amaechi, Rawls, & Lee, 2011). Before the formulation of NEs, its formula is essentially optimized using methods like response surface methodology or software like Box Behnken Design. Therefore, a better understanding of all parameters would help in easy transfer of lab-scale technology to large-scale manufacturing units.

6.4 Mechanism of Action Responsible for Antimicrobial Activity of NEs

A characteristic NE is composed of an inner dispersed phase, surfactants, and cosurfactants at the interface and an outer continuous phase. There are different theories available in literature explaining the mechanism responsible for the antimicrobial action of NEs.

However, all these hypotheses relate with either one of the three phases (dispersed, interface, and continuous phase) present in NEs or with the resulting interaction forces between these phases.

NE itself is responsible for the antimicrobial action due to nanosized droplets. The nanosized particles of NEs have a high surface tension, which easily penetrate in the lipid-containing cell membrane of pathogens and disrupt the membrane of microorganisms and result in cell death (Hamouda & Baker, 2000; Singh, Van Hamme, & Ward, 2007). Moreover, the NEs prepared using amphiphilic surfactants reduce the surface and interfacial tensions of immiscible fluids by accumulating at the interface. These can also increase the solubility of insoluble organic compounds that are essentially present in the outer cell walls of microorganisms. Furthermore, the surfactant present in NE may inhibit the degradation of microorganism by dispersing the pathogens in aqueous phase (Rajalakshmi, Mahesh, & Kumar, 2011). When NE systems come in contact with microorganisms, these will thermodynamically interact with the pathogens, and this interaction is further enhanced by the electrostatic attraction between the NE and bacteria. Further, the energy released by fusion destabilizes the lipid membrane of the pathogens and results in cell lysis and death (Bourne & Dittert, 1996). Moreover, the potential of NEs to work against gram-positive and gram-negative bacteria is reported to be unlike. This may be due to the difference in composition of their outer cell walls. The high content of lipids and proteins in the outer membrane of gram-negative bacteria provides resistance from detergents. Vaara (1992) explained that the lipid-containing cell membrane provides only limited diffusion of hydrophobic molecules from it and is impermeable to a large number of macromolecules due to its lipophilic nature. This nature also makes it resistant to neutral and anionic surfactants that are important components involved in the formulation of NEs.

6.5 Application of NE as Antimicrobial Agents

6.5.1 NEs as Antibacterial Agents

Jerobin, Sureshkumar, Anjali, Mukherjee, and Chandrasekaran (2012) encapsulated a neem (*Azadiracta indica*) metabolite, azadiractin, known to have antibacterial, antifungal, and antiviral properties in an NE. The NE was cross-linked with glutaraldehyde to prepare NE beads and further coated with starch and polyethylene glycol. The beads were found to be of spherical shape with 1.28–1.49 mm diameter size of particles. The % entrapment efficacy was high in starch-coated beads. The rate of swelling of beads was low in starch-coated beads when compared with polyethylene glycol (PEG)-coated beads, showing controlled release of azadiractin. These coated beads were found to be cytotoxic to lymphocytes.

Yu, Ma, Lei, Li, and Tan (2014) developed metronidazole-loaded NEs for treatment of rosacea (skin disease). The NE optimized via D-optimal design had a particle size of 27.31 nm, with a PDI of 0.215. The *in vitro* studies tested on pig skin represented flux values of 7.36% and 6.88% for NE and gel, respectively. Gels showed a parabolic trend after 24 h of skin retention-time profile when compared with NE, which showed a cumulative increase, suggesting that NE had greater skin retention when compared with gel. NE can be retained for a much longer time on the skin than gel without entering the systemic circulation, thus suggesting a good *in vitro in vivo* correlation (IVIVC) correlation. NEs act as a controlled system for the delivery of metronidazole for the treatment of rosacea.

Dental caries formation occurs due to the accumulation of planktonic bacteria to a cellular pellicle coating the oral surface. Ramalingam, Amaechi, Ralph, and Lee (2012) developed a NE and evaluated its antimicrobial effect. The NE was prepared by microfluidizer method at 20,000 psi at room temperature and had a mean diameter of 308 nm. It was revealed through live and dead staining that each component of NE separately had less microbicidal effect when compared with an NE. When compared with chlorhexidine, it was found that NE had better antibacterial activity. It was hypothesized that the observed activity was due to the electrostatic interaction developed between the positive surface charge of planktonic bacteria and negatively charged NE. The NE affected the adherence of bacteria, as indicated through adherence assays.

In a similar study, Ramalingam, Frohlich, and Lee (2013) explored the effect of NE made using cetyl-pyridinium chloride in reducing the bacterial levels in dental problems. The dental unit waterline contamination is a major concern in dental hospitals these days, as bacteria from saliva and plaque of one patient can inoculate other patients via dental unit water syringes and hand pieces. Waterline biofilms treated with NE for 1, 6, 12, 24, 48, and 72 h showed a reduction in bacterial growth at 12 and 24 h (67 cfu/mL). A significant decrease in the bacterial population was seen with a maximum % dead area of up to 99.8% after 48 and 72 h.

Lin et al. (2012) formulated water-in-oil NE of amoxicillin and checked its activity against *Helicobacter pylori*. *H. pylorus* is a gram-negative bacteria responsible for the development of a pathological condition of peptic ulcers. The combination of spans and tweens led to the formation of a stable NE with desired HLB values. NE consisted of chitosan/heparin prepared by using paraffin oil and Span 20 and Tween 20 as surfactant combinations having a particle size of 270.1 ± 9.8 nm, a PDI of 0.19 ± 0.06, and a constant HLB of 10.6. Amoxicillin showed a release of 20.5% ± 1.2% at pH 1.2 for over a time period of 120 min, whereas there was a modest release of 35% at pH 6 and a rapid release of 100% at pH 7 due to instability and burst release at pH 6 and 7, respectively.

Teixeira et al. (2007) observed the antibacterial efficacy of oil-in-water NE (soybean oil and tri-*n*-butylphosphate emulsified with Triton X-100) and oil-in-water microemulsion (ethyl oleate with Tween 80 as emulsifier and *n*-pentanol as a coemulsifier). The antibacterial activity was evaluated against suspensions of *Salmonella* spp. *Escherichia coli* 0157:H7 (VT–), *Pseudomonas aeruginosa*, *Staphylococcus aureus*, and *Listeria monocytogenes*. From findings, it was observed that both microemulsion and NE have prominent antibacterial activity. NE reduced microorganisms by 70% in just 1 min and 100% for *L. monocytogenes* after 15 min of incubation. In contrast, the microemulsion showed activity against all tested pathogens and resulted in a reduction of pathogens more than 99%. Both emulsions reduced the biofilm formation after 30 min of exposure.

In another study, Sugumar et al. (2014) developed eucalyptus oil NE via ultrasonication method and evaluated its antibacterial activity against *Staphylococcus aureus*, a major causative organism present in the infection of skin abrasions and open wounds acquired from hospitals. NE prepared by sonication at 40% amplitude for various time intervals of 0, 5, 10, 15, 20, 25, and 30 min showed a reduction in the size of particles and PDI with increased sonication time. The NE sonicated for 25 min was stable for 3 months. There was immediate reduction in count of cells (0.324 log cfu/mL) after 1 min. After 15 min, a 100% loss of viability was seen. The diluted NE also showed significant antibacterial activity. Animal studies showed no skin irritancy cases. The NE started to treat the wounds and showed considerable contraction from 10th day with 100% wound healing after 16 days.

Hamouda et al. (2001) developed a novel nonionic based NE and studied its biocidal activity against bacteria, fungus, and virus. NE prepared by mixing tributyl phosphate, soybean oil, Triton X-100, and deionized water with a reciprocating syringe pump had a droplet size in the range of 400–800 nm. Herpes simplex and influenza A viruses treated with 1% NE for 15 min resulted in a 6-log reduction in colony forming unit (cfu) The vaccinia virus was less susceptible to NE. *Candida albicans* was resistant to the cidal effect of NE; the resistance could be due to the rigid cell wall structure of yeast.

Respiratory infection is the major infection in patients suffering from cystic fibrosis. Among the various microorganisms responsible for respiratory infection, *Burkholderia cepacia* complex is the most harmful in cystic fibrosis (LiPuma, 2001), as it is among the most antimicrobial-resistant microorganisms. LiPuma et al. (2009) investigated the antibacterial activity of NE against 150 bacterial isolates recovered from cystic fibrosis (CF) respiratory tract specimens. The growth of all selected strains was inhibited by NE with minimum inhibitory concentration (MIC_{50}) of 1.2 µg/mL and MIC_{90} of 125 µg/mL. NB-401 was more active against non-*Burkholderia* strains than *Burkholderia* strains. NE was thus effective in treating respiratory infections related to cystic fibrosis.

Similarly, Hwang et al. (2013) also developed an NE and investigated it for antibacterial activity against a multidrug resistant *Acinetobacter baumannii*. An NE was prepared using microfluidizer. NEs containing 10% v/v Triton X-100, 25% v/v soybean oil, and 1% w/v cetyl pyridinium chloride showed remarkable antibacterial activity against all the strains of *A. baumannii*. NE was active even at higher dilutions, i.e., 1:2,187 for MIC and 1:729–1:2,187 for minimum bactericidal concentration (MBC). At 1:1,333 dilutions, bacterial colony counts were reduced to 2–3 logs at 15 min. Biofilm studies showed that NE at 1:1,000 dilutions reduced the metabolic activity of *A. baumannii* to 80% within 1 h of treatment and to 90% at 1:400 dilutions.

Gupta et al. (2014) also developed an NE loaded with phytochemicals for urinary tract infection and checked it against bacteria *E. coli*, uropathogenic *E. coli* (UPEC). An oil-in-water NE was developed by ultrasonication method with 89.47 nm particle size and a PDI of 0.236. The finalized NE inhibited the growth of bacteria within 5 h of incubation when compared with its aqueous form (15 h). This could be due to the penetration of small particles of NE inside the cell membrane that causes cell lysis and ultimately cell death.

Kaur et al. (2017) also prepared an NE loaded with curcumin and polyphenon 60 against *E.coli* for the treatment of urinary tract infection. The findings confirmed that the developed NE effectively inhibited the bacterial growth within 5 h, whereas aqueous drug solution inhibited the bacteria in 10 h. Moreover, the NE was effectively delivered intravaginally to the rats, which showed maximum uptake in the urinary tract organs.

Kaur et al. (2018) also developed a green tea and ciprofloxacin NE for its antibacterial action. NE was tested on resistant uropathogenic strains for its antibacterial activity, and findings confirmed the effectiveness of NE used against extended spectrum beta lactamase and metallobeta lactamase, producing uropathogens at low concentrations. The higher antimicrobial effect of NE could be due to the development of surface tension on the surface of nanosize particles, which enhances its permeation in the lipid-containing cell membrane to cause cell lysis.

6.5.2 NEs as Antifungal Agents

Fungal infections are the common infections of skin occurring in the human society. The main causative organism responsible for skin infection is dermatophytes from genera: *Trichophyton*, *Epidermophyton*, and *Microsporum* spp. The organism that causes infection of the moist skin parts and anus are *C. albicans*. Pannu et al. (2009) investigated the antifungal activity of a novel NE. The NE was prepared using highly purified oil, ethanol, polysorbate 20, cetyl pyridinium chloride, and water. The developed NE showed a mean droplet size of 180 nm and tested against five clinical isolates of *Trichophytonrubrum*. The MIC and minimum fungicidal concentration (MFC) of novel NE for all isolates were found to be 2–4 and 2–8 µg/mL, respectively, when compared with antibiotic terbinafine having MIC and MFC of greater than 8 µg/mL. NE also showed activity against 12 genera of filamentous fungi with MIC values of 0.06–8 µg/mL. NE tested against *C. albicans* showed an MIC and MFC of 2 and 8 µg/mL, respectively. Electron microscopy revealed disruption of fungal cell surface and subsequent fungal lysis. Thus, the novel NE proved to be a broad-spectrum topical antifungal used for skin and nail diseases.

Myc, Vanhecke, Landers, Hamouda, and Baker (2003) investigated the NE for its fungicidal activity against clinically important yeast, such as *C. albicans* and *C. tropicalis*, and filamentous fungi. The pre-emulsion was prepared by blending 64% oil, 8% solvent, and detergent at three levels of 8%, 1%, and 0.7%. The finalized NE was then formed by mixing with 18.3% water using the Silverson L4RT Mixer for 3 min at 10,000 rpm. It was found that NE changed the shape and integrity of yeast cells. Although the untreated cells remained intact, the pH range affected the activity of NE, with the highest activity being found at a pH range of 7–9. NE showed potential antifungal activity against yeast and filamentous fungi and could be used for topical treatment of skin infections.

Bedoya-Serna, Dacanal, Fernandes, and Pinho (2018) also developed an NE with oregano (*Origanum vulgare*) essential oil and found its antifungal activity both *in vitro* and after application on Minas Padrão cheese. The results proved that NE inhibited the growth of *Cladosporium* sp., *Fusarium* sp., and *Penicillium* sp. The antifungal activity was further verified on Minas Padrão cheese slices. In both tests, the developed NE showed higher antifungal activity against *Penicillium* sp. than *Cladosporium* sp. and *Fusarium* sp.

6.5.3 NEs as Antiviral Agents

Presently used influenza vaccination has limitations of efficacy and safety. The inactivated virion-consisting vaccines administered intramuscularly are unable to produce cell-mediated immune response. The live attenuated vaccines generate a high immune response but are not recommended due to safety reasons in high-risk patients. Thus, new approaches are needed for the delivery of influenza vaccine.

Das et al. (2012) investigated various NEs with different ratios of cationic and nonionic surfactants for their activity as an adjuvant in influenza vaccine to improve the immune responses against influenza. The novel influenza vaccine HINI was composed of inactive influenza virus and NE. The vaccine was administered intranasally. The immune responses were compared with the vaccine containing inactive virus alone prepared in phosphate buffer saline (PBS). All vaccines containing NE elicited a high immunoglobulin G (IgG) concentration in serum when compared with PBS only vaccine. NEs having cationic to nonionic surfactant concentration in the ratio of 1:6 elicited the highest immune response. Mice immunized with NE showed a higher concentration of influenza-specific antigens immunoglobulin A (IgA) in the bronchoalveolar fluid. The vaccine with NE given intramuscular generated a high serum IgG antibody when compared with intranasal administration, whereas the vaccine with NE given intranasal generated a high mucosal IgG antibody when compared with intramucosal administration.

Further, Stanberry et al. (2012) also developed a new NE that checked the safety and immunogenicity by combining it with seasonal influenza antigen (Fluzone®). It was tested on 199 healthy volunteers under human, randomized, controlled, and observer-blind Phase I clinical trial. The NE was given intranasally in the concentration of 5%, 10%, 15%, or 20%, combined with 4 or 10 μg of strain-specific Fluzone and compared with intranasal PBS, intranasal Fluzone, or 15 μg strain-specific intramuscular Fluzone. Adverse events studied were mild and lasted for short duration. The severe adverse events were 5% among NE recipients, lasting for a median duration of 1 day, 4% in Fluzone recipients, and 11% in PBS recipients, both of which lasted for 2 days. Group receiving NE suffered from headache and throat pain. The adjuvant vaccine produced high serum and mucosal immune response, indicating high effectiveness in respiratory infections. The NE adjuvant with inactivated antigen proved to be safe and effective in healthy adults.

Myc et al. (2013) investigated another NE nasal adjuvant for its activity on epithelial and dendritic cells. It was revealed that the antigen containing NE nasal adjuvant could activate both humoral and cell-mediated immunity. Mice immunized intranasal with the antigen+NE elicited an increased production of IgG1 and IgG2b, cytokines, and markers for thyroid antigen cellular response, suggesting increased humoral and cell-mediated immunity responses. The broad spectrum activity of NE could be due to the uptake of antigens by epithelial cells and engulfment of antigen-primed epithelial cells. It was suggested that this could be due to the positive charge on NE antigen particles, allowing binding to the membrane of the cell and engulfment into the interior of the cell by endocytosis. The NE-antigen hydrolyzes the complex by fusing with lysosomes. This reveals the effectiveness of NE as an adjuvant for the enhancement of immune responses in the body.

Donovan et al. (2000) investigated the activity of two novel nonionic surfactant NEs against influenza virus passaged in mice. The two NEs were prepared by soybean oil, tributyl phosphate, and triton X-100. The mice were administered NEs intranasally for the determination of safe dosage. Animals administered with influenza virus mixed with NE for 5 days resulted in no deaths. NEs at concentration of 1.0% produced no toxic effects and were well tolerated. The NE decreased the symptoms of infection, resulting in 80% survival. These studies showed that the developed novel NEs were effective in treating influenza virus infection.

Ebola virus is an extremely stable biological agent, sterilization of which with multiple methods has proven to be unsuccessful. It causes a highly contagious and fatal hemorrhagic fever. Chepurnov et al. (2003) evaluated the antibacterial activity of surfactant NE on two strains of ebola virus EBO (strain Zaire) obtained from Vero cell culture fluid (EBO-zc) and from blood of infected monkeys (EBO-zb). After 20 min of exposure, 10% NE completely inactivated both EBO-zb and EBO-zc. One percent NE was inactive against EBO-zc, whereas in the case of EBO-zb, 96% inactivation was achieved after 24 h. A complete eradication from the surface was seen when studied on glass, metal, and plastic surfaces.

Acquired immunodeficiency syndrome (AIDS) is one of the deadliest epidemics in the world. Human immunodeficiency virus (HIV), a retrovirus, is the causative organism for AIDS (Rios, 2014). HIV mainly affects the host immune system, making the person more susceptible to opportunistic infectious diseases and tumors (Soares, Garbin, Moimaz, & Garbin, 2014). A vast majority of people suffering from AIDS belong to low- and middle-income countries. The antiretroviral therapy includes drugs in various class reverse transcriptase inhibitors nucleoside reverse transcriptase inhibitor (NRTI), nonnucleoside reverse transcriptase inhibitors (NNRTI), protease inhibitor (PI), and fusion inhibitors (FI). Highly active antiretroviral therapy includes a combination of two or more drugs in combinatory action (Chearskul, Rongkavilit, Al-Tatari, & Asmar, 2006). Despite many advances in antiretroviral therapy, there is still no cure for it. New approaches and efforts are needed to address the epidemic.

Saquinavir is a peptide derivative that belongs to a PI class. It binds the protease enzyme active site and prevents cleavage of viral polypeptides, thus inhibiting the maturation of virus (Vyas, Shahiwala, & Amiji, 2008). Vyas et al. (2008) developed novel o/w NEs of saqui-navir to enhance its oral bioavailability and study its brain disposition. NE containing flax seed oil or safflower oil and 400 µg/mL of saquinavir was prepared by sonication at 21% amplitude and 50% cycle for 10 min. Prepared NE showed globule size in nanorange with 100–200 nm and a zeta potential of –40 mV. The plasma and brain concentrations were high for the NE than an aqueous suspension of saquinavir. The average plasma concentration for saquinavir was found to be 17.4 and 11.8 µg/g after 2 h, respectively, for flax seed oil and safflower oil NE. Plasma and brain concentration of saquinavir was found to be higher for NE than the aqueous saquinavir. The oral serum bioavailability of saquinavir was enhanced from 42.19% for drug suspension to 108.1% and 59.73%, respectively, for flaxseed NE and saf-flower NE. The intravenous (i.v.) serum bioavailability was enhanced to 71.09% and 89.82%, respectively, for flaxseed and safflower oil NE. Similarly, bioavailability in serum and brains was enhanced to 86.69% and 364%, respectively, in the case of flaxseed oil NE. Therefore, NE greatly enhanced the oral bioavailability and brain disposition of saquinavir.

Efavirenz is an antiretroviral drug discovered by Merk Research Laboratories. It is mainly used in pediatric and adult patients. It is a highly lipophilic drug falling in class II according to biopharmaceutical classification system (BCS) classification that has a bio-availability of 40% (Madhavi et al., 2011). Kotta, Khan, Ansari, Sharma, and Ali (2014), encapsulated Efavirenz in a NE to increase its bioavailability for HIV therapy. The NE was prepared by phase inversion method and contained Capryol 90 (2.86%, v/v), Gelucire (13.728%, v/v), Transcutol®HP (3.432%, v/v), and double distilled water (79.98%, v/v). The prepared NE showed a droplet size of 26.427 ± 1.960 nm and a PDI of 0.117 ± 0.0034. The drug release was found to be 90%. *In vivo* studies on female albino wistar rats showed an increase in bioavailability up to 2.5 times in NE when compared with drug suspension. The t_{max} for NE was found to be 4 h with a C_{max} of 3.12 ± 0.0596 µg/mL. NE loaded with Efavirenz could act as an effective drug delivery system for the treatment of HIV I.

6.5.4 NEs as Antiparasitic Agents

Parasites such as *Plasmodium vivax*, *P. ovale*, and *Trypanosoma evansi* are the causes of epi-demic diseases such as malaria. These are the major problems behind the mortality and morbidity in developing countries. These parasites are becoming resistant to the pres-ently used antiprotozoals. Therefore, scientists are looking for some alternative therapy to which these organisms remain sensitive for longer duration.

Primaquine belonging to 8-aminoquinoline category is used to treat malaria caused by both *P. vivax* and *P. ovale*. Primaquine causes disruption of the mitochondrial membrane and is the only drug against malaria (Baird & Hoffman, 2004). Singh and Vingkar (2008) devel-oped a NE loaded with primaquine using HPH. The emulsion had a particle size of 96.5 nm, which was stable against creaming, cracking, or phase separation. Encapsulation efficiency of NE was 95% with a drug release of >90.0% within 8–10 h. Animal studies showed that NE reduced the dose up to 25%. It was effective at a dose of 1.5 mg/kg/day when compared with the drug solution that was effective at 2.0 mg/kg/day. Pharmacokinetic studies revealed that the peak plasma concentration for NE was 1.5 times higher (6.27 µg/mL) than the aqueous drug solution. The oral bioavailability of primaquine was enhanced 1.3 times when com-pared with the area under curve (AUC) of NE than the drug solution. The drug level concen-tration in the liver was higher for NE, suggesting better drug targeting than drug solution, proving NE to be a successful delivery system for primaquine for malarial treatment.

Borhade, Pathak, Sharma, and Patravale (2012) evaluated the antimalarial activ-ity of clotrimazole. Clotrimazole is an antifungal drug that acts on the fungal cell wall.

It inhibits the formation of cell wall and thus prevents infection. It is a highly lipophilic drug. The antimalarial activity of clotrimazole encapsulated in NE was checked against *P. berghei*. The "suppressive tests" proved NE to be effective at 10 mg/kg, and in the "onset of activity" and "recrudescence test," NE was effective at 10 mg/kg when compared with a suspension effective at 15 mg/kg. NE showed a dose-dependent inhibition of parasitic growth and proved to be nontoxic.

Baldissera et al. (2013) also investigated the antiparasitic activity of essential oils andiroba (*Carapa guaianensis*) and aroeira (*Schinus molle*) alone and in the form of NE. The antiparasitic activity was tested against *T. evansi*. The tested oils were used in the concentrations of 0.5%, 1%, and 2%. The oils alone and in the form of NE could reduce the number of parasites within 3 h, and no live parasite was observed after 6 h.

6.6 Patents Related to NEs Having Antimicrobial Activity

Dr Baker and his associates at the University of Michigan developed an antimicrobial NE technology that is exclusively licensed to NanoBio (R). NanoBio (R) Corporation has been awarded four patents related to therapeutics, which showed activity against fungal, viral, and bacterial infections of skin and mucosal membranes.

U.S. Patent No. 7767216 claims the composition and method of treating Herpes Simplex I virus infection using a topical NE. This invention consisted of a method of preparation of o/w formulation using oil, emulsifying mixture, and aqueous solution. Additionally, these formulations are nontoxic to human and animals, ensuring their safe use thereof (Baker, Hamouda, Shih, & Myc, 2010).

U.S. Patent Nos. 6635676 and 6559189 have been granted under the same name of "Nontoxic antimicrobial compositions and methods of use." Another patent, U.S. Patent No. 6506803, under the name of "Methods of preventing and treating microbial infections" has been granted to the same company. All the earlier three patents are related with the same claims of method of preventing and composition of formulation used for decontamination of areas infected by pathogens and viruses (Baker, Hamouda, Shih, & Myc, 2003a; Baker, Hamouda, Shih, & Myc, 2003b).

All these patents will be beneficial for humans by their commercialization of an extensive array of applications based on NanoStat (TM) NE technology platforms. Furthermore, long-term products used for the treatment of genital herpes, shingles, and urinary tract infection are under development, which would substantially improve and compliment the nanotechnology field in the coming days.

6.7 Limitations of NEs

In recent years, NEs have acted as reasonable carriers of active ingredients and their delivery at target sites. Various new NEs have been introduced in the market for the treatment of diseases, and many of them are under preclinical and clinical stages. Despite this huge development in the area of nanoformulation, these are still under research and not yet commercialized due to the following reasons:

- Many of the compounds, such as nucleic acid, proteins, and enzymes, are thermolabile in nature. Hence, it is very difficult to encapsulate these in a single nanocarrier system.
- Preparation of NEs requires high-energy methods that require consumption of money and space (Tadros, Izquierdo, Esquena, & Solans, 2004).
- The role of surfactants and cosurfactants in the NE system and the mechanisms behind the submicron size of droplets are not cleared yet.
- Lack of awareness of the benefits of using NEs over classical macroemulsion systems (Aboofazeli, 2010).

6.8 Future Prospective

The NEs showed much better physical and chemical properties than the standard drugs. These are highly stable in nature and also possess antimicrobial activity due to the presence of surfactants and cosurfactants in the formulation. Due to these properties of nanoformulations, these could be developed for their use in the antimicrobial therapy and disinfection industry over standard emulsions. Besides, there are a lot of challenges behind the use of NEs, commercially, in antimicrobial pharmacology owing to the limited knowledge related to the guiding of the choice of processing method. Moreover, the understanding of the possible interaction between the prepared NE and other ingredients would be beneficial for the development of new formulations and their production and optimization in a cost-effective manner at the industrial scale. Considering possible interactions at an early stage could help in choosing the ingredients that avoid any negative interactions during actual application (Bagchi, Moriyama, & Shahidi, 2012).

6.9 Conclusion

NEs have been widely used in research, dosage form design, and delivery of active ingredients at the site of targets. This could be due to the peculiar characteristics of NEs, such as optical clarity, ease of preparation, kinetic stability, and nanosize of particles. The submicron droplet size of the NEs makes them a suitable vehicle for the transport of drugs as well as antimicrobial agents encapsulated in them at the site of action. These are designed to overcome many problems of the traditional medication system, such as low bioavailability and noncompliance. Moreover, the NEs are prepared using less surfactants, so it is likely that NEs will play an important role commercially. This chapter has highlighted the developments of nanoformulations for their use against antimicrobial and antifungal activities. The NEs could be used for delivery of drugs through all routes of drug administration and are used in different fields, including cosmetics, dentistry, or therapeutics. With the invention of new instruments and competition among various manufactures, the cost of production of NE formulations is likely to decrease soon. Therefore, NEs could act as a novel system for the delivery of antimicrobial agents.

References

Abbas, S., Bashari, M., Akhtar, W., Li, W. W., & Zhang, X. (2014). Process optimization of ultrasound-assisted curcumin nanoemulsions stabilized by OSA-modified starch. *Ultrasonics Sonochemistry, 21*(4), 1265–1274.

Abismaïl, B., Canselier, J. P., Wilhelm, A. M., Delmas, H., & Gourdon, C. (1999). Emulsification by ultrasound: Drop size distribution and stability. *Ultrasonics Sonochemistry, 6*(1–2), 75–83.

Aboofazeli, R. (2010). Nanometric-scaled emulsions (nanoemulsions). *Iranian Journal of Pharmaceutical Research: IJPR, 9*(4), 325.

Anton, N., Benoit, J. P., & Saulnier, P. (2008). Design and production of nanoparticles formulated from nano-emulsion templates—A review. *Journal of Controlled Release, 128*(3), 185–199.

Attwood, D., Mallon, C., Ktistis, G., & Taylor, C. J. (1992). A study on factors influencing the droplet size in nonionic oil-in-water microemulsions. *International Journal of Pharmaceutics, 88*(1–3), 417–422.

Bagchi, M., Moriyama, H., & Shahidi, F. (2012). *Bio-Nanotechnology: A Revolution in Food, Biomedical and Health Sciences.* John Wiley & Sons, Hoboken, NJ.

Baird, J. K., & Hoffman, S. L. (2004). Primaquine therapy for malaria. *Clinical Infectious Diseases, 39*(9), 1336–1345.

Baker Jr, J. R., Hamouda, T., Shih, A., & Myc, A. (2003a). U.S. Patent No. 6,635,676. Washington, DC: U.S. Patent and Trademark Office.

Baker Jr, J. R., Hamouda, T., Shih, A., & Myc, A. (2003b). U.S. Patent No. 6,506,803. Washington, DC: U.S. Patent and Trademark Office.

Baker Jr, J. R., Hamouda, T., Shih, A., & Myc, A. (2010). U.S. Patent No. 7,767,216. Washington, DC: U.S. Patent and Trademark Office.

Baldissera, M. D., Da Silva, A. S., Oliveira, C. B., Zimmermann, C. E., Vaucher, R. A., Santos, R. C., Monteiro, S. G.(2013). Trypanocidal activity of the essential oils in their conventional and nanoemulsion forms: In vitro tests. *Experimental Parasitology, 134*, 356–361.

Bałdyga, J., Orciuch, W., Makowski, Ł., Malski-Brodzicki, M., & Malik, K. (2007). Break up of nano-particle clusters in high-shear devices. *Chemical Engineering and Processing: Process Intensification, 46*(9), 851–861.

Bechtel, S., Gilbert, N., & Wagner, H. G. (1999). Grundlagenuntersuchungen zur Herstellung von Öl/Wasser-Emulsionen im Ultraschallfeld. *Chemie Ingenieur Technik, 71*(8), 810–817.

Bedoya-Serna, C. M., Dacanal, G. C., Fernandes, A. M., & Pinho, S. C. (2018). Antifungal activity of nanoemulsions encapsulating oregano (*Origanum vulgare*) essential oil: In vitro study and application in Minas Padrão cheese. *Brazilian Journal of Microbiology, 49*(4), 929–935.

Blair, J. M., Webber, M. A., Baylay, A. J., Ogbolu, D. O., & Piddock, L. J. (2015). Molecular mechanisms of antibiotic resistance. *Nature Reviews Microbiology, 13*(1), 42.

Borhade, V., Pathak, S., Sharma, S., & Patravale, V. (2012). Clotrimazole nanoemulsion for malaria chemotherapy. Part II: Stability assessment, in vivo pharmacodynamic evaluations and toxicological studies. *International Journal of Pharmaceutics, 431*(1–2), 149–160.

Borrin, T. R., Georges, E. L., Moraes, I. C., & Pinho, S. C. (2016). Curcumin-loaded nanoemulsions produced by the emulsion inversion point (EIP) method: An evaluation of process parameters and physico-chemical stability. *Journal of Food Engineering, 169*, 1–9.

Bourne, D. W. A., & Dittert, L. W. (1996). Models for assessing drug absorption and metabolism. In Banker, G. S. and Rhodes, C. T. (eds.) *Modern Pharmaceutics*, 3rd ed., Dekker, New York, ISBN 0-8247-9371-4.

Candau, S. J., Hirsch, E., Zana, R., Safran, S., & Clark, N. (1987). *Physics of Complex Supermolecular Fluids.* John Wiley & Sons Inc., Hoboken, NJ.

Cazabat, A. M., & Langevin, D. (1981). Diffusion of interacting particles: Light scattering study of microemulsions. *The Journal of Chemical Physics, 74*(6), 3148–3158.

Chearskul, P., Rongkavilit, C., Al-Tatari, H., & Asmar, B. (2006). New antiretroviral drugs in clinical use. *The Indian Journal of Pediatrics*, *73*(4), 335–341.

Chepurnov, A. A., Bakulina, L. F., Dadaeva, A. A., Ustinova, E. N., Chepurnova, T. S., & Baker Jr, J. R. (2003). Inactivation of Ebola virus with a surfactant nanoemulsion. *Acta Tropica*, *87*(3), 315–320.

Chesa-Jiménez, J., Peris, J. E., Torres-Molina, F., & Granero, L. (1994). Low bioavailability of amoxicillin in rats as a consequence of presystemic degradation in the intestine. *Antimicrobial Agents and Chemotherapy*, *38*(4), 842–847.

Cook, E. J., & Lagace, A. P. (1985). U.S. Patent No. 4,533,254. Washington, DC: U.S. Patent and Trademark Office.

Das, S. C., Hatta, M., Wilker, P. R., Myc, A., Hamouda, T., Neumann, G., ... Kawaoka, Y. (2012). Nanoemulsion W805EC improves immune responses upon intranasal delivery of an inactivated pandemic H1N1 influenza vaccine. *Vaccine*, *30*(48), 6871–6877.

Donovan, B. W., Reuter, J. D., Cao, Z., Myc, A., Johnson, K. J., & Baker Jr, J. R. (2000). Prevention of murine influenza A virus pneumonitis by surfactant nano-emulsions. *Antiviral Chemistry and Chemotherapy*, *11*(1), 41–49.

Donsì, F., Annunziata, M., Vincensi, M., & Ferrari, G. (2012). Design of nanoemulsion-based delivery systems of natural antimicrobials: effect of the emulsifier. *Journal of Biotechnology*, *159*(4), 342–350.

Floury, J., Desrumaux, A., Axelos, M. A., & Legrand, J. (2003). Effect of high pressure homogenisation on methylcellulose as food emulsifier. *Journal of Food Engineering*, *58*(3), 227–238.

Forgiarini, A., Esquena, J., González, C., & Solans, C. (2001). Formation and stability of nanoemulsions in mixed nonionic surfactant systems. In Koutsoukos, P. G. (eds.) *Trends in Colloid and Interface Science XV* (pp. 184–189). Springer, Berlin, Heidelberg.

Goldberg, A. H., & Higuchi, W. I. (1969). Mechanisms of interphase transport II: Theoretical considerations and experimental evaluation of interfacially controlled transport in solubilized systems. *Journal of pharmaceutical sciences*, *58*(11), 1341–1352.

Gupta, S., Bansal, R., Maheshwari, D., Ali, J., Gabrani, R., & Dang, S. (2014). Development of a nanoemulsion system for polyphenon 60 and cranberry. *Advanced Science Letters*, *20*(7–8), 1683–1686.

Gupta, S., Gabrani, R., Ali, J., & Dang, S. (2011). Exploring novel approaches to vaginal drugdelivery. *Recent Patents on Drug Delivery & Formulation*, *5*(2), 82–94.

Halnor, V. V., Pande, V. V., Borawake, D. D., & Nagare, H. S. (2018). Nanoemulsion: A novel platform for drug delivery system. *Journal of Material Science and Nanotechonology*, *6*(1), 104.

Hamouda, T., & Baker Jr, J. R. (2000). Antimicrobial mechanism of action of surfactant lipid preparations in enteric Gram-negative bacilli. *Journal of Applied Microbiology*, *89*(3), 397–403.

Hamouda, T., Myc, A., Donovan, B., Shih, A. Y., Reuter, J. D., & Baker Jr, J. R. (2001). A novel surfactant nanoemulsion with a unique non-irritant topical antimicrobial activity against bacteria, enveloped viruses and fungi. *Microbiological Research*, *156*(1), 1–7.

Han, M., He, C. X., Fang, Q. L., Yang, X. C., Diao, Y. Y., Xu, D. H., ... Gao, J. Q. (2009). A novel camptothecin derivative incorporated in nano-carrier induced distinguished improvement in solubility, stability and anti-tumor activity both in vitro and in vivo. *Pharmaceutical Research*, *26*(4), 926–935.

Heurtault, B., Saulnier, P., Pech, B., Proust, J. E., & Benoit, J. P. (2002). A novel phase inversion-based process for the preparation of lipid nanocarriers. *Pharmaceutical Research*, *19*(6), 875–880.

Hielscher, T. (2005). Ultrasonic production of nano-size dispersions and emulsions, *Paper Presented at 1st Workshop on Nano Technology Transfer. ENS Paris*. 14–16 December. Paris, France.

Higuchi, W. I., & Misra, J. (1962). Physical degradation of emulsions via the molecular diffusion route and the possible prevention thereof. *Journal of Pharmaceutical Sciences*, *51*(5), 459–466.

Huppertz, T. (2011). Homogenization of milk| other types of homogenizer (high-speed mixing, ultrasonics, microfluidizers, membrane emulsification). *Encyclopedia of Dairy Sciences*, 751–764.

Hwang, Y. Y., Ramalingam, K., Bienek, D. R., Lee, V., You, T., & Alvarez, R. (2013). Antimicrobial activity of nanoemulsion in combination with cetylpyridinium chloride on multi-drug resistant *Acinetobacter baumannii*. *Antimicrobial Agents and Chemotherapy*, *57*(8), 3568–3575.

Jerobin, J., Sureshkumar, R. S., Anjali, C. H., Mukherjee, A., & Chandrasekaran, N. (2012). Biodegradable polymer based encapsulation of neem oil nanoemulsion for controlled release of Aza-A. *Carbohydrate Polymers, 90*(4), 1750–1756.

Jintapattanakit, A. (2017). Preparation of nanoemulsions by phase inversion temperature (PIT) method, *Pharmaceutical Sciences Asia, 42*, 1–12.

Kallen, A. J., Mu, Y., Bulens, S., Reingold, A., Petit, S., Gershman, K. E. N.,...Townes, J. M. (2010). Health care–associated invasive MRSA infections, 2005–2008. *JAMA, 304*(6), 641–647.

Karthikeyan, R., Amaechi, B. T., Rawls, H. R., & Lee, V. A. (2011). Antimicrobial activity of nanoemulsion on cariogenic *Streptococcus mutans. Archives of Oral Biology, 56*(5), 437–445.

Kaur, A., Kapoor, N., Gupta, S., Tyagi, A., Sharma, R., Ali, J., … Dang, S. (2018). Development and characterization of green tea catechins and ciprofloxacin-loaded nanoemulsion for intravaginal delivery to treat urinary tract infection. *Indian Journal of Pharmaceutical Sciences, 80*(3), 442–452.

Kaur, A., Saxena, Y., Bansal, R., Gupta, S., Tyagi, A., Sharma, R. K., … Dang, S. (2017). Intravaginal delivery of Polyphenon 60 and Curcumin Nanoemulsion Gel. *American Association of Pharmaceutical Sciences, 18*(6), 2188–2202.

Kelmann, R. G., Kuminek, G., Teixeira, H. F., & Koester, L. S. (2007). Carbamazepine parenteral nanoemulsions prepared by spontaneous emulsification process. *International Journal of Pharmaceutics, 342*(1–2), 231–239.

Komaiko, J., & McClements, D. J. (2015). Low-energy formation of edible nanoemulsions by spontaneous emulsification: Factors influencing particle size. *Journal of Food Engineering, 146*, 122–128.

Koroleva, M. Y., & Yurtov, E. V. E. (2012). Nanoemulsions: The properties, methods of preparation and promising applications. *Russian Chemical Reviews, 81*(1), 21–43.

Kotta, S., Khan, A. W., Ansari, S. H., Sharma, R. K., & Ali, J. (2014). Anti HIV nanoemulsion formulation: optimization and in vitro–in vivo evaluation. *International Journal of Pharmaceutics, 462*(1–2), 129–134.

Lee, L., & Norton, I. T. (2013). Comparing droplet breakup for a high-pressure valve homogeniser and a microfluidizer for the potential production of food-grade nanoemulsions. *Journal of Food Engineering, 114*(2), 158–163.

Li, P. H., & Chiang, B. H. (2012). Process optimization and stability of D-limonene-in-water nanoemulsions prepared by ultrasonic emulsification using response surface methodology. *Ultrasonics Sonochemistry, 19*(1), 192–197.

Lifshitz, I. M., & Slyozov, V. V. (1961). The kinetics of precipitation from supersaturated solid solutions. *Journal of Physics and Chemistry of Solids, 19*(1–2), 35–50.

Lin, Y. H., Chiou, S. F., Lai, C. H., Tsai, S. C., Chou, C. W., Peng, S. F., & He, Z. S. (2012). Formulation and evaluation of water-in-oil amoxicillin-loaded nanoemulsions using for Helicobacter pylori eradication. *Process Biochemistry, 47*(10), 1469–1478.

LiPuma, J. J. (2001). Burkholderia cepacia complex: A contraindication to lung transplantation in cystic fibrosis? *Transplant Infectious Disease, 3*(3), 149–160.

LiPuma, J. J., Rathinavelu, S., Foster, B. K., Keoleian, J. C., Makidon, P. E., Kalikin, L. M., & Baker, J. R. (2009). In vitro activities of a novel nanoemulsion against Burkholderia and other multidrug-resistant cystic fibrosis-associated bacterial species. *Antimicrobial Agents and Chemotherapy, 53*(1), 249–255.

Liu, W., Sun, D., Li, C., Liu, Q., & Xu, J. (2006). Formation and stability of paraffin oil-in-water nanoemulsions prepared by the emulsion inversion point method. *Journal of Colloid and Interface Science, 303*(2), 557–563.

Lobo, L., & Svereika, A. (2003). Coalescence during emulsification: 2. Role of small molecule surfactants. *Journal of Colloid and Interface Science, 261*(2), 498–507.

Lovelyn, C., & Attama, A. A. (2011). Current state of nanoemulsions in drug delivery. *Journal of Biomaterials and Nanobiotechnology, 2*(05), 626.

Madhavi, B. B., Kusum, B., Chatanya, C. K., Madhu, M. N., Harsha, V. S., & Banji, D. (2011). Dissolution enhancement of efavirenz by solid dispersion and PEGylation techniques. *International Journal of Pharmaceutical Investigation, 1*(1), 29.

Mohr, K. H. (1987). High-pressure homogenization. Part II. The influence of cavitation on liquid–liquid dispersion in turbulence fields of high energy density. *Journal of Food Engineering, 6*(4), 311–324.

Myc, A., Kukowska-Latallo, J. F., Smith, D. M., Passmore, C., Pham, T., Wong, P., ... Baker Jr, J. R. (2013). Nanoemulsion nasal adjuvant W805EC induces dendritic cell engulfment of antigen-primed epithelial cells. *Vaccine, 31*(7), 1072–1079.

Myc, A., Vanhecke, T., Landers, J. J., Hamouda, T., & Baker, J. R. (2003). The fungicidal activity of novel nanoemulsion (X8W 60 PC) against clinically important yeast and filamentous fungi. *Mycopathologia, 155*(4), 195–201.

Nicolaos, G., Crauste-Manciet, S., Farinotti, R., & Brossard, D. (2003). Improvement of cefpodoxime proxetil oral absorption in rats by an oil-in-water submicron emulsion. *International Journal of Pharmaceutics, 263*(1–2), 165–171.

Olson, D. W., White, C. H., & Richter, R. L. (2004). Effect of pressure and fat content on particle sizes in microfluidized milk. *Journal of Dairy Science, 87*(10), 3217–3223.

Ostertag, F., Weiss, J., & McClements, D. J. (2012). Low-energy formation of edible nanoemulsions: factors influencing droplet size produced by emulsion phase inversion. *Journal of Colloid and Interface Science, 388*(1), 95–102.

Padovan, J., Ralić, J., Letfus, V., Milić, A., & Mihaljević, V. B. (2012). Investigating the barriers to bioavailability of macrolide antibiotics in the rat. *European Journal of Drug Metabolism and Pharmacokinetics, 37*(3), 163–171.

Pangeni, R., Sharma, S., Mustafa, G., Ali, J., & Baboota, S. (2014). Vitamin E loaded resveratrol nanoemulsion for brain targeting for the treatment of Parkinson's disease by reducing oxidative stress. *Nanotechnology, 25*(48), 485102.

Pannu, J., McCarthy, A., Martin, A., Hamouda, T., Ciotti, S., Fothergill, A., & Sutcliffe, J. (2009). NB-002, a novel nanoemulsion with broad antifungal activity against dermatophytes, other filamentous fungi, and *Candida albicans. Antimicrobial Agents and Chemotherapy, 53*(8), 3273–3279.

Peshkovsky, A. S., Peshkovsky, S. L., & Bystryak, S. (2013). Scalable high-power ultrasonic technology for the production of translucent nanoemulsions. *Chemical Engineering and Processing: Process Intensification, 69,* 77–82.

Rajalakshmi, R., Mahesh, K., & Kumar, C. K. (2011). A critical review on nanoemulsions. *International Journal of Drug Discovery, 1,* 1–8.

Ramalingam, K., Amaechi, B. T., Ralph, R. H., & Lee, V. A. (2012). Antimicrobial activity of nanoemulsion on cariogenic planktonic and biofilm organisms. *Archives of Oral Biology, 57*(1), 15–22.

Ramalingam, K., Frohlich, N. C., & Lee, V. A. (2013). Effect of nanoemulsion on dental unit waterline biofilm. *Journal of Dental Sciences, 8*(3), 333–336.

Rios, A. (2014). HIV-related hematological malignancies: A concise review. *Clinical Lymphoma Myeloma and Leukemia, 14,* S96–S103.

Salager, J. L., Forgiarini, A., Marquez, L., Pena, A., Pizzino, A., Rodriguez, M. P., & Rondon-Gonzalez, M. (2004). Using emulsion inversion in industrial processes. *Advances in Colloid and Interface Science, 108,* 259–272.

Salvia-Trujillo, L., Rojas-Graü, M. A., Soliva-Fortuny, R., & Martín-Belloso, O. (2013). Effect of processing parameters on physicochemical characteristics of microfluidized lemongrass essential oil-alginate nanoemulsions. *Food Hydrocolloids, 30*(1), 401–407.

Seil, J. T., & Webster, T. J. (2012). Antimicrobial applications of nanotechnology: Methods and literature. *International Journal of Nanomedicine, 7,* 2767.

Ševčíková, P., Kašpárková, V., Vltavská, P., & Krejčí, J. (2012). On the preparation and characterization of nanoemulsions produced by phase inversion emulsification. *Colloids and Surfaces A: Physicochemical and Engineering Aspects, 410,* 130–135.

Shah, P., Bhalodia, D., & Shelat, P. (2010). Nanoemulsion: A pharmaceutical review. *Systematic Reviews in Pharmacy, 1*(1), 24–32.

Singh, A., Van Hamme, J. D., & Ward, O. P. (2007). Surfactants in microbiology and biotechnology: Part 2. Application aspects. *Biotechnology Advances, 25*(1), 99–121.

Singh, K. K., & Vingkar, S. K. (2008). Formulation, antimalarial activity and biodistribution of oral lipid nanoemulsion of primaquine. *International Journal of Pharmaceutics, 347*(1–2), 136–143.

Soares, G. B., Garbin, C. A. S., Moimaz, S. A. S., & Garbin, A. J. Í. (2014). Oral health status of people living with HIV/AIDS attending a specialized service in Brazil. *Special Care in Dentistry, 34*(4), 176–184.

Solans, C., Esquena, J., Forgiarini, A.M., Morales, D., Izquierdo, P., Azemar, N., & Garcia, M. J. (2003). Nano-emulsions: Formation, properties and applications. *Surfactant Science Series, 109,* 525–554.

Solans, C., Izquierdo, P., Nolla, J., Azemar, N., & Garcia-Celma, M. J. (2005). Nano-emulsions. *Current Opinion in Colloid & Interface Science, 10*(3–4), 102–110.

Stanberry, L. R., Simon, J. K., Johnson, C., Robinson, P. L., Morry, J., Flack, M. R.,… Baker Jr, J. R. (2012). Safety and immunogenicity of a novel nanoemulsion mucosal adjuvant W805EC combined with approved seasonal influenza antigens. *Vaccine, 30*(2), 307–316.

Sugumar, S., Ghosh, V., Nirmala, M. J., Mukherjee, A., & Chandrasekaran, N. (2014). Ultrasonic emulsification of eucalyptus oil nanoemulsion: antibacterial activity against Staphylococcus aureus and wound healing activity in Wistar rats. *Ultrasonics Sonochemistry, 21*(3), 1044–1049.

Tadros, T. F. (2009). *Emulsion Science and Technology: A General Introduction* (pp. 1–56). Wiley-VCH Verlag GmbH & Co. KGaA, Weinheim.

Tadros, T., Izquierdo, P., Esquena, J., & Solans, C. (2004). Formation and stability of nano-emulsions. *Advances in Colloid and Interface Science, 108,* 303–318.

Tal-Figiel, B. (2007). The formation of stable w/o, o/w, w/o/w cosmetic emulsions in an ultrasonic field. *Chemical Engineering Research and Design, 85*(5), 730–734.

Tang, S. Y., Manickam, S., Wei, T. K., & Nashiru, B. (2012). Formulation development and optimization of a novel Cremophore EL-based nanoemulsion using ultrasound cavitation. *Ultrasonics Sonochemistry, 19*(2), 330–345.

Tang, S. Y., Shridharan, P., & Sivakumar, M. (2013). Impact of process parameters in the generation of novel aspirin nanoemulsions–comparative studies between ultrasound cavitation and microfluidizer. *Ultrasonics Sonochemistry, 20*(1), 485–497.

Taylor, P. (2003). Ostwald ripening in emulsions: Estimation of solution thermodynamics of the disperse phase. *Advances in Colloid and Interface Science, 106*(1–3), 261–285.

Teixeira, P. C., Leite, G. M., Domingues, R. J., Silva, J., Gibbs, P. A., & Ferreira, J. P. (2007). Antimicrobial effects of a microemulsion and a nanoemulsion on enteric and other pathogens and biofilms. *International Journal of Food Microbiology, 118*(1), 15–19.

Tenover, F. C. (2006). Mechanisms of antimicrobial resistance in bacteria. *American Journal of Infection Control, 34*(5), S3–S10.

Vaara, M. (1992). Agents that increase the permeability of the outer membrane. *Microbiological Reviews, 56*(3), 395–411.

Vatsraj, S., Chauhan, K., & Pathak, H. (2014). Formulation of a novel nanoemulsion system for enhanced solubility of a sparingly water soluble antibiotic, clarithromycin. *Journal of Nanoscience, 2014,* 7.

Vitale, S. A., & Katz, J. L. (2003). Liquid droplet dispersions formed by homogeneous liquid–liquid nucleation: "The Ouzo effect." *Langmuir, 19*(10), 4105–4110.

Vyas, T. K., Shahiwala, A., & Amiji, M. M. (2008). Improved oral bioavailability and brain transport of Saquinavir upon administration in novel nanoemulsion formulations. *International Journal of Pharmaceutics, 347*(1), 93–101.

Wagner, C. (1961). Theorie der alterung von niederschlägen durch umlösen (Ostwald-reifung). *Zeitschrift für Elektrochemie, Berichte der Bunsengesellschaft für physikalische Chemie, 65*(7–8), 581–591.

Washington, C. (1987). Emulsion production by microfluidizer. *Laboratory Equipment Digest, 85,* 69–71.

Wojnarowicz, J., Opalinska, A., Chudoba, T., Gierlotka, S., Mukhovskyi, R., Pietrzykowska, E., … Lojkowski, W. (2016). Effect of water content in ethylene glycol solvent on the size of ZnO nanoparticles prepared using microwave solvothermal synthesis. *Journal of Nanomaterials, 2016,* 1.

Xu, Y., Liu, X., Lian, R., Zheng, S., Yin, Z., Lu, Y., & Wu, W. (2012). Enhanced dissolution and oral bioavailability of aripiprazole nanosuspensions prepared by nanoprecipitation/homogenization based on acid–base neutralization. *International Journal of Pharmaceutics*, 438(1–2), 287–295.

Yu, M., Ma, H., Lei, M., Li, N., & Tan, F. (2014). In vitro/in vivo characterization of nanoemulsion formulation of metronidazole with improved skin targeting and anti-rosacea properties. *European Journal of Pharmaceutics and Biopharmaceutics*, 88(1), 92–103.

Yuan, Y., Gao, Y., Mao, L., & Zhao, J. (2008a). Optimisation of conditions for the preparation of β-carotene nanoemulsions using response surface methodology. *Food Chemistry*, 107(3), 1300–1306.

Yuan, Y., Gao, Y., Zhao, J., & Mao, L. (2008b). Characterization and stability evaluation of β-carotene nanoemulsions prepared by high pressure homogenization under various emulsifying conditions. *Food Research International*, 41(1), 61–68.

Zhang, Y., Liu, J. M., & Yan, X. P. (2012). Self-assembly of folate onto polyethyleneimine-coated CdS/ZnS quantum dots for targeted turn-on fluorescence imaging of folate receptor overexpressed cancer cells. *Analytical Chemistry*, 85(1), 228–234.

Zhao, L., Wei, Y., Huang, Y., He, B., Zhou, Y., & Fu, J. (2013). Nanoemulsion improves the oral bioavailability of baicalin in rats: in vitro and in vivo evaluation. *International Journal of Nanomedicine*, 8, 3769.

Zheng, B., Tice, J. D., & Ismagilov, R. F. (2004). Formation of droplets of alternating composition in microfluidic channels and applications to indexing of concentrations in droplet-based assays. *Analytical Chemistry*, 76(17), 4977–4982.

7

Analysis of Air Quality and Impacts on Human Health

Japsehaj Singh Wahi, Mayank Deepak Thar, Muskan Garg,
Charu Goyal, and Megha Rathi

Jaypee Institute of Information Technology

CONTENTS

7.1 Introduction

In today's world, air pollution has become one of the major reasons of deteriorating health conditions among humans as well as animals (Srinivas and Purushotham, 2013, Ocak and Turalioglu, 2008, 2010). Taking the case of country like India, air condition level has been successively worsened due to human-related sources like increase in population, unhampered increase of industries, increased vehicular emission on road, refuse of construction activities, burning of materials mainly plastic, absence of general consciousness of the public, temporal variations such as wind storms, hurricane, etc. (Srinivas and Purushotham, 2013). Air pollution is a major factor that can cause chronic and acute health effects. According to studies, it has been established that the youth and old-age group of individuals are more likely to get affected by air pollution, since they have a lesser immunity toward various bacterial and fungal infections that polluted air can lead to. Some examples of acute health effects due to polluted unhealthy air include various kinds of eye, skin, and nose infections, headaches, and many chemical reactions in the body. Some chronic health effects include various types of cancer, predominantly lung cancer, brain hemorrhage, liver and kidney malfunction, heart disease, and respiratory problems (Kang et al., 2018). Air pollution is the major contributing factor in the origination of acid rain, which is harmful for humans, wildlife, trees, vegetation, etc. Other negative impacts of air pollution include global warming, which can cause various types of skin diseases. Hence, the rising air pollution level becomes the most important concern (issue) for everyone in this world. From the research study of various air pollutant concentrations from various sources of emission, matter of course, i.e., particulate matter, and sulfur dioxide play the most contributing role in determining the air quality level, thereby leading to bad human health conditions. Meteorological parameters (e.g., solar radiation, speed of wind including its direction, etc.) that play an essential task in determining origination dominate the movement and, moreover, influence oxidation–reduction reactions of air pollutants (Kang et al., 2018). Chemical and physical transformation, long-range transport and deposition of air pollutants vary considerably from year to year and are strongly dependent on meteorological conditions (Andersson et al., 2007). To predict pollutant levels more efficiently and with less complexity, many machine leaning models have been developed to replace traditional methods.

Andersson et al. (2007) made an effort to study the air condition level of Delhi, using air quality index (AQI). AQI is a tool, basically a numerical quantity, used to indicate the level of pollutant concentration in air (Carslaw and Ropkins, 2012). AQI is used as a decision-making tool by various organizations, such as schools and colleges, to plan any outdoor event so that the harmful effects of bad air are kept minimum.

AQI alerts the general public about the alarming concentration of pollutants so that young children and elderly people become more cautious toward their health. The concept of AQI effectively determines the air quality condition. In this study, IND-AQI declared by Central Pollution Control Board (CPCB) was used to measure AQI.

Table 7.1 shows the major pollutants and their effects (see Tables 7.2 and 7.3).

7.2 Related Work

If we have data points from air monitoring stations, then we can calculate the relation between variables by making use of mathematical techniques like regression analysis. We also have statistical models to judge the nearness among the predicted and real-world measurements in exact conditions. The factors that affect pollutant levels are inherently regarded in the air data and are used to make a better use of the model. Another beneficial feature of using the model is that they have low cost and material usage.

The following is comparison of different papers available on the said matter:

- Katsoulis (1996): In this paper, he established that certain pollutants such as CO and O_3 are brought about by the factors such as speed of wind and traffic congestion. This research was conducted in Greece, Athens.

TABLE 7.1

U.S. Environmental Protection Agency Criteria Air Pollutants

Pollutant	Sources	Effects
Carbon monoxide. A colorless gas that is emitted by burning of leaves and fossil fuels.	Carbon monoxide is released when engines burn fossil fuels. CO is also released when vehicles are not properly maintained, which leads to increased vehicular emission. Conventional methods of cooking also results in emission of carbon dioxide. Moreover, emissions from gas stoves and heaters also contribute to increased level of CO.	Carbon monooxide has a huge and deadly impact on human health. Once accumulated in the body, all oxygen is consumed and eventually leads to suffocation and death. Heart attacks and respiratory problems occur. Elderly people and young children are more prone to attacks.
Nitrogen dioxide. A red–brown gas that comes from the burning of fossil fuels. It has a prominent and bad smell at increased concentrations.	Nitrogen dioxide mainly comes from emission of power plants and cars. Nitrogen dioxide is formed in two ways—either when fuel is burned which has high concentrations of nitrogen or when it reacts with compounds of oxygen at high altitudes. Major contribution is in formation of acid rain.	Increased levels of nitrogen dioxide by direct exposure can give people respiratory problems. Higher chance of getting respiratory infection is to those who are in direct contact with nitrogen gas. Major contribution is in the formation of acid rain, which harms vegetation and humans as well.
Particulate matter. Very small-sized particles ranging 0.1 mm wide and can be as small as 0.00005 mm. They can be in solid or liquid form.	There are two types of particulate matter—coarse particles and fine particles. Sources like dust and construction activities are major contributors in the formation of course particles. Burning of fuel in automobiles and power plants leads to the formation of fine particles.	Particulate matter is small enough to cause health problems and respiratory problems. Some of these problems include heart and, respiratory attacks, thereby causing early death.
Sulfur dioxide. A gas that cannot be seen or smelled at low levels but can have a "rotten egg" smell at high levels.	Sulfur dioxide is mainly emitted by burning of coal or oil in power plants. Like nitrogen dioxide, sulfur dioxide reacts with the atmosphere to form acid rain.	Sulfur dioxide on direct exposure mainly affects people who have asthma. Irritation in eyes, skin, and throat are some of the effects. Sulfur dioxide can harm vegetation and humans.

Source: Based on information provided by the Environmental Fact Sheet (2012)

TABLE 7.2

Various Categories of IND-AQI

Air Quality Index Values	Remark	Levels of Health Concern
0–50	Good	Good
51–100	Satisfactory	Moderate
101–200	Moderately polluted	Unhealthy for sensitive groups
201–300	Poor	Unhealthy
301–400	Very poor	Very unhealthy
400–500	Severe	Hazardous

Source: National Air Quality Index (2017).

- Elminir (2005): Wind direction was found to have an influence not only on pollutant concentrations but also on the correlation between pollutants.
- Dueñas et al. (2002): Ozone concentrations are valuable indicators of possible health and environmental impacts.

TABLE 7.3

The Means, Maximum, Minimum, and Standard Deviation of Meteorological Parameters and
Pollutant Concentration between 2016 and 2018

Pollutants and Meteorological Parameters	Mean	Maximum	Minimum	Standard Deviation	Number of Observations
PM_{10} concentration ($\mu g/m^3$)	307.9471	556.1256	0	205.1429	19,207
$PM_{2.5}$ concentration ($\mu g/m^3$)	103.6727	532.9634	0	113.1685	19,207
NO_2 concentration ($\mu g/m^3$)	21.72098	498.2679	0	48.15624	19,207
SO_2 concentration ($\mu g/m^3$)	21.72098	482.5512	0	18.06924	19,207
CO concentration (mg/m^3)	1.276493	490.0934	0	1.54758	19,207
Temperature (°C)	23.52865	46.8500	0	8.264977	19,207
RH (%)	52.63869	93.1700	0	18.54115	19,207
WS (m/s)	0.8995666	144.9012	−5.93	2.253728	19,207
WD	203.591	330.0070	0	58.49976	19,207

Note: Negative sign in WS indicates that the wind is blowing from north to south (north wind).

- Hargreaves et al. (2000): Wind speed (WS) and the pollutant NO_2 are highly negatively correlated.
- Dockery et al. (1993): They conducted a research to find the relation between the amount of particulate pollution and daily mortality rates. They found some correlation between the two irrespective of different demographic factors, such as gender, age, and BMI. Factors such as occupational exposure and smoking status were also found to be correlated.
- Gupta et al. (2008): This study was conducted in the high population density region where the prominent players contributing to the pollution level were the industrial, commercial, and residential factors. A correlation value was to be found out between the contributing factors and the concentration of different pollutants, such as PM_{10}, NO_2, and SO_2. The data about atmospheric factors of wind speed and direction, rainfall, and humidity was found out from India Meteorological Department (IMD). A study of a similar kind during the colder months was done, and it was found that the pollutant level during these months was larger in magnitude irrespective of data gathering technique and time line.
- Corani and Scanagatta (2016): They used the Bayesian classifier to estimate the chances of a pollutant level surpassing a certain predefined value. They also found out that multiple predictions are needed for dependent variables. To correct this, they used a multilabel classifier.
- Xi et al. (2015): They conducted a research in more than 70 cities in China and tried to find a model that best fits each individual city. From conducting their experiments, they found that the best output is obtained when we use different groups of feature selection and model selection.
- Ahmad et al. (2011): This study was conducted in Pakistan. They used the artificial neural network (ANN) model to predict the data. They also found out that during the colder months the pollution level is relatively higher and highlighted the reasons for the same. They also stressed that techniques like ANN will be important for future studies of such kind. ANN falls in the bracket of advanced machine learning algorithm.

7.3 Materials and Methodology

7.3.1 Study Area

Delhi, India's capital territory (Wikipedia, 2019), is a massive metropolitan area in the country's north, with a population of 18.6 million (2017) and an area of 1,484 km^2 and lies on the geographical coordinates of 28.7041° N, 77.1025° E. Delhi has a varied climate with hot summers to cold winters to heavy rainfall. Hence, pollution level is also varied in different seasons.

7.3.2 Data Collection

Air quality data of several air pollutants and meteorological parameters from January 2016 to March 2018 were collected from the CPCB monitoring station. Finer matter PM_{10}, $PM_{2.5}$, sulfur dioxide (SO_2), nitrogen dioxide (NO_2), and carbon dioxide (CO_2) were collected at an interval of 4 hours for four major districts of Delhi: Anand Vihar, situated in east Delhi; Punjabi Bagh, situated in west Delhi; Mandir Marg, situated in central Delhi; and RK Puram, situated in south Delhi. We have selected those meteorological variables that would affect air pollutant concentrations, including atmospheric temperature, relative humidity (RH), and WS. Pollutants are measured in microgram per cubic meter ($\mu g/m^3$), except CO, which is measured in milligram per cubic meter (mg/m^3). WS is measured in meter per second (m/s), wind direction (WD) measured in degree from the north, temperature measured in degree Celsius (°C), RH measured in percentage (%), and rainfall measured in millimeter per hour (mm/h).

7.3.3 Data Preprocessing

Column of date was divided into different columns of date and time according to date and time format to make our analysis easier. However, data collected contained missing values for various pollutants as well as meteorological parameters. For initial preprocessing of the data collected, we replaced the missing values of numeric attributes by their mean month value (Figure 7.1).

7.3.4 Analysis

Using the R programming language software (R Development Core Team) and its package openair (Carslaw and Ropkins, 2012), the data analysis is done. Several methods and equations are used for determination of the AQI (R Development Core Team) in different countries. AQI can be calculated from the concentration of different pollutants using the following formula (Anderson et al., 2016):

$$AQI = \left[\frac{\begin{array}{l} \text{concentration}\,(PM_{10})/\text{standard}\,(PM_{10}) + \text{concentration}\,(PM_{2.5})/\text{standard}\,(PM_{2.5}) \\ + \text{concentration}\,(SO_2)/\text{standard}\,(SO_2) + \text{concentration}\,(NO_2)/\text{standard}\,(NO_2) \\ + \text{concentration}\,(CO)/\text{standard}\,(CO) \end{array}}{5} \right]$$

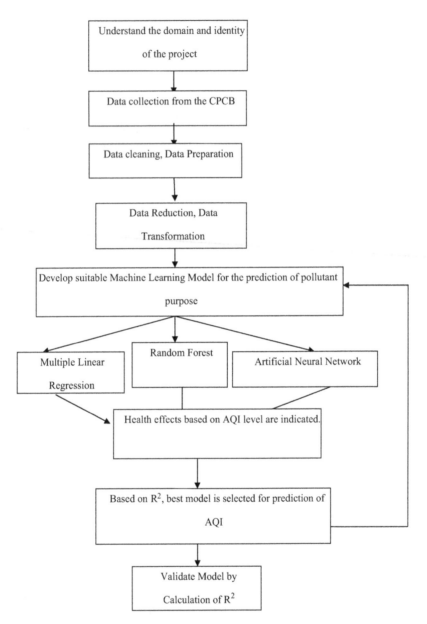

FIGURE 7.1
Flowchart of the proposed methodology.

7.4 Machine Learning Techniques Used

For doing the analysis on air pollution and predicting future, AQI comparative study of the following techniques was done: (1) multiple linear regression (MLR), (2) ANN, and (3) random forest. These three techniques were chosen due to the variation in their methodology in predicting data.

7.4.1 Multiple Linear Regression

Regression techniques are used to study the relationships between different variables that are independent as well as dependent. When there are more than one independent variable, analysis is done using multiple linear regression. By fitting a linear relationship to the given data, Multiple Linear Regression makes a model to establish a relationship between independent and dependent variables. Multiple linear regression models are trained based on existing measurements and are used to predict future concentrations of air pollutants in the future according to the corresponding meteorological variables (Zhang and Ding, 2017).

The equation is as follows:

$$Z = A + B_1X_1 + B_2X_2 + B_3X_3 + B_4X_4 + Q \tag{7.1}$$

where A symbolizes the constant of regression and B symbolizes the coefficient of regression. Using the least error square method, the values of coefficients and constants are calculated. Unit of measurement R^2 (root mean square error (RMSE)) is used to compare the results. Less the value of R^2, the more appropriate it is.

$$R^2 = 1 - \left(SS_{res} \div SS_{total}\right) \tag{7.2}$$

Value of R^2 is 1 if each and every observation of the data lie on the line fitted between independent and dependent variables. The value of R^2 is 0 when no relationship is found in between the two types of variables and none of them fall on the fitted line.

Values of R^2 that have negligible values have been eliminated, since no relationship between independent and dependent variables were found. Eliminating values also helps us in analyzing the regression more efficiently. Since one pollutant had a significant correlation with more than one meteorological factor, Multiple Linear Regression analysis has been used in which major contributing pollutants like particulate matter PM_{10} and $PM_{2.5}$ and various gases such as CO, NO_2, and SO_2 were treated as dependent variables, while previous day's pollutant concentration and meteorological parameters, such as direction of wind and its speed, were treated as individual variables.

The observed regression equation for air pollutants is given by

$$PM_{10} = 137.58 + \left(-7.8 * \text{previous day value of AT}\right) + \left(-1.9 * \text{previous day value of RH}\right)$$
$$+ \left(-0.59 * \text{previous day value of WD}\right) + \left(57.4 * \text{previous day value of WS}\right) \tag{7.3}$$

From the earlier equation, it can be concluded that the concentration of PM_{10} was decreased with a small increase of temperature, RH, and WD , and with the increase of speed of wind, it increased.

$$R^2 = 0.48$$

$$NO_2 = 102.96 + \left(4.9 * \text{previous day value of AT}\right) + \left(-1.3 * \text{previous day value of RH}\right)$$
$$+ \left(-1.42 * \text{previous day value of WD}\right) + \left(-7.04 * \text{previous day value of WS}\right) \tag{7.4}$$

$$R^2 = 0.77$$

This equation tells us that with a slight increase in atmospheric temperature, the concentration of NO_2 increases. It starts to decrease with a slight increase in concentration of humidity, speed of wind, and its direction. From the regression model, it could be seen that there is a good significant relationship between values predicted from model and experimental values.

7.4.2 Random Forest

Various combinations of tree predictors make a random forest. These random trees depend on random values of each independent variable. Strength of the individual trees and the correlation factor determines the generalization error of the tree. In this model, several trees are built on the dataset. Through the method of averaging, many small trees so formed are combined to make a final result tree. To construct a random tree, three choices need to be fulfilled. These are (i) to split the leaves, a method needs to be chosen, (ii) define the type of predictor variable used, and (iii) to inject randomness into the tree what method is to be chosen (Denil et al., 2014).

7.4.3 Artificial Neural Network

ANN can be defined as a computational network based on biological networks. The aim is to duplicate the functionality of actual brain. The nodes in neural network can be considered as neurons for transferring the information. A neuron receives input through its dendrites, processes the information, and transfers it if the output signal is above the electrical threshold to the dendrite of the new neuron. A neuron can take multiple inputs, but each time it is assigned a unique weight that is dependent on the strength of input message. Activation function is applied to give an output signal. The architecture of neural networks consists of nodes that generate a signal or remain silent as per a sigmoid activation function in most cases (Kang et al., 2018). It is used in various applications like prediction of stock markets, for climate control, for medicinal purposes, etc. We have used neural net package in R to train our model for the prediction of AQI. We first normalized our data using min–max normalization technique to scale our data between 0 and 1. Data was divided into 70–30 ratio for training and testing for maximum efficiency.

7.4.4 Relationship between Pollutants and Meteorological Factor

With reference to Table 7.4, an input layer was selected for each pollutant to build the ANN model. Only those meteorological parameters that had positive correlation with the corresponding pollutant were selected. For example, for predicting the next-day concentration level for $PM_{2.5}$, RH and WD were selected along with previous-day concentration level for $PM_{2.5}$.

A four-layer ANN model was built for each pollutant (ANN model for $PM_{2.5}$ is given later). The input layer for $PM_{2.5}$ contained three neurons, including meteorological parameters that are RH, WD, and PD_$PM_{2.5}$ (previous-day value). Weights to the neurons and the

TABLE 7.4

Correlation (r) between Daily Average Pollutants and Daily Average Meteorological Parameters

Pollutants	Atmospheric Temperature (AT)	RH	WS	WD
PM_{10}	−0.1575122	−0.06671861	0.01900569	0.0694724
$PM_{2.5}$	−0.3028522	0.09167271	−0.0722094	0.05758892
NO_2	−0.1114934	−0.1000005	0.00013236	0.03227619
SO_2	0.01312308	−0.1744609	0.02793046	0.001219993
CO	0.2760514	0.1310469	−0.0175773	0.004771014

number of hidden layers were chosen to maximize the efficiency of the neural network. The output layer contained only one variable, i.e., the target variable $PM_{2.5}$. For further analysis and to check the efficiency of the model, the values were denormalized. RMSE was chosen as the performance metric.

Similar models were built for each pollutant to predict their concentration level (Figures 7.2 and 7.3).

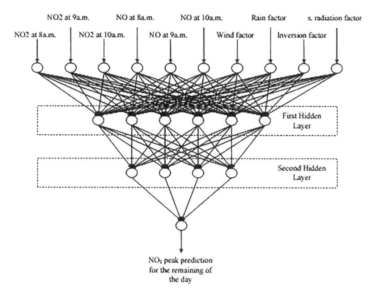

FIGURE 7.2
ANN model for air quality.

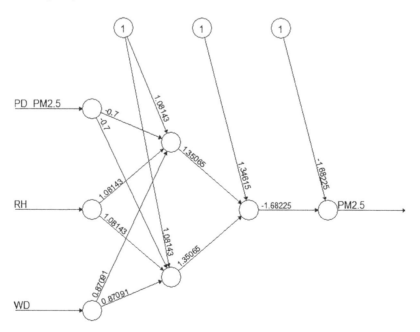

FIGURE 7.3
ANN outcome for pollutant's prediction. The RMSE was used to check the performance and error rate for the model.

7.4.5 Predicting AQI Using ANN Model

AQI is a number used to analyze the quality of air on any specific day. It basically tells you how clean the air is. Since the ANN for predicting the concentration of next-day pollutants gave comparatively less error as multiple liner regression, ANN-predicted values were selected as the input layer for the prediction of AQI (Spellman, 1999).

A four-layer ANN model was built for each pollutant (ANN model for AQI is given later). AQI is found to be dependent on all the concentration levels of pollutant. So, the input layer of the model consisted of five neurons, including the pollutants $PM_{2.5}$, PM_{10}, CO, NO_2, and SO_2. Weights to the neurons and the number of hidden layers were chosen to maximize the efficiency of neural network. The output layer contained only one variable, i.e., the target variable AQI. The values were then denormalized so that it can be used for further analysis and to check the performance of the model (Figure 7.4).

Exposure to pollutants such as particulate matter and sulfur dioxide has been associated with many types of respiratory and cardiovascular diseases. The predicted levels of pollutants have hazardous impacts on human health, as shown in the earlier table. AQI is divided into ranges, in which each range provides a number from level 0 to level 500 to show the level of health risk associated with air quality. Respiratory diseases have a higher probability of occurrence when the concentration level of $PM_{2.5}$ and PM_{10} are higher, as it is a major contributing factor. Studies have shown that skin diseases are more likely to occur when the concentration levels of NO_2 and SO_2 are higher (Table 7.5).

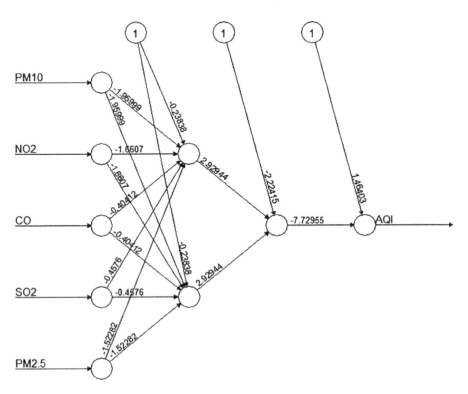

Error: 0.15746   Steps: 4010

FIGURE 7.4
Final outcome of AQI being predicted.

TABLE 7.5

Associated Health Impacts with the Level of AQI

AQI	Associated Health Impacts
Good (0–50)	Very little impact
Satisfactory (51–100)	Low-immunity people might face breathing problems
Moderately polluted (101–200)	Breathing-related illness to young children and adults who have various types of heart and lung diseases
Poor (201–300)	On extended exposure, it causes slight pain in breathing to those who have heart disease
Very poor (301–400)	Respiratory problems to people on extended exposure, mainly by indulging more in outdoor activities
Severe (401–500)	Adverse health impacts on healthy people as well.

7.5 Data Visualization

7.5.1 Correlation Plot

The correlation plot shows the correlation of different air pollutant concentrations and respective meteorological parameters. Three unique methods by shape, color, and values are used to depict the correlation (Figure 7.5).

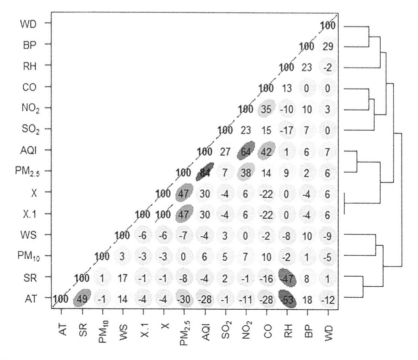

FIGURE 7.5
Correlation between pollutants and meteorological parameters.

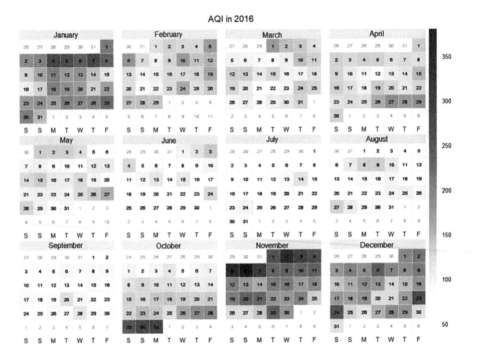

FIGURE 7.6
Calendar plot for 2016.

7.5.2 Calendar Plot

This plot is effective in analyzing pollutant concentration for a particular month. Dark color shade signifies that the concentration of pollutant is higher for that day. From the plot, it can be observed that colder months have higher AQI means more polluted air due to formation of smog. Diwali months of October and November have a higher concentration of pollutants (Figure 7.6).

7.5.3 Normalized Line Plot

The time Variation() function gives the variation of various pollutant concentrations by hours and days of the week (Figures 7.7 and 7.8).

7.6 Results

The chosen dataset was trained using three models, namely Multiple Liner Regression, random forest, and ANN, on a daily data chosen from January 2016 to March 2018. The forecasted values of pollutants were measured with the actual ones. The respective values of R and R^2 are shown in Table 7.6. The statistical analysis of the models, as shown in the table, reveals that since ANN has least R^2, it is more efficient than other models for the prediction. Moreover, since R^2 of ANN model is in the acceptable range, the model is best suited for AQI prediction and can be used for real-time analysis.

Table 7.6 gives the conclusion of the results.

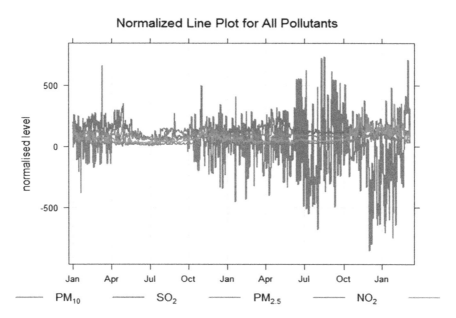

FIGURE 7.7
This graph shows the normalized line plot for all pollutants. The graph shows the amount of variation from the normal level of these pollutants.

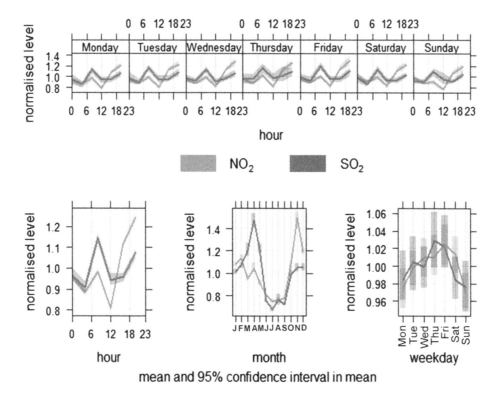

mean and 95% confidence interval in mean

FIGURE 7.8
The variations of pollutants in hour, month, and weekday are shown.

TABLE 7.6

Errors in Different Models of Machine Learning

S. No.	Model	R	R^2
1.	Multiple linear regression	0.6928	0.48
2.	ANN	0.7937	0.63
3.	Random Forest	0.7141	0.51

7.7 Novelty

In this chapter, we analyzed air quality and predicted the same. Novelty lies at the point where we have compared the three models, namely regression analysis, random forest, and ANN, based on the value of R^2. Forecasted value of pollutants has been analyzed by all three methods. Based on comparison, finding out which model is best is then used for predicting AQI. Moreover, associated health impacts of AQI are indicated.

7.8 Conclusions

From the study, the relationship between different air quality predictors and various meteorological parameters could be established. They were analyzed using three models, i.e., regression analysis, random forest, and ANN. The maximum concentration of pollutants was observed during the peak hours in the morning as well as during the night, mainly in the winter months (December, January), because of the formation of smog. Increased vehicular emissions were the main contributors to air pollution. Meteorological parameters simulated an indicative role in affecting the quality level of air.

A statistical model was developed for the prediction of the next day's air pollutant concentrations with respect to relevant meteorological parameters (seeing the maximum correlation factor) and preceding day's pollution level. The correlation factor between preceding day's PM_{10}, NO_2, and SO_2 pollutant and true PM_{10}, NO_2, and SO_2 pollutant levels were measured to be 0.77, 0.59, and 0.61, respectively. Temperature, humidity, and WS showed good correlation between pollutants like $PM_{2.5}$ and NO_2. Hence, it can be concluded that daily polluting concentrations are not only affected by different meteorological variables but also with the past day's pollutant concentration levels as well. The neural network model for the estimation of air pollution level is sufficiently effective than the regression technique and random forest.

References

Ahmad, S. S., Biiker, P., Emberson, L., & Shabbir, R. (2011). Monitoring nitrogen dioxide levels in urban areas in Rawalpindi, Pakistan. *Water, Air, & Soil Pollution, 220*(1–4), 141–150.

Andersson, C., Langner, J., & Bergstroumm, R. (2007). Interannual variation and trends in air pollution over Europe due to climate variability during 1958–2001 simulated with a regional CTM coupled to the ERA40 reanalysis. *Tellus B: Chemical and Physical Meteorology, 59*(1), 77–98.

Carslaw, D. C., & Ropkins, K. (2012). Openair—an R package for air quality data analysis. *Environmental Modelling & Software, 27*, 52–61.

Corani, G., & Scanagatta, M. (2016). Air pollution prediction via multi-label classification. *Environmental Modelling & Software, 80*, 259–264.

Denil, M., Matheson, D., & De Freitas, N. (2014, January). Narrowing the gap: Random forests in theory and in practice. In *International Conference on Machine Learning* (pp. 665–673). Beijing, China.

Dockery, D. W., Pope, C. A., Xu, X., Spengler, J. D., Ware, J. H., Fay, M. E., ... & Speizer, F. E. (1993). An association between air pollution and mortality in six US cities. *New England Journal of Medicine, 329*(24), 1753–1759.

Dueñas, C., Fernández, M. C., Cañete, S., Carretero, J., & Liger, E. (2002). Assessment of ozone variations and meteorological effects in an urban area in the Mediterranean Coast. *Science of the Total Environment, 299*(1–3), 97–113.

Elminir, H. K. (2005). Dependence of urban air pollutants on meteorology. *Science of the Total Environment, 350*(1–3), 225–237.

Environmental Fact Sheet, New Hampshire Department of Environmental Sciences, 2012.

Gupta, K. (2016). Mining of air pollution and visualization. *International Journal of Computer Trends and Technology (IJCTT), 35*(4), 193–197.

Gupta, A. K., Karar, K., Ayoob, S., & John, K. (2008). Spatio-temporal characteristics of gaseous and particulate pollutants in an urban region of Kolkata, India. *Atmospheric Research, 87*(2), 103–115.

Hargreaves, P. R., Leidi, A., Grubb, H. J., Howe, M. T., & Mugglestone, M. A. (2000). Local and seasonal variations in atmospheric nitrogen dioxide levels at Rothamsted, UK, and relationships with meteorological conditions. *Atmospheric Environment, 34*(6), 843–853.

Kang, G. K., Gao, J. Z., Chiao, S., Lu, S., & Xie, G. (2018). Air quality prediction: Big data and machine learning approaches. *International Journal of Environmental Science and Development, 9*(1), 8–16.

Katsoulis, B. D. (1996). The relationship between synoptic, mesoscale and microscale meteorological parameters during poor air quality events in Athens, Greece. *Science of the Total Environment, 181*(1), 13–24.

Kumar, S. S., & Sharma, K. (2016). Ambient air quality status of Jaipur city, Rajasthan, India. *International Research Journal of Environmental Sciences, 5*, 43–48.

National Air Quality Index, CPCB Report, 2017.

Ocak, S., & Turalioglu, F. S. (2008). Effect of meteorology on the atmospheric concentrations of traffic-related pollutants in Erzurum, Turkey. *Journal of International Environmental Application & Science, 3*(5), 325–335.

Ocak, S., & Turalioglu, F. S. (2010). Relationship between air pollutants and some meteorological parameters in Erzurum, Turkey. In Dincer, I., Hepbasli, A., Midilli, A., Karakoc, T. (eds) *Global Warming* (pp. 485–499). Springer, Boston, MA.

Spellman, G. (1999). An application of artificial neural networks to the prediction of surface ozone concentrations in the United Kingdom. *Applied Geography, 19*(2), 123–136.

Srinivas, J., & Purushotham, A. V. (2013). Determination of air quality index status in industrial areas of Visakhapatnam, India. *Research Journal of Engineering Sciences, 2*(6), 13–24.

Team, R. C. R Development Core Team (2012) *R: A Language and Environment for Statistical Computing.* R Foundation for Statistical Computing. Vienna, Austria.

Wikipedia. (2019). Delhi. Retrieved from wikipedia.org/wiki/Delhi. Last modified June 23, 2019.

Xi, X., Wei, Z., Xiaoguang, R., Yijie, W., Xinxin, B., Wenjun, Y., & Jin, D. (2015, November). A comprehensive evaluation of air pollution prediction improvement by a machine learning method. In *2015 IEEE International Conference on Service Operations and Logistics, and Informatics (SOLI)* (pp. 176–181). IEEE, Hammamet, Tunisia.

Zhang, J., & Ding, W. (2017). Prediction of air pollutants concentration based on an Extreme Learning Machine: The case of Hong Kong. *International Journal of Environmental Research and Public Health, 14*(2), 114.

8

Brain Tumor Detection and Classification in MRI: Technique for Smart Healthcare Adaptation

Asmita Dixit and Aparajita Nanda
Jaypee Institute of Information Technology

CONTENTS

8.1 Introduction

Brain tumor is termed as an unnatural cell growth and division of brain tissues, which may be cancerous or noncancerous. Yet, these tumor cells, being uncommon, are very fatal in nature. Hence, early detection leads to a greater probability to cure completely. These advancements in medical technology promote suitable cost-effective development in smart healthcare. Computed tomography, magnetic resonance imaging (MRI), single-photon emission computed tomography, magnetic resonance spectroscopy, and positron emission tomography work upon extracting different parameters (location, size, shape) of tumor cells. However, wide availability of MRI tags it as a standard technique. MRI is harmless and is able to differentiate the neural architecture of brain. MRI technique uses radio wave signal with a very strong magnetic field that intensifies the target region to produce its intrinsic structure. At the time of image acquisition, the levels of excitation are tuned to result in different MRI sequences. MRI technique uses radio wave signal with a very strong magnetic field that intensifies the target region to produce its intrinsic structure. At the time of image acquisition, the levels of excitations are tuned to result in different MRI sequences. MRI with different modalities yields different levels of contrast images, which further depicts structural information. Basically, four basic MRI modalities such as T1-weighted MRI, T2-weighted MRI, T1-weighted MRI with gadolinium contrast enhancement (T1-Gd), and fluid attenuated inversion recovery (FLAIR) are taken into consideration for brain tumor classification. T1 MRI differentiates normal tissues; T2 images depict the tumor region that produces a bright effect on the image. T1-Gd easily differentiates boundary of region of interest, whereas FLAIR images help to distinguish the edema region by suppressing the water molecule. Figure 8.1 describes the four modalities of MRI (Figure 8.2).

Every tumor cell development is different and varies from patient to patient. Tumor is grouped into primary and secondary categories. The tumor cells that tend to arise inside brain tissue and remain there are categorized as primary. More than 120 different categories of brain and nervous structure tumors prevail, ranging from being less aggressive, benign to more aggressive, harmful, malignant (Işin et al., 2016). The rate of growth of tumor cells can be depicted through different grades, as described in Table 8.1. The other category of tumor cells that generate somewhere else in the body and make a progress toward the brain is being metastatic. Malignant tumor has seven broad types: gliomas, medulloblastoma, metastatic brain tumors, brain stem glioma, meningioma, pituitary tumors, and lymphoma.

Technically, classification of brain tumor cells in MRI is judged by a step-by-step approach like preprocessing, segmentation, and classification. It contributes in collecting

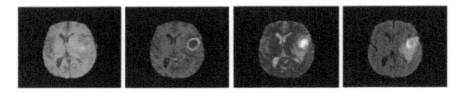

FIGURE 8.1
MRI modalities starting from left: T1, T1-Gd, T2, and FLAIR. (Reprinted with permission: Işin et al., 2016.)

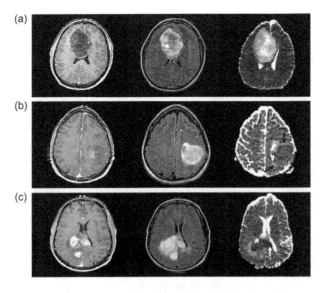

FIGURE 8.2
Different tumor stages: grade II: (a), grade III: (b), and grade IV: (c). The *first column* represents axial postcontrast T1-weighted images, the *second column* presents FLAIR images, and the *third column* projects apparent diffusion coefficient and depicts models of three nonidentical grades of astrocytoma.

TABLE 8.1

Characterizing Attributes of Different Grades

Grade I	Slow in growth, tumor cells more or less look like normal brain cells
Grade II	Have chance to expand to nearest tissues, malignant on expansion
Grade III	Shows abnormalities and may occur repeatedly; rapid tendency of dividing and spreading
Grade IV	Most abnormal with maximum spreading speed

neighborhood information about the variations in tumor cells' size, shape, and other intensity values (Liao et al., 2010), and this may include histogram equalization and median filtering. Volumetric entropy of the brain tumor images is determined as the entropy of the brain provides an informative tool to study brain functions and states (Wang et al., 2014). Similarly, segmentation is performed by integrating the local and global properties of an image (Wang, 2017). Image segmentation algorithms are preferred to be performed on grayscale images, as the existing difficulties of gray scale images is less than that of color images. Two-dimensional format of an image provides easier detection of edges, textures, brightness, contrast, edges, shape, contour, textures, shadows, etc. Also, through grayscale images, measurement of intensity of light in images is easily possible (Salamh, 2017). Classifier classifies the tumor cells accurately with less computational speed, which may include support vector machine (SVM), AdaBoost, random forest, etc. With faster computational speed, the complexity of code is reduced, and a complex algorithm can be easily implemented, since the image is converted from a three-dimensional format to a two-dimensional format.

The following are most challenges in classifying tumor cells by brain MRI:

a. The noise removal in the preprocessing step is generated by the fluctuations of magnetic field (Mohan & Subashini, 2018)

b. Bias field correction of the images having low-frequency need to be corrected before performing segmentation or classification (Juntu et al., 2005)

c. Selection of the best classifier for accurate results with less computational speed (Lefkovits et al., 2017)

d. Edge detection of active contours (Unde et al., 2012)

e. Partial volume effect correction to improve calculation

f. Collection of datasets from several MRI machines, resulting in different categories of noise, problems in tumor alignment, and image registration.

Thus, a healthcare adaptation system needs to be formulated to overcome all these challenges. It is observed that most of the problems must be resolved at the preprocessing step itself before the image is fed into a classifier for classification of tumor as normal or abnormal tissues. Preprocessing may include removal of background, skull, and any region that is not part of the tumor mask, and a simple brain surface extractor algorithm can be applied (Mohan & Subashini, 2018). Many approaches on segmentation and feature extraction are applied so that result analysis leads to better findings and early detection. The innovations in the field of medical science are motivating engineering technology to develop automated machinery for early detection of cancer cells. Recent trends concentrate on the growth of completely automatic tumor segmentation techniques using deep neural network (Havaei et al., 2017). Most popular 2013 BRATS datasets (Havaei et al., 2017) are available for MRI brain tumor classification.

8.2 Related Work

Classification of brain tumor cells as benign and malignant involves various traditional and recent approaches. The related work is broadly categorized into three areas: feature-based, segmentation-based, and classifier-based approaches.

Nayak et al. (2016) perform successful segmentation and detection of cancer cells, obtaining 99.53% and 100% accuracy with the use of algorithm Discrete Wavelet Transform + probabilistic principal component analysis + AdaBoost Random Forest. The use of probabilistic principal component analysis enables computation of low-dimensional depiction of data with a proportionate probability distribution of large dimensional data. AdaBoost for classification is simple and robust to noise and outliers and also measures missing data. Dataset-66 and Dataset-160 obtain 100% accuracy. Dataset 66 consists of seven types of diseases of both normal and abnormal brains: glioma, meningioma, Alzheimer's, Pick's, sarcoma, and Huntington's disease (Mohan & Subashini, 2018). Dataset-255 obtains 99.53% accuracy, including chronic subdural hematoma, cerebral toxoplasmosis, herpes encephalitis, and multiple sclerosis (Nayak et al., 2016). Similarly, Işin et al. (2016) describe a study of traditional methods of segmentation as well as the recent trends of deep learning using BRATS dataset. Their approach focuses on the difference between semiautomatic and automatic methods. Automatic segmentation is discriminative and generative as well. Ibrahim et al. (2018) implemented segmentation by Fractional Wright Energy Function (FWF) as an energy depreciation parameter to substitute the recognized gradient-descent technique. The proposed FWF detects the borderline of an object by measuring the internal and external properties of the contour. The objective being differentiation between segmented images being processed and ground truth by a dataset of statistical measures of accuracy, including true positive (TP), true negative (TN), false positive (FP), and false negative (FN). They have validated a formulated approach on BRATS 2013 (Menze et al., 2015) image dataset and achieved 94.8% ± 4.7% as an average sensitivity score for tumor segmentation.

Shree and Kumar (2018) include noise removal methods, gray-level co-occurrence matrix (GLCM), and feature extraction. Also, DWT-based region growing segmentation is used to decrease the complexity and enhance the performance. Followed by morphological filtering, the noise probability of being developed after segmentation is eradicated. The probabilistic neural network classifier trains and tests the performance accuracy in tumor cell detection by brain MRI. Results after experiment attain nearly 100% accuracy in depicting normal and abnormal tissues from brain MRI, indicating the effectiveness of the suggested technique. The suggested methodology involves utilization of brain MRI of pixel size 256×256 and 512×512. It is transformed into gray scale for further improvement. Menze et al. (2015) suggested a generative brain tumor segmentation model including 20 different segmentation algorithms. These algorithms are applied to a 65 multicontrast MRI, including lower- and higher-grade glioma images. An accuracy of 74%–85% is achieved on a BRATS image dataset. Unde et al. (2018) termed a new way of edge detection for agile contours on the basis of local adaptive threshold technique through fluctuating energy minimization for contour stoppage at a required object borderline. It is able to perform tumor segmentation using thresholding segmentation algorithm. Performance analysis is measured on 512×512 size of image of 16-bit Digital Imaging and Communications in Medicines (DICOM) (Shree & Kumar, 2018). Their approach clearly defines the boundaries on images, without any loss of changing curve at object edge and correct segmentation. Comparison of accuracy with various methodologies is displayed in Table 8.2.

TABLE 8.2

Accuracy Comparison

Approach	Accuracy (%)
DWT	95 (Shree & Kumar, 2018)
Generative model	82 (Mohan & Subashini, 2018)
Clustering	80 (Wang et al., 2014)
AdaBoost with random forest	99.53 (Nayak et al., 2016)
Fractional wright function	98.5 (Ibrahim et al., 2018)

8.3 Basic Methodology

The basic methodology of brain tumor MRI classification follows subsequent procedures such as preprocessing, segmentation, feature extraction, and classification. The detail of each step is described in the following subsections. The overview of classic techniques is described in Figure 8.3.

8.3.1 Preprocessing

Preprocessing is required for quality enhancement of input MRI. Preprocessing contributes in enhancing aspects like signal-to-noise ratio (Bahadure et al., 2017) and improves visual appearance. A large variety of preprocessing methods, such as homogeneity correction, registration, noise reduction, skullstripping, and intensity normalization, are performed in different circumstances (Mohan & Subashini, 2018). In preprocessing steps, MRI bias-field correction, image registration, and nonbrain tissue removal are the most important requisites. Algorithms like simplified multiplicative model, surface fitting method, and low-pass filtering methods are applied with automatic segmentation (Haralick et al., 1973). Similarly, edge refinement, hole-loop clearance, and contrast adjustment are used to separate the foreground image from the background. Further, morphological operation (dilation, erosion) processes are used for reducing the noise in the preprocessing step (Liao et al., 2010). It has been observed that median filter is preferred over linear filter for edge-based noise removal (George & Karnan, 2012). The other important step in preprocessing is intensity normalization, histogram equalization, and histogram normalization. Similarly, Wiener filter is used for noise removal and SPM5 method is used to differentiate brain tissue pixels with nonbrain pixels. Besides these approaches, image registration is employed in preprocessing step for spatial alignment of multiple images captured at different times and is computed through affine transformation (Zitova & Flusser, 2003).

8.3.2 Segmentation

Segmentation process is categorized into manual, semiautomatic, and completely automatic (Mohan & Subashini, 2018). Segmentation performed manually is a

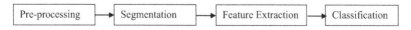

FIGURE 8.3
Overview of basic techniques for brain tumor classification.

time-consuming process, but it gives accurate results and is done by an expert radiologist. Manual segmentation is processed by a tool named ITKSNAP, which displays
three-dimensional images in sagittal, coronal, and axial two-dimensional orthogonal
view (Mohan & Subashini, 2018). Semiautomatic segmentation involves both user interaction and computing for defining Region Of Interest, which is used for further processing of detecting edge using region-based active contours and level set approach (Liu
et al., 2014). Traditional segmentation techniques like region-growing algorithm, edge
detection, active contours, thresholding segmentation, histogram-based segmentation,
model-based segmentation, and semiautomatic segmentation still prevails (Mohan &
Subashini, 2018). Automatic segmentation is done to avoid human intervention and
obtain accuracy. Algorithms such as Markov random field model use atlas-based segmentation (Lefkovits et al., 2016). Another discriminative model approach is random
forest classifier (Bauer et al., 2010). Automatic segmentation is also done by K-nearest
neighbor (K-NN) classifier, artificial neural networks (ANNs), Bayesian classifier, and
clustering algorithms, including K-means clustering and fuzzy C-means clustering
(Haralick et al., 1973). Classification-based segmentation includes SVM, neural networks,
and self-organizing map (Zacharaki et al., 2009). Tumor segmentation plays a crucial
role in analysis of image as the process improves step-by-step interpretation of isolated
regions, which collectively form a comprehensive image. Segmentation also involves
methods of region enhancement, deformation of templates, border-lining, and other pattern recurrence recognition techniques of pixel clustering.

8.3.3 Feature Extraction

Feature extraction represents an image into a group of features and helps to find the distinct features present in tumor location (Mohan & Subashini, 2018). It focuses on contrast,
homogeneity, correlation, entropy, shape, energy, texture, color, and intensity (Bauer et al.,
2010). GLCM (Nayak et al., 2016), Gabor features, wavelet transformation, DWT, probabilistic
neural network (Shree & Kumar, 2018), and spectral mixture analysis (Mohan & Subashini,
2018) are used for feature extraction. Haralick et al. (1973) introduces GLCM and texture
calculation, which are most widely implemented applications for image analysis. Similarly,
set methodology approach follows a two-segment protocol for feature extraction from
biomedical images. The first one being the depiction of gray-level matrices followed by
feature calculation based on GLCM (Bahadure et al., 2017). Feature extraction is a vital step
for which classification results are computed directly based on extracted features. Certain
feature extraction parameters for textural feature extraction are summarized as follows:

- Contrast: It measures pixel intensities and neighborhood of images, defined as

$$\text{Contrast} = \sum_{m=0}^{p-1} \sum_{n=0}^{q-1} (m-n)^2 f(m,n) \tag{8.1}$$

- Energy: Represents the range of repetitions of pixels defined as

$$\text{Energy} = \sqrt{\sum_{p=0}^{k-1} \sum_{q=0}^{j-1} f^2(p,q)} \tag{8.2}$$

- Entropy: Randomness present in textural image is defined as

$$\text{Entropy} = -\sum_{x=0}^{s-1}\sum_{y=0}^{t-1} f(x,y)\log_2 f(x,y)$$

(8.3)

- Homogeneity: Measures the quality of being homogeneous for finding whether the image is textured or nontextured defined as

$$\text{HOG} = \sum_{i,j=0}^{m-1} \frac{P_{ij}}{1+(i-j)^2}$$

(8.4)

8.3.4 Classification

After segmentation, classification is performed for analyzing and quantifying the abnormalities or tumor present in the brain MRI. Classification involves supervised methods like ANN, K-NN, SVM (Mohan & Subashini, 2018), etc. Similarly, self-organizing map and fuzzy C-means are the unsupervised classification techniques (Mohan & Subashini, 2018). The classification method relies on a vast dataset of brain scan images. A highly trained classifier provides correct classification results by identifying type of tumor, i.e., benign or malignant. Recently, automatic classification methods such as Harmony Crow Search are introduced, which trains the classifier with multisupport vector neural network (Raju et al., 2018).

8.3.5 Deep Learning Methodology

Conventional methods depend on feature extraction, which is a vital step for classification. The better the feature extraction, better is the classification accuracy. Convolutional neural network is the emerging trend based on deep learning, which enables self-mining of features and learning from the datasets available. Recent evolution of deep learning methods (Işin et al., 2016) has gained widespread popularity and speeds up the process of learning from examples. Convolutional neural network follows a two-pathway layout extracting local and global (Havaei et al., 2017) details of the brain. Deep learning includes various hidden layers that are applicable for extracting details of data. Feed forward neural network (Rani & Vashisth, 2017) easily classifies different types of tumor grade. Deep learning-based approaches give comparatively faster and accurate results than do the traditional methods.

8.4 Datasets and Evaluation Criteria

A dataset comprises a large number of MRIs of human brain, which are captured from various cross-sectional views. The sample images in dataset represent various challenges like illumination variation, different contrast-level images, and irregular and unclear tumor boundary.

For each dataset, MRI scan imposes intensity biasness in different portions of images due to the drastic variations in parameters used in MRI acquisition device. Various widely accepted benchmark datasets such as BRATS dataset (Işin et al., 2016) and DICOM dataset

TABLE 8.3

Dataset Descriptions

Modalities	Dataset Description	Database
T1w	20 normals_T1 8-bit (60 patients, positionally normalized 16-bit slices, 256 ×256	NeuroImaging informatics Tools and Resources Clearinghouse
T1w	20 patients segmented with brain images	NITRC
T1-weighted contrast-enhanced images	233 patients, meningioma (708 slices), glioma (1,426 slices), and pituitary tumor (930 slices)	figshare
T2w axial	256 × 256, 66 patients	Harvard

(Shree & Kumar, 2018) with multimodal images (T1 weighted, T2 weighted, FLAIR) are available to validate the tumor classification accuracy. The details of datasets are briefly stated in Table 8.3.

BRATS dataset is designed for automatic segmentation of brain tumor, and presently, it is also used for comparing the performance of different tumor segmentation methods. Various versions of BRATS datasets are available. BRATS 2015 comprises 274 multimodality MRI of patients with high- and low-modality gliomas. It also includes ground truth segmentations for evaluation, and 110 MRIs are present with unidentified grades, which are used for the test. Another version of BRATS dataset is MICCAI BRATS 2015, available by virtual skeleton database. The dataset includes T1-weighted, contrast-improved T1 MRIs, also T2-weighted and T2-FLAIR MRIs. Similarly the other available open-source dataset for analysis would be the DICOM dataset collected from Shree and Kumar (2018). The dataset includes sample images of almost all glioma modalities of five patients. Dataset comprises 25 images, out of which 18 are infected.

8.4.1 Evaluation Criteria

The performance is usually verified using confusion matrix on the basis of sensitivity, specificity, and accuracy. Results of the prediction are drawn from the computation of TP, FP, TN, and FN (Bahadure et al., 2017). Normal images are categorized as TN, and tumor images are categorized as TP (Chinnu, 2015). The criterions are defined as follows:

- Sensitivity: It calculates the amount of exact positive predictions for tumor detection distinguished by the complete number of positives. It can also be termed as recall (REC) or TP rate.

$$\text{Sensitivity} = \frac{TP}{TP + FN} \tag{8.5}$$

- Specificity: It calculates the number of correct negative predictions, i.e., absence of tumor upon total negative predictions.

$$\text{Specificity} = \frac{TN}{TN + FP} \tag{8.6}$$

- Accuracy: It calculates the count of exact predictions divided by the total number of datasets, i.e., correct classification of MRIs.

$$\text{Accuracy} = \frac{TP + TN}{TP + TN + FP + FN} \tag{8.7}$$

8.5 Conclusion

MRI processing is greatly benefitted by the enhanced usage of machine learning and deep learning. A smart healthcare adaption system can be designed by combining all these crucial steps in a device that scans MRIs of the brain and classify, locate, or detect the tumor region. The early detection of the diseases helps to take steps to cure it. The available datasets on brain MRI with its ground truth easily validate the experiments over the sample images. It not only speeds up the diagnosis process but also is painless for patients. The only challenge is writing a comprehensive algorithm for combining classification and segmentation techniques, concluding a speedy reference from them for diagnosis.

References

Bahadure, N.B., Ray, A.K. and Thethi, H.P., (2017). Image analysis for MRI based brain tumor detection and feature extraction using biologically inspired BWT and SVM. *International Journal of Biomedical Imaging*, 2017, 12.

Bauer, S., Seiler, C., Bardyn, T., Buechler, P. and Reyes, M., (2010, August). Atlas-based segmentation of brain tumor images using a Markov random field-based tumor growth model and non-rigid registration. In *Annual International Conference of the IEEE Engineering in Medicine and Biology Society (EMBC), 2010* (pp. 4080–4083). IEEE.

Chinnu, A., (2015). MRI brain tumor classification using SVM and histogram based image segmentation. *International Journal of Computer Science and Information Technologies*, 6(2), 1505–1508.

George, E.B. and Karnan, M., (2012). MRI brain image enhancement using filtering techniques. *International Journal of Computer Science & Engineering Technology (IJCSET)*, 3, 2229–3345.

Haralick, R.M., Shanmugam, K. and Dinstein, I.H., (1973). Textural features for image classification. *IEEE Transactions on Systems, Man, and Cybernetics*, 3(6), 610–621.

Havaei, M., Davy, A., Warde-Farley, D., Biard, A., Courville, A., Bengio, Y., Pal, C., Jodoin, P.M. and Larochelle, H., (2017). Brain tumor segmentation with deep neural networks. *Medical Image Analysis*, 35, 18–31.

Ibrahim, R.W., Hasan, A.M. and Jalab, H.A., (2018). A new deformable model based on fractional wright energy function for tumor segmentation of volumetric brain MRI scans. *Computer Methods and Programs in Biomedicine*, 163, 21–28.

Işın, A., Direkoğlu, C. and Şah, M., (2016). Review of MRI-based brain tumor image segmentation using deep learning methods. *Procedia Computer Science*, 102, 317–324.

Juntu, J., Sijbers, J., Van Dyck, D. and Gielen, J., (2005). Bias field correction for MRI images. In Kurzyński, M., Puchała, E., Woźniak, M., Żołnierek, A. (eds.) *Computer Recognition Systems* (pp. 543–551). Springer, Berlin, Heidelberg.

Lefkovits, L., Lefkovits, S. and Vaida, M.F., (2016). Brain tumor segmentation based on random forest. *Memoirs of the Scientific Sections of the Romanian Academy*, 39(1), 83–93.

Lefkovits, L., Lefkovits, S., Vaida, M.F., Emerich, S. and Măluțan, R., (2017). Comparison of classifiers for brain tumor segmentation. In *International Conference on Advancements of Medicine and Health Care through Technology; 12th–15th October 2016*, Cluj-Napoca, Romania (pp. 195–200). Springer, Cham.

Liao, Z., Hu, S. and Chen, W., (2010). Determining neighbourhoods of image pixels automatically for adaptive image denoising using nonlinear time series analysis. *Mathematical Problems in Engineering*, 2010, 14.

Liu, J., Li, M., Wang, J., Wu, F., Liu, T. and Pan, Y., (2014). A survey of MRI-based brain tumor segmentation methods. *Tsinghua Science and Technology*, 19(6), 578–595.

Menze, B.H., Jakab, A., Bauer, S., Kalpathy-Cramer, J., Farahani, K., Kirby, J., Burren, Y., Porz, N., Slotboom, J., Wiest, R. and Lanczi, L., (2015). The multimodal brain tumor image segmentation benchmark (BRATS). *IEEE Transactions on Medical Imaging*, 34(10), 1993.

Mohan, G. and Subashini, M.M., (2018). MRI based medical image analysis: Survey on brain tumor grade classification. *Biomedical Signal Processing and Control*, 39, 139–161.

Nayak, D.R., Dash, R. and Majhi, B., (2016). Brain MR image classification using two-dimensional discrete wavelet transform and AdaBoost with random forests. *Neurocomputing*, 177, 188–197.

Raju, A.R., Suresh, P. and Rao, R.R., (2018). Bayesian HCS-based multi-SVNN: A classification approach for brain tumor segmentation and classification using Bayesian fuzzy clustering. *Biocybernetics and Biomedical Engineering*, 38, 646–660.

Rani, N. and Vashisth, S., (2017). Brain tumor detection and classification with feed forward backprop neural network. arXiv preprint arXiv:1706.06411.

Salamh, A.B.S., (2017) Investigation the effect of using gray level and RGB channels on brain tumor image.

Shree, N.V. and Kumar, T.N.R., (2018). Identification and classification of brain tumor MRI images with feature extraction using DWT and probabilistic neural network. *Brain informatics*, 5(1), 23–30.

Uden, L., Pérez, J., Herrera, F. and Rodrıguez, J., (2018) Advances in intelligent systems and computing: Preface. *Advances in Intelligent Systems and Computing*, 172.

Unde, A.S., Premprakash, V.A. and Sankaran, P., (2012, March). A novel edge detection approach on active contour for tumor segmentation. In *Students Conference on Engineering and Systems (SCES), 2012* (pp. 1–6). IEEE.

Wang, Z., (2017). Image segmentation by combining the global and local properties. *Expert Systems with Applications*, 87, 30–40.

Wang, Z., Li, Y., Childress, A.R. and Detre, J.A., (2014). Brain entropy mapping using fMRI. *PLoSOne*, 9(3), e89948.

Zacharaki, E.I., Wang, S., Chawla, S., Soo Yoo, D., Wolf, R., Melhem, E.R. and Davatzikos, C., (2009). Classification of brain tumor type and grade using MRI texture and shape in a machine learning scheme. *Magnetic Resonance in Medicine*, 62(6), 1609–1618.

Zitova, B. and Flusser, J., (2003). Image registration methods: A survey. *Image and Vision Computing*, 21(11), 977–1000.

9

Deep Strategies in Computer-Assisted Diagnosis and Classification of Abnormalities in Medical Images

Ankit Vidyarthi
Jaypee Institute of Information Technology

Shilpa Gundagatti
Deewan Group of Institutions

Nisha Chaurasia
Jaypee Institute of Information Technology

CONTENTS

9.1 Introduction

Digital diagnosis based on computer-assisted technologies is a procedure that provides another objective consultation to radiologist beyond their knowledge for the assistance of medical image in terms of proper diagnosis and their interpretation. In recent studies, the digital diagnosis became a handful implementation in various imaging forms, such as magnetic resonance imaging (MRI), mammography, Computed Tomography (CT) scan, histopathology imaging, and ultrasound diagnostic. The incorporation of such intelligent systems into the diagnostic process improves the performance by reducing interobserver variation and providing the qualitative and quantitative support for clinical decisions such as malignancy prediction, arteries blockage, cancer prediction, and biopsy recommendations.

The conventional design of digital diagnosis for abnormality identification is often composed of several steps: feature extraction, feature selection, segmentation, prediction, and classification. These steps need to be separately fine-tuned and well addressed, which were later integrated together for the overall performance tuning. The art of extraction of discriminative features is of key concern, because it could potentially ease the latter steps of machine learning for accurate prediction. Nevertheless, the art of extraction of effective and informative features is problem-oriented and needs assistance from various external parameters, including clinical knowledge and radiological experience of image handling. Thus, the final decision of digital diagnosis has found full dependency on how well the proper related informative features were extracted, which were later used for machine learning followed by automatic prediction and analysis of medical images.

For the past several years, the impact of deep learning is found in almost every application field of machine learning. The layered network structure techniques potentially change the design paradigm of the machine learning framework that gives several advantages over the traditional network structure. The main advantages of deep network are classified into threefold: First, deep architecture learning can automatically unbox features from the training data, and hence, the effort of fetching features based on imaging characteristics can be significantly alleviated. Second, the feature selection process will be significantly simplified due to the feature interaction that can be exploited jointly within the internal deep architecture of a neural network. Third, the three-step processes of neural architecture, i.e., feature extraction, selection, and classification, can be self-optimized within a singular deep architecture. Thus, the inclusion of such a systematic architecture in machine learning model will tune the performance easily in a systematic fashion.

After gaining success of deep learning architecture in other real-world application, it becomes a style of choice for analyzing medical images. It provides exciting solutions with superior accuracy rate for medical imaging and is seen as a key method for future applications of radiology. In this chapter, the state-of-the-art deep learning architecture used for medical image analysis is presented. Next, the optimization techniques in deep architecture used for medical image processing are discussed. Later, several challenges of deep learning-based methods for medical imaging are presented.

9.2 Trends for Deep Architecture Learning

A deep neural network architecture is a hierarchical computation of multiple layers of neuron stacks. In literature, the trend of modification of neural architecture used for medical image analysis is seen from the past decade. Various types of deep learning algorithms that are in use for disease prediction are presented in Table 9.1. The table shows the various parameters of network architecture along with their strengths and limitations.

Among all the variants of deep learning architecture, the most widely used network for medical imaging is convolutional neural network (CNN) [7]. In literature, there exists several other deep layered variants of CNN as well which are used for medical image analysis for representation learning. In Ref. [8] and [9], authors provide a thorough review of techniques that were used for clustering of image patches, dictionary approaches, and many more. Based on the submitted manuscripts of digital repositories, there are several tasks of medical image in which deep architecture is used, which is shown in Figure 9.1.

These variant of deep architectures are used for almost every medical imaging modality, i.e., from MRI to pathological imaging. Based on the medical imaging modalities in the literature of digital repositories such as Institute of Electrical and Electronics Engineers (IEEE), Springer, Science Direct, and other state-of-the-art sources, machine-assisted diagnosis and prediction using deep learning architecture are presented in Figure 9.2.

These imaging modalities, when given input to deep layers, will resolve the requirement of manual feature extraction, which requires a higher degree of precision and domain

TABLE 9.1

Evolution of Deep Learning Architecture in Medical Image Analysis

Author	Network	Network Basics	Strength	Limitation
Igor [1]	Deep neural network	Complex nonlinear relationship	Simple architecture	Slow learning process
Fukushima [2]	CNN	Convolutional filter-based transformation	Fast model learning	Worked on labeled 2D data
Faustino [3]	Recurrent neural network	Time sequence learning architecture	Handles real-time data sequences	Gradient vanishing dependent
Shan [4]	Deep convolution extreme learning	Learning basis is Gaussian probability	Handles both 2D and 3D data	Prior probability is required
Ruslan [5]	Deep Boltzmann machine	Undirectional connections in between hidden layers	Works for ambiguous datasets	Parameter optimization fails for huge datasets
Hinton [6]	Deep belief network	Every hidden layer will be visible to the next layer	Uses greedy approach for learning Expectation Maximization (EM) algorithm	Training process is really expensive

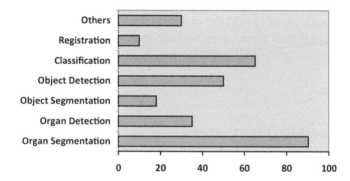

FIGURE 9.1
Category-wise percentage of papers existing in digital repositories.

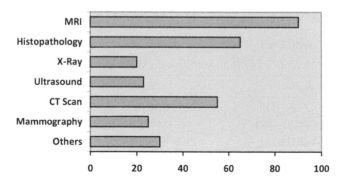

FIGURE 9.2
Imaging modality-wise percentage of papers that exist in digital repositories.

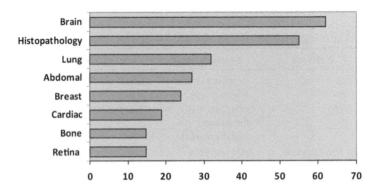

FIGURE 9.3
Percentage of papers existing in digital repositories associated with human organs.

expertise. The automatic analysis of features using convolutional network and learning of the model based on different hidden layers will help the machine learning model to predict the abnormality based on trends present in imaging modality. Since every imaging modality has different characteristics and different associated features, the deep model will definitely resolve the burden of feature description of a variety of diseases. In addition, these imaging modalities are associated with different body parts covering some specific organ of human body. The trends of the associated work on medical images present in literature have focused on some of the benign and malignant images in terms of segmentation, classification, and prediction of malignancy using World Health Organization (WHO) scale. The associated work based on human body parts that exist in literature and used in this chapter is shown in Figure 9.3.

9.3 Deep CNN Architecture Variants

Given the pervasiveness of CNN in medical image analysis, some of the mostly used CNN model variant architectures and their differences are elaborated. These networks are extensions of the existing CNN network with some specific parameters associated with the network. These networks have been used in a variety of applications, including clinical diagnosis to online challenges, conducted by authentic medical organizations like BRATS, MICCAI, ImageNet, and more. These variants of CNN are shown in Table 9.2.

TABLE 9.2

Evolution of CNN Architecture Variants

Author	Network	Year
LeCun [10]	LeNet	1998
Krizhevsky [11]	AlexNet	2012
Lin [12]	InceptionNet	2013
Simonyan [13]	OxfordNet	2014
Szegedy [14]	GoogleNet	2014
He [15]	ResNet	2015
Kamnitsas [16]	DualpathNet	2017

From Table 9.2, it is identified that, from 2012 onwards, the small change in deep layer engineering can increase the performance from "good" to "better," and year-by-year, the slight change in tuning parameters will result in more sophisticated architectures of CNN. Uses of these architectures are found in lots of medical research articles for providing specific solutions for some of the major complicated problems, including tumor detection [17], cancer prediction [18], cancer cell identification [19], retinopathy [20], and more.

9.4 Deep Architectures in Radiology for Problem-Solving

Some of the applications of deep architectures for various radiological applications are discussed in Figure 9.1. The most commonly used applications are classification, segmentation, and detection of abnormalities in imaging formats. These applications are tested on several organs of the human body, which is listed in Figure 9.3 for computer-assisted diagnosis and prognosis. Based on the literature study, the detail of each application is indicated with their pros and cons in this section.

A. Operations on brain imaging: The deep architecture on brain imaging will resolve some of the major problems of radiology like segmentation of abnormal regions, classification of brain slices, and diagnosis of diseases like Alzheimer. The literature on brain disease diagnosis is presented in Table 9.3. In general, it is found that brain images that are used for computer-aided diagnosis are in the form of 3D voxels in all literature works, but most of the given methods worked for 2D images only. Thus, the analyses of 3D voxels are performed by analysis of 2D images slice-by-slice. The use of deep architecture has also seen some of the standard brain imaging challenges from 2013 to the present in BRATS, multiple sclerosis lesion segmentation challenge, Ischemic Stroke Lesion Segmentation (ISLES), MICCAI, and MRBrains. They have used different variants of deep architectures and won top ranks for various objectives of diagnosis like segmentation, identification, classification, and prediction.

B. Operations on Ophthalmic Imaging: Ophthalmic imaging is the imaging associated with eye. For the past years, deep architecture has done great work in the analysis of ophthalmic images. The associated work with ophthalmic images with deep learning architectures are shown in Table 9.4. The literature suggests that, among the existing variants of deep architecture, the most commonly used architecture is CNN for various applications like segmentation and detection of retina-based abnormalities, diagnosis of infections associated with eye, and more. In addition, there are several challenges conducted by various Research and Development (R&D) and organizations for finding solutions for specific problems like Kaggle challenge of diabetic retinopathy detection. Even in such challenges, the trend of use of deep architectures is found where the performance claimed is far better than the human perception with naked eye.

C. Operations on mammographic imaging: One of the areas of medical society where a lot of research is focused on detection and segmentation of tumors regions is mammography imaging, followed by the classification of mammographic images. For the past several years, the rate of growth in terms of patient count for this severe disease increases worldwide. A lot of initiatives were taken by various researchers

TABLE 9.3

Survey of Papers Using Deep Architecture Learning for Brain Imaging

Focused Domain	Network	Description
Abnormality classification	Deep belief network [21–23]	Deep belief network is used for automatic classification of abnormality regions from MRI/Functional Magnetic Resonance Imaging (fMRI) brain images.
	Autoencoder [24,25]	Latent feature extraction mechanism for large sets from MRI and Positron Emission Tomography (PET) imaging, with fine-tuning based stacked autoencoders.
	Boltzmann machines [26]	Classification of Alzheimer's disease using Boltzmann network machines on MRI and PET modalities.
	Convolution network [27–30]	Training with sparse autoencoders on 3D imaging with the use of 3D convolutional autoencoder on fMRI data and adapted Lenet-5 architecture on fMRI data and regression models for sparse representations of Alzheimer disease classification.
Abnormality segmentation	Autoencoder [31,32]	Hippocampus and visual pathway segmentation on MRI andother medical images and encoder-based representation learning used for patch similarity measurement. Also, encoder-based learning appearance features for segmentation of steering the shape models of medical images.
	Recurrent network [33,34]	Used for cell and tissue segmentation of clinical disorders in MRIs.
	Convolution network [35–43]	Used for the segmentation oftumor cells and brain structures in adults and child. Also, used for anatomical segmentation with 2D and 3D imaging of MRI andfMRI.
Abnormality identification and analysis	Convolution network [44–46]	Using 2D/3D imagings with convolutional network for Lacune andMicrobleed detection and automatic tumor grading.
Other	Belief network [47]	Deep Belief Network (DBN) with conventional Restricted Boltzmann machine (RBM) layers for modeling the variability in brain morphology and lesion distribution in multiple sclerosis using manifold learning.
	Boltzmann machines [48]	Use of RBM for both internal and functional interaction-induced latent sources detection on fMRI images with blind source separation.
	Convolution network [49,50]	Used for similarity measurement on 3D images with estimating similarity between reference and moving images. Also used for medical image registration.

for early diagnosis of breast cancer cells and segmentation. Traditional methods are based on the manual extraction of features and biomarkers for the identification of malignancy in mammogram images. These methods gave significant results, but the art of extracting relevant and informative features was a tedious task. The impact of deep architecture in mammographic imaging resolves the big burden of researchers for feature extraction complications. Due to the power of automatic extraction of features from images by deep network, it becomes the first choice of the medical society for image computations. After the impact of deep learning on other domains, the use of deep architecture is largely found in various research articles. The summarized use of deep architectures for mammographic images is shown in Table 9.5. One of the major observations found in literature is the use of limited size of databases, which is freely available, and the use of old screened images. The digital repositories that have such imaging datasets have not updated the imaging modalities and thus, even after incorporating deep architectures, the

TABLE 9.4

Survey of Papers Using Deep Architecture Learning for Ophthalmic Imaging

Focused Domain	Network	Description
Segmentation	Recurrent network [51]	Segmentation of the blood cells in eye using conditional random forest as recurrent network
	Convolution network [52–55]	Segmentation of the blood cells and classification using saliency maps with convolution architecture. Also, optic disk and optic cup segmentation aredone using booting-based convolution network
	Very deep CNN [56]	Blood cell segmentation in human eye images using 19-layered deep network with convolution-based filter.
Detection	Convolution network [57–61]	Detection of glaucoma using end-to-end CNN in ophthalmic images.
		Detection of retina for diabetic patient'sophthalmic images and analysis of abnormality using freely available dataset.
		Special focus on area segmentation of ophthalmic images like age-based macular degeneration. Hemorrhage detection with selective data sampling in CNN.
	GoogLeNet [62]	Detection of retinopathy of prematurity using ImageNet trained GoogLeNet to find disease automatically.

TABLE 9.5

Survey of Papers Using Deep Architecture for Mammographic Imaging

Focused Domain	Network	Description
Segmentation	Convolution network [63–65]	Used for the segmentation of breast and fibroglandular tissue with a convolution network for training and localization of malignant masses.
	Autoencoder [66]	Autoencoder-based segmentation of breast density and parameter estimation usingmammographic images.
Detection	Convolution network [67–69]	First impact of CNN for abnormality detection in mammographic images, with predefined manual and automatic feature extraction mechanism to find abnormality regions.
Classification	Adaptive deconvolution network [70]	Classification of abnormality-detected masses using four-layered adaptive network.
	Convolution network [71–76]	Classification of abnormal tissues and malignant masses with automatic feature extraction mechanism using CNN.
	Boltzmann machine [77]	Binary classification of malignant to benign cells for mammographic images.

percentage of accuracy for identification, segmentation, and classification of mammography images is very limited. Once the large-scaled imaging datasets are available for deep architecture, which is one of the requirement of training in deep neural network architecture, then the existing accuracies will be improved.

D. Operations on abdominal imaging: The source of diagnosis for gastroenterologists is abdominal imaging. The general abdominal imaging includes genitals, urinary organs, and intestines for diagnosis and treatment of abnormalities. The radiological imaging of abdominal is also used for several other diagnosis of organs like liver, kidney, gall bladder, prostate, colon, and pancreas. The traditional methods, except medical test based diagnosis, depend on fetching human-centric features from imaging modalities like CT, MRI, and ultrasounds. This process requires a lot of human interventions and expertise in a specific domain. Later, for past some years, after the evolution of deep architectures in medical domain, especially convolution-based deep architecture, the automatic feature extraction made the task as easy as possible. The power of the network to learn and predict the informative features from imaging itself would really boost the performance of disease diagnosis, proper abnormality region detection and segmentation, and automatic classification of organs using computer-assisted machines. The survey on deep architectures that were used for abdominal images is presented in Table 9.6. The literature suggests the use of convolution-based deep network for computer-aided diagnosis system.

E. Operations on histopathology imaging: Histopathology imaging, or microscopic imaging, is the source of current generation imaging, where computer-assisted intervention is focused. Due to the growing availability of whole-slide images of cells, this digital pathology and microscopic imaging analysis become a very interesting research domain for deep architecture researchers. This imaging is also considered as more challenging due to the unavailability of specific hand-crafted feature generation algorithms. Thus, in such a case, the deep architecture provides the desired solution for histopathology images. The literature present on histopathology imaging focuses on three main aspects: (i) identification and segmentation of nuclei, (ii) segmentation and classification of human organs, and (iii) classification of the disease using whole-slide imaging. The detailed review analysis of deep architecture based on histopathology imaging is presented in Table 9.7. This imaging modality has differentiation with other medical imaging formats. As seen in radiological imaging of MRI, CT, and ultrasound, where the image is of gray color despite three color bands (Red, Green, Blue (RGB)), histopathology images are mostly colored. The most commonly used imaging is hematoxylin and eosin staining (H&E). The literature used in Table 9.7 is related to H&E for detection, segmentation, and classification of abnormalities, organs, and nuclei.

TABLE 9.6

Survey of Papers Using Deep Architecture for Segmentation in Abdominal Imaging

Focused Domain	Network	Description
Liver	Convolution network [78–80]	Segmentation of liver 2D abnormality patches of dynamic and fixed size 17 ×17 patches using CNN. Also, implemented in online challenge SLIVER07.
	Convolution network [81–84]	Segmentation of liver 3D liver images using conditional random field with convolution network. The implementation is also seen in online challenges with great accuracy.
Kidney	Convolution network [85–87]	Segmentation of the kidney regions using hybrid local patch and slice based features with convolution network on small databases of around 20–60 images.
Pancreas	Convolution network [88–90]	Segmentation of the pancreas using superpixel approach with convolutional network. Also, the pancreas was segmented using conditional random field and random forests.
Prostate	Autoencoder [91]	Feature extraction using autoencoder from patches that were taken as input to network for segmentation of prostate diseases.
	Hybrid network [92–94]	2D and 3D image segmentation using the hybrid architecture of CNN with ResNet and UNet. The architecture is also used in online competition of PROMISE12.

TABLE 9.7

Survey of Papers for Histopathology and Microscopic Imaging with H&E

Focused Domain	Subdomain	Description
Nucleus	Mitosis detection [95–99]	Convolution-based pixel classifier network that combines shape and handcrafted features with CNN and its ensemble networks.
	Nucleus detection [100–105]	Use of structured regression model with automatic and handcrafted features with CNN and sparse autoencoders.
	Nucleus segmentation [106,107]	Implementation of the resolution-adaptive deep hierarchical learning scheme in CNN.
	Cell segmentation [108–110]	Use of f-CNN for bounding box with single and multiscale CNN for segmentation.
	Nucleus classification [111,112]	Transfer learning-based classification of cells into tumor, lymphocyte, Hep2, and stromal classes.
Human Organs	Colon glands segmentation [113–118]	Used two or more convolution network and Fully Convolutional Neural Network (fCNN) network to segment glands and their separating structures.
	Muscle regions segmentation [119]	Used conditional random field with fCNN that is jointly trained for segmentation of regions.
	Perimysium segmentation [120]	Implemented 2D spatial clockwork Recurrent Neural Network (RNN) for patch segmentation.
Specific Disease	Carcinoma detection [121]	Normal convolution-based classifier-based abnormal cell detection.
	Colon cancer classification [122]	Multiple instance learning framework with CNN features.
	Colorectal cancer prediction [123]	Extracted CNN features from epithelial tissue for prediction.
	Gliomas classification [124]	Ensemble of CNN is used for gliomas grade classification.
	Thyroid cytopathology classification [125]	Implementation of fine-tuning pretrained AlexNet for thyroid cell classification.
	Breast cancer detection [126,127]	The proposed model uses shearlet features with CNN and fCNN for cancer cell detection.

9.5 Issues, Limitations, and Dependencies on Medical Imaging Research

One of the limitations or requirements of deep learning is the large amount of training dataset, which is required as a classification accuracy of deep networks is solely reliant on the size of the dataset. Moreover, unavailability of free and open access dataset is one the biggest obstacle in the successful implementation of deep learning in radiological applications. On the dual side, it is also true that the development of large medical imaging data is quite difficult, as annotation requires multiple expert opinions to overcome the human error, which is a time-consuming task.

The next issue in computer-assisted medical image analysis is the legal and privacy parameter. It is found in the literature that most of the experimented datasets are with the authors only and not devoted to open access for later research perspectives. The sharing of the dataset is much more complicated and difficult when compared with other real-world images. In medical imaging, privacy of the data has both sociological and technical issues, which must be handled jointly. The issues are related to provide legal rights to patients regarding their individual identity information and obligations for disclosure openly.

With the use of medical imaging datasets, machine-assisted data analytics researchers found it challenging to abstract the patient information to prevent its use or disclosure in research.

9.6 Discussion on the Presented Work

This chapter covers the state-of-the-art literature of around 127 articles, either published or archived, for the domain of deep learning in various digital repositories. The selected papers are in such a form that it pervaded every aspect of medical image analysis using deep architectures and learning. It is noted from the class of articles that a maximum of selected articles are latest, i.e., published within last 4 years (2015–2018). Using these selected articles, a large diversity of deep architectures is covered, which is shown in Table 9.1.

The traditional method of computer-assisted medical diagnosis system involves the use of manual handcrafted feature extraction methods, which requires a lot of expertise and domain knowledge. After incorporation of the deep architectures in medical imaging, the process becomes simpler and much more accurate as earlier methods. The art of automatic feature extraction and learning of deep architecture based network had made this machine learning approach as first choice for various radiological applications. Based on the existing survey, the list of papers used for domain-specific problems of machine learning is presented in Figure 9.1, while the trend in the use of specific medical imaging with specific organ-based analysis is presented in Figures 9.2 and 9.3.

In the last few years, it is identified that, among the various deep architectures (Table 9.2), the most commonly used architecture for deep learning is the end-to-end trained convolutional network that has become the first choice for medical imaging of disease identification, segmentation, and classification. Based on survey analysis, it is found that convolutional networks are followed by the largest group of papers in this survey and claimed that accuracy achieved is much more as desired when compared with traditional methods.

After studying and analyzing around 127 papers, we found that the deep learning method and architecture for individual task and medical application prove trustworthy in the diagnosis of abnormalities in medical imaging and radiology. But one of the important conclusions is that the use of deep architecture is not at all the most important factor in getting an absolute result. The use of similar architecture with same imaging systems in different places will give different results. This trend is noticed in several online competitions where participants used existing deep architectures for problem-solving. However, the variation in terms of accuracy prediction is noticed in almost every case. Thus, rather than architecture, it is methodology and domain expertise that both play a role in diagnosis system. One of the examples is introduction of the AlexNet and VCC-19 deep architecture network, where different methodologies are introduced to find a solution with higher precision.

It is concluded that deep architecture based learning application provided positive feedbacks in terms of accuracy and diagnosis. However, due to the sensitivity of radiological dataset imaging and challenges, the requirement of more sophisticated deep architectures is still in demand and can deal with complex imaging structures efficiently. Lastly, we conclude that there are unlimited opportunities to improve deep architectures for medical system.

References

1. Igor, N., et al., *Multi Valued and Universal Binary Neurons: Theory, Learning and Applications*, Kluwer Academic Publisher, Norwell, MA, 2000.
2. Fukushima, K., Neocognitron: A self-organizing neural network model for a mechanism of pattern recognition unaffected by shift in position, *Biol. Cybern.*, vol. 36(4), 193–202, 1980.
3. Faustino, J., et al., Co-evolving recurrent neurons learn deep memory POMDPs, *7th Annual Conference on Genetic and Evolutionary Computation*, Washington DC, USA, pp. 491–498, 2005.
4. Shan, P., Xinyi, Y., Deep convolutional extreme learning machine and its application in hand-written digit classification, *Comput. Intell. Neurosci.*, vol. 2016(6), 6, 2016.
5. Ruslan, S., et al., Efficient learning of deep Boltzmann machine, *Mach Learn. Res.*, vol. 9(1), 693–700, 2010.
6. Hinton, G., et al., Deep belief networks, *Scholarpedia*, vol. 4(5), 5947, 2009.
7. Lo, S.C., et al., Artificial convolution neural network techniques and applications for lung nodule detection, *IEEE Trans. Med. Imaging*, vol. 14, 711–718, 1995.
8. Bengio, Y., Courville, A., Vincent, P., Representation learning: A review and new perspectives, *IEEE Trans. Pattern Anal. Mach. Intell.*, vol. 35(8), 1798–1828, 2013.
9. Ravi, D., et al., Deep learning for health informatics, *IEEE J. Biomed. Health Inf.*, vol. 21, 4–21, 2017.
10. LeCun, Y., Bottou, L., Bengio, Y., Haffner, P., Gradient-based learning applied to document recognition, *Proc. IEEE*, vol. 86, 2278–2324, 1998.
11. Krizhevsky, A., Sutskever, I., Hinton, G., Imagenet classification with deep convolutional neural networks, *Adv. Neural Inf. Processing Syst.*, vol. 1, 1097–1105, 2012.
12. Lin, M., Chen, Q., Yan, S., Network in network, arXiv: 1312.4400, 2013.
13. Simonyan, K., Zisserman, A., Very deep convolutional networks for large-scale image recognition, arXiv: 1409.1556, 2014.
14. Szegedy, C., et al., Going deeper with convolutions, arXiv: 1409.4842, 2014.
15. He, et al., Deep residual learning for image recognition, arXiv: 1512.03385, 2015.
16. Kamnitsas, K., et al., Efficient multi-scale 3D CNN with fully connected CRF for accurate brain lesion segmentation, *Med. Image Anal.*, vol. 36, 61–78, 2017.
17. Kashif, M., et al., Hand crafted features with convolutional neural networks for detection of tumor cells in histology images, *IEEE International Symposium on Biomedical Imaging*, Prague, Czech Republic, pp. 1029–1032, 2016.
18. Esteva, A., et al., Dermatologist-level classification of skin cancer with deep neural networks, *Nature*, vol. 542, 115–118, 2017.
19. Liu, Y., et al., Detecting cancer metastases on gigapixel pathology images, arXiv: 1703. 02442, 2017.
20. Gulshan, V., et al., Development and validation of a deep learning algorithm for detection of diabetic retinopathy in retinal fundus photographs, *JAMA*, vol. 316, 2402–2410, 2016.
21. Brosch, T., Tam, R., Manifold learning of brain MRIs by deep learning, *Med Image Comput. Comput. Assist. Interv.*, vol. 8150, 633–640, 2013.
22. Ortiz, A., et al., Ensembles of deep learning architectures for the early diagnosis of the Alzheimer's disease, *Int. J. Neural Syst.*, vol. 26, 1650025, 2016.
23. Plis, S.M., et al., Deep learning for neuroimaging: A validation study, arXiv:1312.5847, 2014.
24. Suk, H.-I., Shen, D., Deep learning-based feature representation for AD/MCI classification, *Med Image Comput. Comput. Assist. Interv.*, vol. 8150, 583–590, 2013.
25. Suk, H.-I., et al., Hierarchical feature representation and multi- modal fusion with deep learning for AD/MCI diagnosis, *Neuroimaging*, vol. 101, 569–582, 2014.
26. Suk, H.-I., Lee, S.-W., Shen, D., Hierarchical feature representation and multi- modal fusion with deep learning for AD/MCI diagnosis, *Neuroimaging*, vol. 101, 569–582, 2014.
27. Payan, A., Montana, G., Predicting Alzheimer's disease: A neuroimaging study with 3D convolutional neural networks, arXiv: 1502.02506, 2015.

28. Hosseini-Asl, E., Gimel'farb, G., El-Baz, A., Alzheimer's disease diagnostics by a deeply supervised adaptable 3D convolutional network, arXiv: 1607.00556, 2016.

29. Sarraf, S., Tofighi, G., Classification of Alzheimer's disease using FMRI data and deep learning convolutional neural networks, arXiv: 1603.08631, 2016.

30. Suk, H.-I., Shen, D., Deep ensemble sparse regression network for Alzheimer's disease diagnosis, In *International Workshop on Medical Image Computing and Computer Assisted Intervention*, 113–121, 2016, Springer, Cham.

31. Guo, Y., et al., Segmenting hippocampus from infant brains by sparse patch matching with deep-learned features, In *International Conference on Medical Image Computing and Computer Assisted Intervention*, pp. 308–315, 2014, Springer, Cham.

32. Mansoor, A., et al., Deep learning guided partitioned shape model for anterior visual pathway segmentation, *IEEE Trans. Med. Imaging*, vol. 35(8), 1856–1865, 2016.

33. Stollenga, M.F., et al., Parallel multi-dimensional LSTM, with application to fast biomedical volumetric image segmentation, *Advances in Neural Information Processing Systems*, Montreal, Canada, pp. 2998–3006, 2015.

34. Andermatt, S., Pezold, S., Cattin, P., Multi-dimensional gated recurrent units for the segmentation of biomedical 3D-data, *Deep Learning in Medical Image Analysis (DLMIA)*, pp. 142–151, 2016, Springer, Cham.

35. Brosch, T., et al., Deep 3D convolutional encoder networks with shortcuts for multiscale feature integration applied to multiple sclerosis lesion segmentation, *IEEE Trans. Med. Imaging*, vol. 35(5), 1229–1239, 2016.

36. Chen, H., et al., Voxresnet: Deep voxelwise residual networks for volumetric brain segmentation, arXiv: 1608.05895, 2016.

37. Ghafoorian, M., et al., Non-uniform patch sampling with deep convolutional neural networks for white matter hyperintensity segmentation, *IEEE International Symposium on Biomedical Imaging*, Prague, Czech Republic, pp. 1414–1417, 2016.

38. Havaei, M., et al., HeMIS: Hetero-modal image segmentation, In *International Conference on Medical Image Computing and Computer Assisted Intervention*, pp. 469–477, 2016, Springer, Cham.

39. Kamnitsas, K., et al., Efficient multi-scale 3D CNN with fully connected CRF for accurate brain lesion segmentation, *Med. Image Anal.*, vol. 36, 61–78, 2017.

40. Kleesiek, J., et al., Deep MRI brain extraction: A 3D convolutional neural network for skull stripping, *Neuroimaging*, vol. 129, 460–469, 2016.

41. Milletari, F., et al., Hough-CNN: Deep learning for segmentation of deep brain regions in MRI and ultrasound, arXiv: 1601.07014, 2016.

42. Pereira, S., et al., Brain tumor segmentation using convolutional neural networks in MRI images, *IEEE Trans. Med. Imaging*, vol. 35(5), 1240–1251, 2016.

43. Shakeri, M., et al., Sub-cortical brain structure segmentation using FCNNs, *IEEE International Symposium on Biomedical Imaging*, Prague, Czech Republic, pp. 269–272, 2016.

44. Pan, Y., et al., Brain tumor grading based on neural networks and convolutional neural networks, *IEEE Engineering in Medicine and Biology Society*, Milan, Italy, pp. 699–702, 2015.

45. Dou, Q., et al., Automatic detection of cerebral microbleeds from MR images via 3D convolutional neural networks, *IEEE Trans. Med. Imaging*, vol. 35, 1182–1195, 2016.

46. Ghafoorian, M., et al., Deep multi-scale location-aware 3d convolutional neural networks for automated detection of lacunes of presumed vascular origin, *NeuroImage Clin.*, vol. 14, 391–399, 2017.

47. Brosch, T., et al., Modeling the variability in brain morphology and lesion distribution in multiple sclerosis by deep learning, In *International Conference on Medical Image Computing and Computer Assisted Intervention*, pp. 462–469, 2014, Springer, Cham.

48. Huang, H., et al., Latent source mining in FMRI data via deep neural network, *IEEE International Symposium on Biomedical Imaging*, Prague, Czech Republic, pp. 638–641, 2016.

49. Simonovsky, M., et al., A deep metric for multimodal registration, In *International Conference on Medical Image Computing and Computer Assisted Intervention*, pp. 10–18, 2016, Springer, Cham.

50. Yang, X., Kwitt, R., Niethammer, M., Fast predictive image registration, *Deep Learning in Medical Image Analysis (DLMIA)*, pp. 48–57, 2016, Springer, Cham.

51. Fu, H., et al., Deepvessel: Retinal vessel segmentation via deep learning and conditional random field, In *International Conference on Medical Image Computing and Computer Assisted Intervention*, pp. 132–139, 2016, Springer, Cham.

52. Fu, H., et al., Retinal vessel segmentation via deep learning network and fully-connected conditional random fields, *IEEE International Symposium on Biomedical Imaging*, Prague, Czech Republic, pp. 698–701, 2016.

53. Mahapatra, D., et al., Retinal image quality classification using saliency maps and CNNs, In *International Workshop on Machine Learning in Medical Imaging*, pp. 172–179, 2016, Springer, Cham.

54. Wu, A., et al., Deep vessel tracking: a generalized probabilistic approach via deep learning, *IEEE International Symposium on Biomedical Imaging*, Prague, Czech Republic, pp. 1363–1367, 2016.

55. Zilly, J., et al., Glaucoma detection using entropy sampling and ensemble learning for automatic optic cup and disc segmentation, *Comput. Med. Imaging Graph*, vol. 55, 28–41, 2017.

56. Maninis, K., et al., Deep retinal image understanding, In *International Conference on Medical Image Computing and Computer Assisted Intervention*, pp. 140–148, 2016, Springer, Cham.

57. Chen, X., et al., Glaucoma detection based on deep convolutional neural network, *IEEE Engineering in Medicine and Biology Society*, Milan, Italy, pp. 715–718, 2015.

58. Abràmoff, M., et al., Improved automated detection of diabetic retinopathy on a publicly available dataset through integration of deep learning, *Invest. Ophthalmol. Vis. Sci.*, vol. 57(13), 5200–5206, 2016.

59. Gulshan, V., et al., Development and validation of a deep learning algorithm for detection of diabetic retinopathy in retinal fundus photographs, *J. Am. Med. Assoc.*, vol. 316, pp. 2402–2410, 2016.

60. Burlina, P., et al., Detection of age related macular degeneration via deep learning, *IEEE International Symposium on Biomedical Imaging*, Prague, Czech Republic, pp. 184–188, 2016.

61. van, G., et al., Fast convolutional neural network training using selective data sampling: application to hemorrhage detection in color fundus images, *IEEE Trans. Med. Imaging*, vol. 35(5), 1273–1284, 2016.

62. Worrall, D., et al., Automated retinopathy of prematurity case detection with convolutional neural networks, *Deep Learning in Medical Image Analysis (DLMIA)*, pp. 68–76, 2016, Springer, Cham.

63. Dalmis, M., et al., Using deep learning to segment breast and fibroglandular tissue in MRI volumes, *Med. Phys.*, vol. 44, pp. 533–546, 2017.

64. Hwang, S., et al., Self-transfer learning for fully weakly supervised object localization, arXiv: 1602.01625, 2016.

65. Kisilev, P., et al., Medical image description using multi-task-loss CNN, *International Workshop on Large-Scale Annotation of Biomedical Data and Expert Label Synthesis*, Athens, Greece, pp. 121–129, 2016.

66. Kallenberg, M., et al., Unsupervised deep learning applied to breast density segmentation and mammographic risk scoring, *IEEE Trans. Med. Imaging*, vol. 35, 1322–1331, 2016.

67. Sahiner, B., et al., Classification of mass and normal breast tissue: a convolution neural network classifier with spatial domain and texture images, *IEEE Trans. Med. Imaging*, vol. 15, 598–610, 2016.

68. Dhungel, N., et al., The automated learning of deep features for breast mass classification from mammograms, *International Conference on Medical Image Computing and Computer Assisted Intervention*, pp. 106–114, 2016, Springer, Cham.

69. Kooi, T., et al., Discriminating solitary cysts from soft tissue lesions in mammography using a pretrained deep convolutional neural network, *Med. Phys.*, vol. 44(3), 1017–1027, 2017.

70. Jamieson, A., et al., Breast image feature learning with adaptive deconvolutional networks, *SPIE on Medical Imaging*, vol. 8315, 831506, 2012.

71. Fonseca, P., et al., Automatic breast density classification using a convolutional neural network architecture search procedure, *SPIE on Medical Imaging*, vol. 9413, 941428, 2015.

72. Akselrod, A., et al., A region based convolutional network for tumor detection and classification in breast mammography, *Deep Learning in Medical Image Analysis (DLMIA)*, pp. 197–205, 2016, Springer, Cham.

73. Arevalo, J., et al., Representation learning for mammography mass lesion classification with convolutional neural networks, *Comput. Methods Program. Biomed.*, vol. 127, 248–257, 2016.

74. Dubrovina, A., et al., Computational mammography using deep neural networks, *Comput. Methods Biomech. Biomed. Eng. Imaging Vis.*, pp. 1–5, 2016.

75. Qiu, Y., et al., An initial investigation on developing a new method to predict short-term breast cancer risk based on deep learning technology, *SPIE on Medical Imaging*, vol. 9785, p. 978521, 2016.

76. Sun, W., et al., Enhancing deep convolutional neural network scheme for breast cancer diagnosis with unlabeled data, *Comput. Med. Imaging Graph*, vol. 57, 4–9, 2017.

77. Zhang, Q., et al., Deep learning based classification of breast tumors with shear-wave elastography, *J. Ultrasonics*, vol. 72, 150–157, 2016.

78. Li, W., et al., Automatic segmentation of liver tumor in CT images with deep convolutional neural networks, *J. Comput. Commun.*, vol. 3(11), 146–151, 2015.

79. Vivanti, R., et al., Automatic liver tumor segmentation in follow-up CT studies using convolutional neural networks, *Patch-Based Methods in Medical Image Processing Workshop*, Quebec City, QC, Canada, pp. 54–61, 2015.

80. Ben-Cohen, A., et al., Deep learning and data labeling for medical applications, *International Workshop on Large-Scale Annotation of Biomedical Data and Expert Label Synthesis*, Athens, Greece, pp. 77–85, 2016.

81. Dou, Q., et al., 3D deeply supervised network for automatic liver segmentation from CT volumes, *IEEE Trans. Biomed. Eng.*, vol. 64(7), 1558–1567, 2016.

82. Hu, P., et al., Automatic 3D liver segmentation based on deep learning and globally optimized surface evolution, *Phys. Med. Biol.*, vol. 61, 8676–8698, 2016.

83. Lu, F., et al., Automatic 3D liver location and segmentation via convolutional neural network and graph cut, *J. Comput. Assist. Radiol. Surg.*, vol. 12, 171–182, 2017.

84. Christ, P., et al., Automatic liver and lesion segmentation in CT using cascaded fully convolutional neural networks and 3D conditional random fields, In *International Conference on Medical Image Computing and Computer-Assisted Intervention*, pp. 415–423, 2016, Springer, Cham.

85. Lu, X., et al., Robust 3d organ localization with dual learning architectures and fusion, *Deep Learning in Medical Image Analysis*, pp. 12–20, 2016, Springer, Cham.

86. Ravishankar, H., et al., Understanding the mechanisms of deep transfer learning for medical images, *Deep Learning in Medical Image Analysis*, pp. 188–196, 2016, Springer, Cham.

87. Thong, W., et al., Convolutional networks for kidney segmentation in contrast-enhanced CT scans, *Computer. Methods Biomech. Biomed. Eng. Imag. Vis.*, Vol. 6(3), 1–6, 2018.

88. Roth, H., et al., DeepOrgan: Multi-level deep convolutional networks for automated pancreas segmentation, In *International Conference on Medical Image Computing and Computer-Assisted Intervention*, pp. 556–564, 2015, Springer, Cham.

89. Cai, J., et al., Pancreas segmentation in MRI using graph-based decision fusion on convolutional neural networks, In *International Conference on Medical Image Computing and Computer-Assisted Intervention*, pp. 442–450, 2016, Springer, Cham.

90. Roth, H., et al., Spatial aggregation of holistically nested networks for automated pancreas segmentation, In *International Conference on Medical Image Computing and Computer-Assisted Intervention*, pp. 451–459, 2016, Springer, Cham.

91. Guo, Y., Gao, Y., Shen, D., Deformable MR prostate segmentation via deep feature learning and sparse patch matching, *IEEE Trans. Med. Imaging*, vol. 35(4), 1077–1089, 2016.

92. Cheng, R., et al., Active appearance model and deep learning for more accurate prostate segmentation on MRI, *SPIE on Medical Imaging*, vol. 9784, p. 978421, 2016.

93. Milletari, F., et al., VNet: Fully convolutional neural networks for volumetric medical image segmentation, arXiv: 1606.04797, 2016.
94. Yu, L., et al., Volumetric ConvNets with mixed residual connections for automated prostate segmentation from 3D MR images, *31st AAAI Conference on Artificial Intelligence*, San Francisco, California, USA, USA, pp. 1–7, 2017.
95. Cire, S., Mitosis detection in breast cancer histology images with deep neural networks, *Med. Image Comput. Comput. Assist. Interv.*, vol. 16, 411–418, 2013.
96. Malon, C.D., Cosatto, E., Classification of mitotic figures with convolutional neural networks and seeded blob features, *J. Pathol. Inform.*, vol. 4, 1–9, 2013.
97. Wang, H., et al., Mitosis detection in breast cancer pathology images by combining hand-crafted and convolutional neural network features, *J. Med. Imaging*, vol. 1, 34003, 2014.
98. Albarqouni, S., et al., Aggnet: Deep learning from crowds for mitosis detection in breast cancer histology images, *IEEE Trans. Med. Imaging*, vol. 35, 1313–1321, 2016.
99. Chen, H., et al., Automated mitosis detection with deep regression networks, *IEEE International Symposium on Biomedical Imaging*, Prague, Czech Republic, pp. 1204–1207, 2016.
100. Xie, Y., et al., Deep voting: A robust approach toward nucleus localization in microscopy images, *Med. Image Comput. Comput. Assist. Interv.*, vol. 9351, 374–382, 2015.
101. Kashif, M.N., et al., Hand crafted features with convolutional neural networks for detection of tumor cells in histology images, *IEEE International Symposium on Biomedical Imaging*, Prague, Czech Republic, pp. 1029–1032, 2016.
102. Romo-Bucheli, D., et al., Automated tubule nuclei quantification and correlation with Oncotype DX risk categories in ER+ breast cancer whole slide images, *Nat. Sci. Rep.*, vol. 6, 32706, 2016.
103. Sirinukunwattana, K., et al., Locality sensitive deep learning for detection and classification of nuclei in routine colon cancer histology images, *IEEE Trans. Med. Imaging*, vol. 35(5), 1196–1206, 2016.
104. Xu, J., et al., Stacked sparse autoencoder (SSAE) for nuclei detection on breast cancer histopathology images, *IEEE Trans. Med. Imaging*, vol. 35, 119–130, 2016.
105. Xie, W., et al., Microscopy cell counting and detection with fully convolutional regression networks, *Comput. Methods Biomech. Biomed. Eng. Imaging Vis.*, pp. 1–10, 2016.
106. Janowczyk, A., et al., A resolution adaptive deep hierarchical (RADHical) learning scheme applied to nuclear segmentation of digital pathology images, *Comput. Methods. Biomech. Biomed. Eng. Imag. Vis.*, pp. 1–7, 2016.
107. Xing, F., et al., An automatic learning based framework for robust nucleus segmentation, *IEEE Trans. Med. Imaging*, vol. 35(2), 550–566, 2016.
108. Akram, S., et al., Cell segmentation proposal network for microscopy image analysis, *Deep Learning in Medical Image Analysis (DLMIA)*, pp. 21–29, 2016, Springer, Cham.
109. Song, Y., et al., Accurate cervical cell segmentation from overlapping clumps in pap smear images, *IEEE Trans. Med. Imaging*, vol. 36, 288–300, 2017.
110. Wang, S., et al., Subtype cell detection with an accelerated deep convolution neural network, In *International Conference on Medical Image Computing and Computer Assisted Intervention*, pp. 640–648, 2016, Springer, Cham.
111. Yao, J., et al., Imaging biomarker discovery for lung cancer survival prediction, In *International Conference on Medical Image Computing and Computer Assisted Intervention*, pp. 649–657, 2016, Springer, Cham.
112. Phan, H., et al., Transfer learning of a convolutional neural network for HEp-2 cell image classification, *IEEE International Symposium on Biomedical Imaging*, Prague, Czech Republic, pp. 1208–1211, 2016.
113. Kainz, P., et al., Semantic segmentation of colon glands with deep convolutional neural networks and total variation segmentation, arXiv: 1511.06919, 2015.
114. BenTaieb, A., Hamarneh, G., Topology aware fully convolutional networks for histology gland segmentation, In *International Conference on Medical Image Computing and Computer Assisted Intervention*, pp. 460–468, 2016, Springer, Cham.

115. BenTaieb, A., et al., Multi loss convolutional networks for gland analysis in microscopy, *IEEE International Symposium on Biomedical Imaging*, Prague, Czech Republic, pp. 642–645, 2016.

116. Chen, H., et al., DCAN: Deep contour-aware networks for accurate gland segmentation, *Med. Image Anal.*, vol. 36, 135–146, 2017.

117. Li, W., et al., Gland segmentation in colon histology images using hand crafted features and convolutional neural networks, *IEEE International Symposium on Biomedical Imaging*, Prague, Czech Republic, pp. 1405–1408, 2016.

118. Xu, Y., et al., Gland instance segmentation by deep multichannel side supervision, arXiv: 1607.03222, 2016.

119. Wang, J., et al., A deep learning approach for semantic segmentation in histology tissue images, In *International Conference on Medical Image Computing and Computer Assisted Intervention*, pp. 176–184, 2016, Springer, Cham.

120. Xie, Y., et al., Spatial clockwork recurrent neural network for muscle perimysium segmentation, In *International Conference on Medical Image Computing and Computer Assisted Intervention*, pp. 185–193, 2016, Springer, Cham.

121. Cruz-Roa, A., et al., Automatic detection of invasive ductal carcinoma in whole slide images with convolutional neural networks, *SPIE on Medical Imaging*, vol. 9041, p. 904103, 2014.

122. Xu, Y., et al., Deep learning of feature representation with multiple instance learning for medical image analysis, *IEEE International Conference on Acoustics, Speech and Signal Processing (ICASSP)*, San Diego, California, USA, pp. 1626–1630, 2014.

123. Bychkov, D., et al., Deep learning for tissue microarray image-based outcome prediction in patients with colorectal cancer, *SPIE on Medical Imaging*, vol. 9791, p. 979115, 2016.

124. Günhan Ertosun, M., Rubin, D.L., Automated grading of gliomas using deep learning in digital pathology images: a modular approach with ensemble of convolutional neural networks, *AMIA Annual Symposium*, pp. 1899–1908, 2015.

125. Kim, E., et al., A deep semantic mobile application for thyroid cytopathology, *SPIE on Medical Imaging*, San Diego, California, USA, vol. 9789, p. 97890A, 2016.

126. Litjens, G., et al., Deep learning as a tool for increased accuracy and efficiency of histopathological diagnosis, *Nat. Sci. Rep.*, vol. 6, 26286, 2016.

127. Rezaeilouyeh, H., et al., Microscopic medical image classification framework via deep learning and shearlet transform, *J. Med. Imaging*, vol. 3(4), 044501, 2016

10

Major Histocompatibility Complex Binding and Various Health Parameters Analysis

Abhinav Gautam, Arjun Singh Chauhan, Ayush Srivastava, Chetan Jadon, and Megha Rathi

Jaypee Institute of Information Technology

CONTENTS

10.1 Introduction

The problem of developing vaccines for a particular disease is an old one, but with the advancement of computational power and research in the field of data analysis using machine tools, the scientist community has not only speeded up the process of creating vaccines but, at the same time, has also managed to save a lot of lives.

10.1.1 Vaccines and T-Cells

The conventional methods of making vaccines include these types:

- Live attenuated vaccines: Live attenuated vaccines are vaccines that have live pathogen cells but are present in extremely small amounts, such that they can be controlled and can be tamed if need be. In certain cases, where the recipient's immune system is extremely weak, like in case of old people, the live attenuated vaccines can turn lethal, because they can end up infecting the person with the same instead of preparing the body for apt immune response.

Inactive vaccines: Inactive vaccines are the ones with dead cells of the pathogen. Since the pathogen cells are already dead, they cannot harm the recipient's body, but they trigger an almost similar response as that of live ones and—in this way—the immune system ends up recording this activity and keeps itself prepared for any such future attacks from the same pathogen.

Since inactive vaccine has dead pathogen cells, even people with a weak immune system can be treated with such vaccines. However, the only problem with such vaccines is that they are not very efficient, since the dead pathogen cells can only trigger a response from a few T-cells.

- Subunit vaccine: Subunit vaccines are not a part of a wholesome vaccine family. Subunit vaccines are composed of a part of pathogen cell—called the antigen. It's the function of antigen to simulate the immune system for antibody response. Antigens can be further filtered out into smaller components like proteins and polysaccharides, which can then be used for treating a particular kind of disease related to that sequence of proteins.

These vaccines are efficient and safe even for recipients with a weak immune system, because only a part of the pathogen cell is used for vaccination, and the antigen part is not harmful to the recipient's body.

Toxoid vaccines: Toxoid vaccines are vaccines with either extremely low bacterial toxin or no activated toxin. Toxoid vaccines do not have wholesome pathogen cells present in them, and it's just the extremely low quantity of toxins.

DNA vaccines: Deoxyribonucleic Acid (DNA) vaccines are the future of vaccination. It's yet to be tested on human beings, but it has worked quite well in case of animal testing, and a veterinary DNA vaccine has been approved for curing horses with West Nile Virus. DNA vaccines work on the principle of modifying the genes in such a way that they trigger a particular type of response when needed again in the encoded pathogen protein. DNA vaccines are sometimes called the future of vaccination, because they are cost effective, have no risk of infection, target response thus lower side effects, and the response time is comparatively lower than those of conventional ways.

Most of the common vaccines work on a simple logic, i.e., training the immune system by making it fight the weakened or dead pathogen cells. Immune system can then retain this in its memory and fight any other cases of similar pathogen cells that it encounters in the future. But in case of certain viruses like Human Immunodeficiency Virus (HIV) or cancer, human body faces immunodeficiency, i.e., our body simply does not know how to react to such pathogen cells and ends up doing nothing. Making vaccines for such virus is altogether a different challenge, since a response has to be first created in the immune system, and then it's trained to trigger when needed.

All the aforementioned procedures of developing a vaccine can be made fast if we can actually predict how various pathogen proteins bind with the cells. This research work is done in labs by pharmaceutical companies, but it can take a lot of time. Another way of doing it with advanced tools that we have is to get a rough idea about how various pathogens will change the body cell dynamics once they come in contact with them.

Once a pathogen cell comes in contact with the body, they form bonds with major histocompatibility complex (MHC). The strength of this bond determines the response of T-cells. T-cells are the antibodies generated by the body to fight any kind of foreign invasion it sees as harmful. T-cells are majorly of two types:

- Helper T-cells: Helper T-cells are the first ones to come in contact with the infected cells, and they are the ones that further lead to generation of killer T-cells and other immunological responses.

- Cytotoxic or killer T-cells: Killer T-cells are the fighter cells. Killer T-cells are the ones that actually fight the bacterial or infected cells and destroy them.

10.1.2 MHC: Class I and Class II

Antigen presenting cells include macrophage, dendritic cells, and B-cells. These cells engulf a foreign material or pathogens through phagocytosis and then respond to the whole immune system of body with the help of a special molecule known as MHC. This molecule works as a receptor. MHCs are of two types MHC I and MHC II. MHC I is tissue specific, and all nucleated cells in our body contain MHC I; on the other hand, only antigen presenting cells contain MHC II. MHC is also known as glycoprotein. When pathogens enter our body, they start spreading and killing our body cell so as to keep the whole body unaffected. MHC I loaded with pathogenic portion interacts with T-cell receptor and cytotoxic killer cells (CD8$^+$) and kills target body cells. MHC I is composed of heavy chain and light chain. Heavy chain consists of three extracellular components and intracytoplasmic carboxyl terminus, wherein light chain consists of B2 microglobulin and transports MHC I to cell surface. MHC II consists of alpha and beta chains and is bound to helper T-cells (CD4$^+$) and use exogenous pathways for MHC binding.

10.1.3 SMM: Stabilized Matrix Method

Stabilized matrix method (SMM) is the key algorithm that is being used for predicting the bond length between the peptide and the MHC. SMM is one of the most sought after immunology analysis algorithm, because it compares its result by using data from 14 human MHC Human Leukocyte Antigen – DR isotype (HLA-DR) and 3 Mouse Alleles (H2-IA). It has been proved to be better than other algorithms like Gibbs Sampler, Support Vector Machine - Regression (SVR)MHC, and Major Histocompatibility Prediction (MHCpred) methods (Nielsen et al., 2007). SMM has been trained and tested for the largest data set on HLA-DR and H2-IA (Nielsen et al., 2007). The SMM method generates quantitative models of sequence specificity of biological processes, which in turn can be used to predict and understand these processes (Peters & Sette, 2005). SMM can eventually help in better understanding and finding the exact epitopes of a given pathogen, thereby leading to a faster development of the vaccine.

10.1.4 BLOSUM: Block Substitution Matrix

Block substitution matrix (BLOSUM): The use of BLOSUM arises when we have to process a sample set of a protein that does not have similarities. BLOSUM is a list of sequences that are aligned with each other without any gap. There are many kinds of these. BLOSUM-62 means those matrices whose similarities between sequences are not greater than 62%, that's why BLOSUM-62 is a kind of middle ground and a commonly used matrix. Now here the question arises that which matrix to use and how we would rationalize a particular matrix. When you want to do sequence searching which is relatively divergent then you should go with number that comes from lower family and having lower percentage of similarities.

10.1.5 PMBEC: Peptide MHC Binding Energy Covariance Matrix

Peptide MHC binding energy covariance matrix (PMBEC) is an advanced version of SMM but different in that it scatters a peptide sequence coverage that is often found in binding datasets by using PMBEC. PMBEC matrix is defined on covariance values. When residues contribute similar to binding of free energy in the same environment, they have a positive covariance, whereas a negative covariance when no residue contributes.

10.2 Literature Review

Peters et al. (2006) talk about various methods that are already in place and are being used by various scientists to predict the peptide and MHC interaction. It clearly states that average relative binding (ARB) methods gave much better results than the general methods, possibly due to lack of sufficient training data for the general methods. On the other hand, Peters et al. (2006) talk about how the neural network-based general methods outperform matrix-based predictions mainly due to its ability to generalize even on a small amount of data, and the paper also retrieved predictions from tools publicly available on the internet. With the use of cell lines that express a single allele, Abelin et al. (2017) found out 16 different HLAs of class I with the help of an application-specific spectral search algorithm that includes training of neural network algorithm with large datasets.

Soria-Guerra et al. (2015) give us the tools for epitope prediction and vaccine development and also state how to make hypervariable vaccines. They give us a broader view of vaccine development and epitope-based vaccination. Sanchez-Trincado et al. (2017) describe that the immune system of body is controlled by B- and T-cells that develop pathogen-specific memory that protects our body. Basically, we analyze the aspects of T-antigen recognition of B-cell used in epitope prediction. T-cells CD4 and CD8 that are able to stimulate a shortest peptide within an antigen is the main function of T-cell epitope prediction. B-cell epitope prediction replaces the antigen for antibody production.

Koup and Douek (2011) state that T-cell vaccine is known to limit HIV and other virus infections. It also provides an overview of the methods that are used for T-cell vaccine approach and also shows the results on the future of T-cell vaccine research. Nielsen et al. (2007) describe the prediction of MHC class II with matrix alignment method and predict the MHC binding affinities with the help of SMM. The performance of prediction method using SMM is much superior to other methods such as Gibbs. Interactions of MHCs played a major role in the discovery of epitopes. In Zhang et al. (1992), MHC class I contains a single bounded peptide, and this paper describes its structure and preparation and also discusses peptide binding and T-cell receptor.

The paper by Liao and Arthur (2011) is based on the study that used Fresno semiempirical scoring function to predict peptide MHC binding using open-source software, and it is also shown that why we cannot use structure-based prediction methods. The performance of the method used is dependent on the crystal structure. Cochran and Stern (2000) describe the interaction of T-cell receptor. T-cell activation process is initiated by various MHC dimers, trimers, and tetramers that are bound to T-cell. It also concludes that T-cell receptors rearrange in the plane of the membrane concurrent with oligomer binding. Buus et al. (2003) talk about quantitative prediction of peptide MHC binding class I molecule with the help of artificial neural network (ANN), which trained for binding as well as nonbinding MHCs.

Wu et al. (2002) discuss about T cell receptor (TCR)-to-peptide MHC binding. This process is described on a physical basis by analyzing residues involved in both processes. He et al. (1999) describe that hepatitis C virus destroys liver and causes liver cell injury. Using two molecules, we are able to detect specific CD8$^+$ concentration in blood.

10.3 Methodology

A lot of work has been already done in vaccine or drug manufacturing field, but this chapter further tries to improve the way things work in the vaccine manufacturing process. This chapter is broadly based on two different branches that are not highly correlated to each other, and thus the methodology for each of the two branches has been explained separately. The first branch being the "life prediction" branch, where dataset from "The 10,000 Immunomes Project" is being processed based on its features, with "age" being the target variable.

The other branch that this chapter broadly talks about is the "MHC Binding Prediction" that deals with how a given amino acid sequence of a virus will bind with MHC of human body. Before beginning with the model-fitting part on the given data, one must understand that this chapter considers the default Inhibitory concentration (IC50) threshold to be 500 nm and the default sequence length as 9. So, for any given length of sequence, multiple smaller sequences each of length 9 will be extracted, i.e., a sequence like ABCDEFGHIJ will be broken into two parts—ABCDEFGHI and BCDEFGHIJ. This way, we make sure that no combination of peptides is left out. The second branch of this chapter takes only two inputs: first one is the MHC class, and the second one is the sequence that has to be tested for binding with the given MHC.

To make things as much user friendly as possible, this chapter has been further implemented using "shiny" package for R and has been deployed on Shiny Server for anyone to use.

Both the branches have been separately explained later, starting off straight from the dataset that we had beforehand and how we further moved ahead with it and came up with our results. It has been represented in the numbered-list format to make it more understandable. For life prediction, we apply the following data mining tasks:

1. Features: study_accession, age, gender, race, subject_accession, B_cells, CD16_neg_monocytes, CD16_pos_monocytes, CD4_T_cells, CD8_T_cells, Central_Memory_CD4_T_cells, Central_Memory_CD8_T_cells, Effector_CD4_T_cells, Effector_CD8_T_cells, Effector_Memory_CD4_T_cells, Effector_Memory_CD8_T_cells, Gamma_Delta_T_cells, Lymphocytes Memory_B_cells, Monocytes, Naive_B_cells, Naive_CD4_T_cells, Naive_CD8_T_cells, NK_cells, NKT_cells, Plasmablasts, T_cells, Transitional_B_cells, Tregs

2. Preprocessing: For the preprocessing part, all the useless features like subject_accession and study_accession were dropped from the imported data frame, since

they were not related to the target variable. Then, na.omit() function was used to remove all the rows that had "NA" values. Lastly, attributes "gender" and "race" were changed into factors of 1 and 2, where

$$\text{Gender}\left(1 = \text{Female}, 2 = \text{Male}\right)$$

$$\text{Race}\left(1 = \text{Asian}, 2 = \text{African or American}, 3 = \text{Others}, 4 = \text{White}\right)$$

What followed this factor conversion was the clustering of age attribute. Since age is our target variable and multiple values of age could lead to an underfit model, it was decided to cluster age with two centers. Two centers were created: 31.6 years and 73.44 years. Now we could classify people into two main groups—people who'll have a short life span that will be clustered around 31.6 years and people who will have a longer life span that will be clustered around 73.44 years.

Principal component Analysis (PCA) was applied on the given dataset, but that wasn't of much help since the attributes used were not correlated to each other—so the whole idea of applying PCA was later dropped.

3. Data split: createDataPartition() function was used to create a partition of data on the basis of age with 80% for training and 20% for testing.

4. Algorithms: Random forest: Random forest algorithm was used on a preprocessed dataset. The number of randomly sampled variables has been kept at 5, with the total number of trees being grown at 500. Five hundred trees were chosen, because leaving out any of the total attributes from the dataset would lead to poor results.

Support Vector Machine (SVM): SVM algorithm was applied on the dataset for getting a rough idea on how well the dataset will perform with other classifiers.

5. Results and accuracies: Random forest showed much better results with the testing dataset when compared with SVM. Confusion matrix from both the classifiers clearly shows that the accuracy for random forest comes at around 96.4%, and for SVM, it comes around 85.9% (Figures 10.12 and 10.13).

MHC binding prediction followed the following steps (Figure 10.1):

1. Features present in each dataset:
   a. Basic dataset (bdata.20130222.mhci.txt): species, mhc, peptide_length, sequences, inequality, bond length (meas).
   b. Dataset: SEQ_IQ, SEQ_PEPTIDE, SEQ_SEQUENCE, Residue, Pos, MHCs with binding energies (e.g. HLA A*0201).
   c. Aminopos: species, mhc, peptide_length, inequality, bond length (meas), binder, pos1,pos2, pos3, pos4, pos5, pos6, pos7, pos8, pos9.

2. Data preprocessing: For the preprocessing part, all MHCs that were part of the dataset were considered, since this combination of MHCs gives the best possible results, as shown by other researchers. Also, the values of bond length of each MHC taken were changed to numeric values, which were initially not a number.

For the Aminopos dataset, separate nine columns were added. Each of these represents the position of the amino acid given in the protein sequence of the corresponding sequence row. These columns are named from pos1 to pos9.

The sequence of length 9 was only taken and less than 9 was ignored.

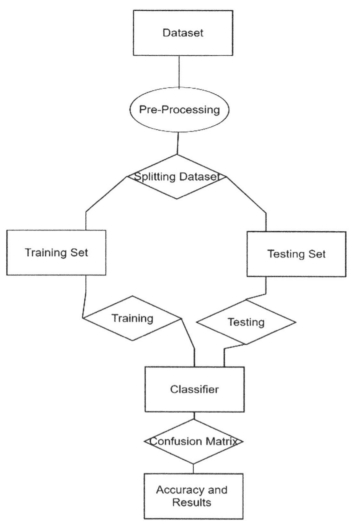

FIGURE 10.1
Explaining the life-prediction working model.

3. Training and testing: Three different training methods are implemented on these datasets: SMM, random forest, and naïve Bayes-based probability addition method. SMM matrix is a conventional prediction method that has been extensively used by researchers doing sequence analysis in this field. Random forest algorithm was applied on each MHC type from the Aminopos dataset, making it a group of random forest based trained model—with each position being a defining value and "binding" as a target variable. This ensured that each MHC is being given equal importance and none of the MHC is left out. Lastly, naïve Bayes-based probability addition method was used, which added up the probability of each sequence character for a given MHC and checked if the sum of probabilities was greater than 0.5 or not (0.5 being considered an average case here and can be changed as and

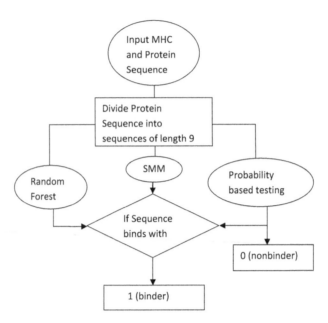

FIGURE 10.2
Flowgraph of a proposed algorithm.

when needed). If the sum for any sequence comes out to be greater than 0.5, it'll be considered a binding sequence, else not (Figure 10.2).

10.4 Technology Used

A detailed description of all techniques and algorithms used in the study is presented in this section. This section provides a brief summary of all the techniques deployed in the proposed work.

10.4.1 R Language

R is a language and environment for statistical computing and graphics. It is a GNU project that is similar to the S language and environment, which was developed at Bell Laboratories. It is being collaboratively developed by various developers from across the globe. The R project was first started in 1997 by Robert Gentleman and R Ihaka, both professors of the University of Auckland. As of today, R is one of the most powerful machine learning languages that is being used by industry giants and is even being provided by clouds-based programs to developers—International Business Machines Corporation (IBM) Watson being one of them.

10.4.2 Stabilized Matrix Method

As mentioned in the Introduction, SMM is neither an integrated part of R language nor one of the conventional machine learning algorithms. Thus, SMM is more of a new technology than an algorithm in itself. More on SMM can be found in Peters and Sette (2005).

10.4.3 IBM Watson

IBM Watson's Data platform Software as a Service (SaaS) has been extensively used throughout the implementation of this chapter due to its better computing abilities and easier graphical user interface (GUI). Further implementation of this chapter on the Shiny Server has been done using IBM Watson, and the heavy computing parts like data preprocessing for MHC binding prediction have been done on IBM Watson.

10.4.4 Shiny Apps Server

Shiny Apps Server has been used to host the web application online on https://arjunchauhan24.shinyapps.io/mhc_binding_analysis/.

10.5 Results

Numerous experiments are conducted to find out the length of bond between the epitope and MHC, and hence assist vaccine developers to gain a better understanding of how various unique virus protein sequences actually interact with human body. For the same, we have implemented two Machine Learning (ML) algorithms, where the output of the developed web interface is presented in the form of screenshots.

In Figure 10.3, it can be seen that a new csv file is created, which would be used to create models for random forest algorithm. Here, every amino acid in the sequence is put in the column corresponding to its position (Figure 10.4).

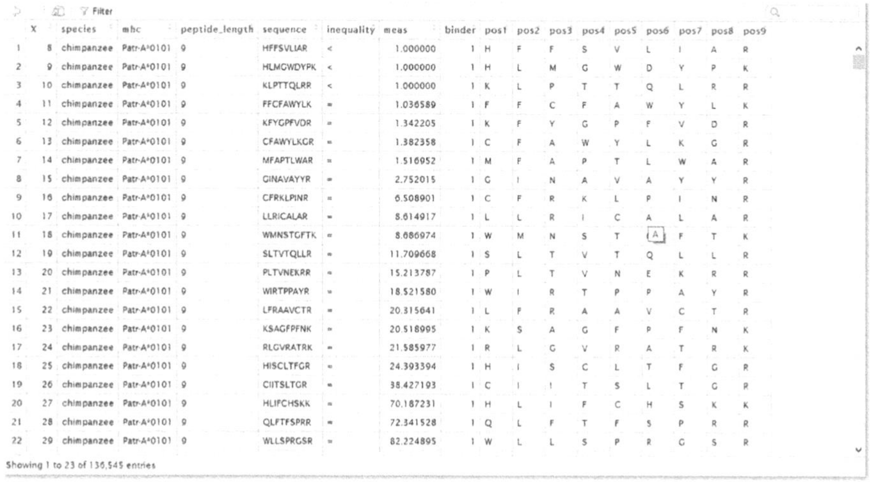

	X	species	mhc	peptide_length	sequence	inequality	meas	binder	pos1	pos2	pos3	pos4	pos5	pos6	pos7	pos8	pos9
1	8	chimpanzee	Patr-A*0101	9	HFFSVLIAR	<	1.000000	1	H	F	F	S	V	L	I	A	R
2	9	chimpanzee	Patr-A*0101	9	HLMGWDYPK	<	1.000000	1	H	L	M	G	W	D	Y	P	K
3	10	chimpanzee	Patr-A*0101	9	KLPTTQLRR	<	1.000000	1	K	L	P	T	T	Q	L	R	R
4	11	chimpanzee	Patr-A*0101	9	FFCFAWYLK	=	1.036589	1	F	F	C	F	A	W	Y	L	K
5	12	chimpanzee	Patr-A*0101	9	KFYGPFVDR	=	1.342205	1	K	F	Y	G	P	F	V	D	R
6	13	chimpanzee	Patr-A*0101	9	CFAWYLKGR	=	1.382358	1	C	F	A	W	Y	L	K	G	R
7	14	chimpanzee	Patr-A*0101	9	MFAPTLWAR	=	1.516952	1	M	F	A	P	T	L	W	A	R
8	15	chimpanzee	Patr-A*0101	9	GINAVAYYR	=	2.752015	1	G	I	N	A	V	A	Y	Y	R
9	16	chimpanzee	Patr-A*0101	9	CFRKLPINR	=	6.508901	1	C	F	R	K	L	P	I	N	R
10	17	chimpanzee	Patr-A*0101	9	LLRICALAR	=	8.614917	1	L	L	R	I	C	A	L	A	R
11	18	chimpanzee	Patr-A*0101	9	WMNSTGFTK	=	8.686974	1	W	M	N	S	T	[A]	F	T	K
12	19	chimpanzee	Patr-A*0101	9	SLTVTQLLR	=	11.709668	1	S	L	T	V	T	Q	L	L	R
13	20	chimpanzee	Patr-A*0101	9	PLTVNEKRR	=	15.213787	1	P	L	T	V	N	E	K	R	R
14	21	chimpanzee	Patr-A*0101	9	WIRTPPAYR	=	18.521580	1	W	I	R	T	P	P	A	Y	R
15	22	chimpanzee	Patr-A*0101	9	LFRAAVCTR	=	20.315641	1	L	F	R	A	A	V	C	T	R
16	23	chimpanzee	Patr-A*0101	9	KSAGFPFNK	=	20.518905	1	K	S	A	G	F	P	F	N	K
17	24	chimpanzee	Patr-A*0101	9	RLGVRATRK	=	21.585977	1	R	L	G	V	R	A	T	R	K
18	25	chimpanzee	Patr-A*0101	9	HISCLTFGR	=	24.393394	1	H	I	S	C	L	T	F	G	R
19	26	chimpanzee	Patr-A*0101	9	CIITSLTGR	=	38.427193	1	C	I	I	T	S	L	T	G	R
20	27	chimpanzee	Patr-A*0101	9	HLIFCHSKK	=	70.187231	1	H	L	I	F	C	H	S	K	K
21	28	chimpanzee	Patr-A*0101	9	QLFTFSPRR	=	72.341528	1	Q	L	F	T	F	S	P	R	R
22	29	chimpanzee	Patr-A*0101	9	WLLSPRGSR	=	82.224895	1	W	L	L	S	P	R	G	S	R

Showing 1 to 23 of 136,545 entries

FIGURE 10.3
Aminopos created using Generate Data.

```
Console C:/Users/Ayush Srivastava/Desktop/Minor/
[1] "training for HLA-B*15:03"
[1] "training for HLA-B*15:09"
[1] "training for HLA-B*15:17"
[1] "training for HLA-B*15:42"
[1] "training for HLA-B*18:01"
[1] "training for HLA-B*27:01"
[1] "training for HLA-B*27:05"
[1] "training for HLA-B*27:20"
[1] "training for HLA-B*35:01"
[1] "training for HLA-B*35:03"
[1] "training for HLA-B*37:01"
[1] "training for HLA-B*38:01"
[1] "training for HLA-B*39:01"
[1] "training for HLA-B*40:01"
```

FIGURE 10.4
Training different models for MHCs.

In Figure 10.5, it can be seen that the accuracy of different MHCs is in the range of 70%–74.50%.

The predicted object for HLA101 can be seen in Figure 10.6. It can be seen from this that the class variable is a binder with a value 0 or 1, where 0 means that the MHC and the sequence will not bind and 1 means that the MHC and sequence will bind.

Accuracy from probability method can be found to be 73.06%, as shown in Figure 10.7.

In Figure 10.8, it can be seen that protein sequences from hepatitis C virus are being tested through our program. The sequence is broken into sequences of length 9 and then tested for its binding capability.

In Figure 10.9, it can be seen that the program has returned the sequences of proteins that will bind with the given MHC. Out of 183 sequences, 28 were selected by random forest for binding and 12 were selected by SMM for the same (Figures 10.10–10.13).

```
Console C:/Users/Ayush Srivastava/Desktop/Minor/
[1] "predicting for HLA-B*44:02"
[1] "accuracy is : 72.948764413938"
[1] "predicting for HLA-B*44:03"
[1] "accuracy is : 70.298915841657"
[1] "predicting for HLA-B*45:01"
[1] "accuracy is : 71.780872248962"
[1] "predicting for HLA-B*45:06"
[1] "accuracy is : 73.9916040394551"
[1] "predicting for HLA-B*46:01"
[1] "accuracy is : 74.5094701315234"
[1] "predicting for HLA-B*48:01"
[1] "accuracy is : 73.5618898982612"
[1] "predicting for HLA-B*51:01"
```

FIGURE 10.5
Random forest fitting models for different MHCs.

```
Console C:/Users/Ayush Srivastava/Desktop/Minor/

3122 samples
   9 predictor
   2 classes: '0', '1'

No pre-processing
Resampling: Bootstrapped (25 reps)
Summary of sample sizes: 3122, 3122, 3122, 3122, 3122, 3122, ...
Resampling results across tuning parameters:

  mtry  Accuracy   Kappa
  2     0.8963823  0.6123065
  5     0.8944585  0.6159183
  9     0.8857639  0.5876089
```

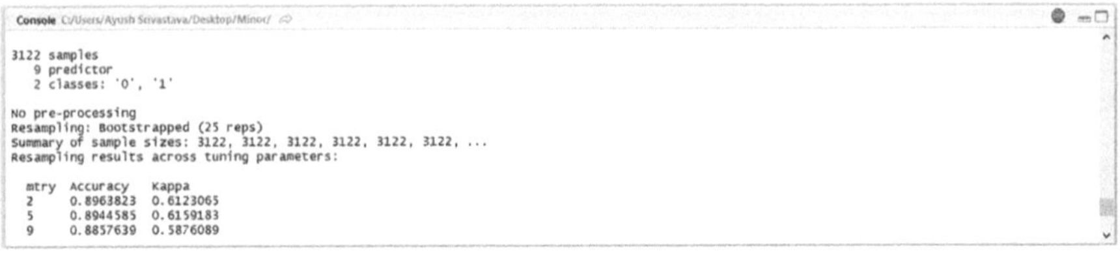

FIGURE 10.6
Accuracy for hlaA101.

```
Console C:/Users/Ayush Srivastava/Desktop/Minor/
> setwd("C:/Users/Ayush Srivastava/Desktop/Minor")
> source("main.R")
> main()
[1] "accuracy is: 0.730662174040434"
      [,1]  [,2]
[1,]  300 19650
[2,]  467  6887
```

FIGURE 10.7
Accuracy and confusion matrix using probability method.

```
Console C:/Users/Ayush Srivastava/Desktop/Minor/
[1] "testing for AQPGYPWPL"
[1] 78
[1] "testing for QPGYPWPLY"
[1] 79
[1] "testing for PGYPWPLYG"
[1] 80
[1] "testing for GYPWPLYGN"
[1] 81
[1] "testing for YPWPLYGNE"
[1] 82
[1] "testing for PWPLYGNEG"
[1] 83
[1] "testing for WPLYGNEGC"
```

FIGURE 10.8
All methods tested for a given organism.

```
Console C:/Users/Ayush Srivastava/Desktop/Minor/
[1] 176
[1] "testing for IFLLALLSC"
[1] 177
[1] "testing for FLLALLSCL"
[1] 178
[1] "testing for LLALLSCLT"
[1] 179
[1] "testing for LALLSCLTV"
[1] 180
[1] "testing for ALLSCLTVP"
[1] 181
[1] "testing for LLSCLTVPA"
[1] 182
[1] "testing for LSCLTVPAS"
[1] 183
[1] "testing for SCLTVPASA"
[1] "from smm"
     peptide
1   GQIVGGVYL
2   QIVGGVYLL
3   AQPGYPWPL
4   NLGKVIDTL
5   TLTCGFADL
6   DLMGYIPLV
7   YIPLVGAPL
8   ALAHGVRVL
9   VLEDGVNYA
10  NLPGCSFSI
11  FLLALLSCL
12  LLSCLTVPA
[1] "from random forest"
 [1] "PQDVKFPGG" "GQIVGGVYL" "QIVGGVYLL" "LLPRRGPRL" "AQPGYPWPL" "PLYGNEGCG" "GCGWAGWLL" "LLSPRGSRP" "NLGKVIDTL"
[10] "KVIDTLTCG" "TLTCGFADL" "TCGFADLMG" "GFADLMGYI" "DLMGYIPLV" "LMGYIPLVG" "YIPLVGAPL" "PLVGAPLGG" "PLGGAARAL"
[19] "ALAHGVRVL" "GVRVLEDGV" "VLEDGVNYA" "NLPGCSFSI" "GCSFSIFLL" "FLLALLSCL" "LLALLSCLT" "ALLSCLTVP" "LLSCLTVPA"
[28] "SCLTVPASA"
>
```

FIGURE 10.9
Results from different algorithms.

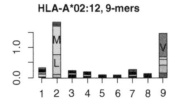

FIGURE 10.10
Binding of amino acid at different positions for HLA-A*02:12.

```
Console ~/ ⌂
Error in view(tab) : could not find function "view"
> tab
x
                        age                              B_cells
                          1                                    1
        CD16_neg_monocytes              CD16_pos_monocytes
                          1                                    1
                 CD4_T_cells                          CD8_T_cells
                          1                                    1
  Central_Memory_CD4_T_cells   Central_Memory_CD8_T_cells
                          1                                    1
          Effector_CD4_T_cells             Effector_CD8_T_cells
                          1                                    1
 Effector_Memory_CD4_T_cells  Effector_Memory_CD8_T_cells
                          1                                    1
          Gamma_Delta_T_cells                            gender
                          1                                    1
 Lymphocytes\tMemory_B_cells                         Monocytes
                          1                                    1
               Naive_B_cells              Naive_CD4_T_cells
                          1                                    1
           Naive_CD8_T_cells                          NK_cells
                          1                                    1
                  NKT_cells                        Plasmablasts
                          1                                    1
                       race               subject_accession
                          1                                    1
                    T_cells            Transitional_B_cells
                          1                                    1
                      Tregs               study_accession
                          1                                    1
```

FIGURE 10.11
Feature list of all features of the life-prediction dataset.

>cm

	1	2
1	40	7
2	5	55

FIGURE 10.12
Confusion matrix 1 for random forest on life prediction analysis.

>cm2
  y_pred2

	1	2
1	36	11
2	4	56

FIGURE 10.13
Confusion matrix 2 for SVM on life prediction analysis.

10.6 Conclusion and Future Scope

The evolution of modern medicine has led to the evolution of disease-causing microorganisms. This evolution is taking place at a very rapid rate, and so to keep up with it, traditional ways of creating vaccines cannot be depended on as they are rather slow. Computational methods are a better way as they can provide results in a short time, thereby enhancing the speed of traditional methods.

In this project, we have created an app that takes in MHC and protein sequence of the microorganism and returns the protein sequence that can be used to create vaccines with satisfactory accuracy.

The project has a vast future scope, simply starting from basic quality of life indicators straight to drug prediction. The "life-prediction" program can be more generically used to indicate how well a person is performing and how long he/she is expected to live under the given circumstances. Since life prediction is not an easy task, it just cannot be quantized to something that only depends on all blood-related features. So, more work can be put into finding other features from other medical tests that can be linked to something as important as life expectancy. In its current state, it can just be considered as a good metric of how healthy a person is and not as an accurate life-expectancy measuring tool.

The "epitope and major histocompatibility complex binding" program can be separately used by various drug manufacturing companies all across the globe to find out how any amino acid sequence of any virus will interact with various human MHCs. With this knowledge, they can make drugs in a more quicker and effective way than ever before. The program reduces the laboratory work of manually checking how each amino acid sequence will interact with human MHCs. For the future scope, the current program can be trained with better machine learning algorithms that can give better accuracies.

References

Abelin, J. G., Keskin, D. B., Sarkizova, S., Hartigan, C. R., Zhang, W., Sidney, J., … Clauser, K. R. (2017). Mass spectrometry profiling of HLA-associated peptidomes in mono-allelic cells enables more accurate epitope prediction. *Immunity*, 46(2), 315–326.

Buus, S., Lauemøller, S. L., Worning, P., Kesmir, C., Frimurer, T., Corbet, S., … Brunak, S. (2003). Sensitive quantitative predictions of peptide-MHC binding by a 'Query by Committee' artificial neural network approach. *Tissue Antigens*, 62(5), 378–384.

Cochran, J. R., & Stern, L. J. (2000). A diverse set of oligomeric class II MHC-peptide complexes for probing T-cell receptor interactions. *Chemistry & Biology*, 7(9), 683–696.

He, X. S., Rehermann, B., López-Labrador, F. X., Boisvert, J., Cheung, R., Mumm, J., … Greenberg, H. B. (1999). Quantitative analysis of hepatitis C virus-specific CD8+ T cells in peripheral blood and liver using peptide-MHC tetramers. *Proceedings of the National Academy of Sciences*, 96(10), 5692–5697.

Koup, R. A., & Douek, D. C. (2011). Vaccine design for CD8 T lymphocyte responses. *Cold Spring Harbor Perspectives in Medicine*, 1(1), a007252.

Liao, W. W., & Arthur, J. W. (2011). Predicting peptide binding affinities to MHC molecules using a modified semi-empirical scoring function. *PLoS One*, 6(9), e25055.

Nielsen, M., Lundegaard, C., & Lund, O. (2007). Prediction of MHC class II binding affinity using SMM-align, a novel stabilization matrix alignment method. *BMC Bioinformatics*, 8(1), 238.

Peters, B., Bui, H. H., Frankild, S., Nielsen, M., Lundegaard, C., Kostem, E., ... Wilson, S. S. (2006). A community resource benchmarking predictions of peptide binding to MHC-I molecules. *PLoS Computational Biology*, 2(6), e65.

Peters, B., & Sette, A. (2005). Generating quantitative models describing the sequence specificity of biological processes with the stabilized matrix method. *BMC Bioinformatics*, 6(1), 132.

R-Project. https://www.r-project.org/about.html.

Sanchez-Trincado, J. L., Gomez-Perosanz, M., & Reche, P. A. (2017). Fundamentals and Methods for T-and B-Cell Epitope Prediction. *Journal of Immunology Research*, 2017. doi: 10.1155/2017/2680160.

Soria-Guerra, R. E., Nieto-Gomez, R., Govea-Alonso, D. O., & Rosales-Mendoza, S. (2015). An overview of bioinformatics tools for epitope prediction: implications on vaccine development. *Journal of Biomedical Informatics*, 53, 405–414.

Wu, L. C., Tuot, D. S., Lyons, D. S., Garcia, K. C., & Davis, M. M. (2002). Two-step binding mechanism for T-cell receptor recognition of peptide–MHC. *Nature*, 418(6897), 552.

Zhang, W., Young, A. C., Imarai, M., Nathenson, S. G., & Sacchettini, J. C. (1992). Crystal structure of the major histocompatibility complex class I H-2Kb molecule containing a single viral peptide: Implications for peptide binding and T-cell receptor recognition. *Proceedings of the National Academy of Sciences*, 89(17), 8403–8407.

11

Partial Digest Problem

Urvi Agarwal, Sanchi Prakash, Harshit Agarwal,
Prantik Biswas, Suma Dawn, and Aparajita Nanda
Jaypee Institute of Information Technology

CONTENTS

11.1 Introduction: Background and Driving Forces

Partial Digest Problem, commonly addressed via its abbreviation "PDP," came into existence long back in 1930, when it first appeared in the field of X-ray crystallography (Patterson, 1935). Later, various techniques belonging to different domains of computer science have been proposed to solve PDP, but all have their own pros and cons. In 1970, Hamilton Smith, an American microbiologist discovered the fact that enzymes cleave a particular Deoxyribonucleic Acid molecule at each occurrence of a distinct sequence (Jones et al., 2004). The locations of these cuts are commonly referred to as restriction sites. The restriction site mapping, which will be elaborated further in this chapter, is a salient application of PDP (Bellon, 1988; Stefik, 1978). A digest experiment in biology is a way of preparing the DNA for processing. Two of the widely known variants of the digest experiments are (i) Complete Digest and (ii) Partial Digest. The Complete Digest problem considers the distance between consecutive sites, whereas PDP observes the distance of each pair of restriction site. Gel electrophoresis technique helps find the distances between every pair of restriction site that acts as the building block for reconstruction of DNA. PDP has many applications in computational biology, like DNA cloning, DNA sequencing (Baker, 2011), and genome cloning (Dear, 2001).

11.2 The Partial Digest Problem

A brief overview of PDP is provided in the earlier section. To provide a better understanding of PDP, we describe it thoroughly in this section. We begin with defining a multiset L that contains pairwise distances between any two restriction sites. These distances can be found using gel electrophoresis, in which the DNA fragments resulting from partial digest experiment are moved through an electric field. The smaller the fragment, the more distance it would be able to travel through the field. This gives the lengths of different DNA fragments; pairwise distances can be inferred from these lengths (Figure 11.1). For example, $L = \{1, 2, 3, 4, 7, 9, 10, 11, 13, 14\}$. Restoring the set X containing original values of restriction sites from L is the PDP. This set is vital for performing restriction site mapping (Bellon, 1988; Błażewicz et al., 2001; Hall, 1956), which can be interpreted as a process for studying extremely long DNA sequences, which otherwise becomes rather exhaustive. Restriction maps are used for further significant biological techniques like DNA manipulation, comparing the DNA of different species and determining gene order (Bellon, 1988; Stefik, 1978; He et al., 2015). Restriction mapping can be used for both long and short DNA sequences (Fitch et al., 1983; Rhee, 1988; Dear, 2001; Narayanan, 2006).

A DNA molecule's composition includes four nucleotides: adenine (A), thymine (T), cytosine (C), and guanine (G). Extensive research on the genome through many years has given major contributions. For example, the complete DNA sequence of the human genome is available as a free resource (Pääbo, 2001). Even after such developments, studying individual DNA molecules is an impractical task, and thus there exist several biological techniques that supply the information about restriction sites. Partial Digest, Double Digest (Sur-Kolay et al., 2009; Ganjtabesh et al., 2012), and Shotgun Sequencing (Venter et al., 1998) are some unique examples of such technique. Partial Digest itself has many classes:

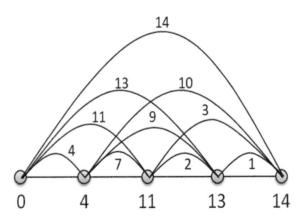

FIGURE 11.1
Representation of pairwise distances.

Simplified Partial Digest (Blazewicz et al., 2007), Labeled Partial Digest (Pandurangan and Ramesh, 2002), and Probed Partial Digest (Karp and Newberg, 1995; Newberg and Naor, 1993) to name a few. Many more problems include various kinds of difference sets. A detailed survey was given by Hall (1956). Our focus is on the Partial Digest technique. A restriction enzyme, when added to a DNA solution, cuts the DNA at specific positions. This results in DNA fragments of all possible distances between restriction sites. Obtaining the original set X containing the restriction sites requires considerable brainstorming, which makes the PDP an engaging problem, and no doubt, it has gained worldwide attention. An analogy to PDP exists in the sphere of computer science, known as the turnpike problem (Dakic, 2000), which is also an extensively researched topic. Another similar problem is the beltway problem that considers these locations as placed in a loop (Fomin, 2018). The inverse problem of Partial Digest is often referred as Chord's Problem (Daurat et al., 2005).

The hardness of PDP is a subject of wide discussion since it is an open problem, and no concrete answer is provided to it yet. In addition to this, no algorithm is able to solve the PDP in polynomial time, increasing the curiosity of researchers. We have a limited knowledge about the problem set X, which includes the number of elements n, that will certainly be equal to positive root of the equation $^nC_2 = k$, where k represents the number of elements of set L. This could be alternatively understood such that if the set X has n elements, L will contain $n(n-1)/2$ cardinality. Methods to acquire the solutions of PDP require an exhaustive search, and as a result, many of the existing algorithms for PDP have exponential running time.

If the restriction sites are {0, 4, 11, 13, 14, 24, 25}, set L can be visualized as shown in Figure 11.2, since the pairwise distances between each number is required, a matrix-based representation would be convenient. As can be seen from Figure 11.1, distances between every pair are calculated and $L = \{1, 1, 2, 3, 4, 7, 9, 10, 10, 11, 11, 11, 12, 13, 13, 14, 14, 20, 21, 24, 25\}$. PDP requires obtaining the set X from set L. Computationally, there exist more than one result to this set L that are $X_1 = \{0, 4, 11, 13, 14, 24, 25\}$ and $X_2 = \{0, 1, 11, 12, 14, 21, 25\}$. When their respective pairwise distance sets are obtained, both of them are equivalent to L (shown in Figures 11.2 and 11.3). The situations that result in more than one solution sets are usual, and the resultant sets are referred to as homometric sets (Bullough, 1961).

Notations: Further, in this chapter, we name the difference set as L and solution set as X. The difference set L, which will be provided as input, is represented as $(l_1, l_2, l_3...l_k)$. The highest element of set L is often referred to as the width of the set. Complement of an element l_i means the element with which the sum of l_i results in a width of L. The solution sets are represented as $X = (x_1, x_2... x_n)$.

	0	4	11	13	14	24	25
0		4	11	13	14	24	25
4			7	9	10	20	21
11				2	3	13	14
13					1	11	12
14						10	11
24							1
25							

FIGURE 11.2
Homometric set 1.

	0	1	11	12	14	21	25
0		1	11	12	14	21	25
1			10	11	13	20	24
11				1	3	10	14
12					2	9	13
14						7	11
21							4
25							

FIGURE 11.3
Homometric set 2.

11.3 Datasets

The problem defined earlier is given a set L, and we need to find a point set X such that pairwise amongst them is equal to elements in L. The algorithms for PDP need to deal with different kinds of dataset possessing certain properties. There exist ideal datasets, simulated datasets, erroneous data, and Zhang datasets. The ideal and simulated datasets, as one can infer from their names, refer to original and computationally generated instances, respectively. Erroneous data means the datasets that either lack some of the distances or include some extra distances occurring because of experimental errors (Dix and Kieronska, 1988). In real world, it is impossible to obtain ideal or error-free data for PDP. Cieliebak and Eidenbenz, through their work, proved that PDP is NP-hard where NP stands for Nondeterministic Polynomial time for cases of erroneous data (Cieliebak and Eidenbenz, 2004). Based on the kind of error that can occur while performing the experiment, Cieliebak classified the problems into Min Partial Digest Superset, t-Partial Digest Superset, Max Partial Digest Subset, Partial Digest with Additive Errors, and Partial Digest with Relative Error. For each of the class, he has provided appropriate proof about the hardness of the problem. The Min Partial Digest Superset is concluded as NP-hard, and the maximization problem Max Partial Digest Subset as hard to approximate. Cieliebak and Eidenbenz (2004) also show that PDP is strongly NP-complete for cases where all measurements are prone to the same additive or multiplicative error. Many algorithms work by incorporating cases of false omissions or additions in input data and run perfectly for both ideal as well as erroneous data.

There also exist hard instances of data for which algorithms take exponential time to obtain the results. These cases were introduced by Zhang in 1994 and are popularly known as Zhang datasets (Zhang, 1994). These datasets are worst case instances, because groups of elements of the original set for these are in arithmetic progression. Conclusively, the resultant difference set consists of largely similar values. This many equal values mislead the algorithm and hence the exponential time. An example is L = {42, 42, 42, 42, 84, 84, 84, 126, 126, 4,748, 4,790, 4,832, 4,832, 4,874, 4,874, 4,874, 4,916, 4,916, 4,958, 4,958, 5,000}. Solutions to the given set are as follows: {{0, 42, 84, 126, 4,874, 4,958, 5,000}, {0, 42, 126, 4,874, 4,916, 4,958, 5,000}}.

11.4 Existing Approaches

PDP is an arduous problem, and as a result, a widely studied and well -researched topic. As PDP is a problem with high combinatorial bounds, researchers strive hard to determine solutions for it. Because of the advances in technology and easier access to genome sequence, there have been significant developments in the techniques for PDP. Despite encouraging progress in algorithms for PDP, it remains a complex challenge for scientists and biologists. All the algorithms present result in at least one solution, but all of them either provide the solutions correctly and take large chunks of time to solve it or fail to provide appropriate solutions.

The algorithms proposed for this topic range from brute force to latest technologies. Over time, several modifications have been made in the already existing algorithms to improve their performance. In parallel, new algorithms with optimized performance have been proposed. Here, we provide a detailed analysis of some of the most prominent algorithms for solving PDP. Some of the prominent works include a pseudopolynomial time algorithm by Lekme and Werman (1988), a backtracking algorithm by Skiena and Sundaram (1994), and a semidefinite programming-based approach by Dakic (2000), optimizing the present algorithm using breadth first search by Abbas and Bahig (2016), a genetic algorithm (Ahrabian et al., 2013) and an algorithm based on multicore systems (Bahig et al., 2017). All the algorithms discussed have their own advantages and disadvantages. We have described some of these in a chronological fashion in the following sections, and more optimized algorithms are presented as one moves further through the sections. Before diving into these algorithms, one must be thorough and clear with all the concepts of PDP. These algorithms use diverse and complex tools to solve the problem, and therefore, an incomplete understanding of PDP would not help in evaluating them.

11.4.1 Naïve Algorithm

The brute force or naïve approach to PDP is an exhaustive search technique. Knowing the difference set L, we infer the highest element that exists and also the size of solution set X. The algorithm randomly picks up $n-2$ elements (irrespective of elements present in set L) lesser than the highest element. The pairwise distances of the elements in X create a difference set S. Resulting set X is the required solution if the difference set S matches L. The same function repeats until the complete search space is traversed. The algorithm results into all possible solutions for the given problem set L. The pseudocode for this algorithm is given later.

A major setback of brute force algorithm is the time complexity of the algorithm. While searching for solutions, it traverses all $^nC_2$ combinations, and thus, usually, takes excessive time to obtain all solutions.

11.4.1.1 Pseudocode—Naïve Algorithm

1. *Naïve_Algorithm* (L, n):
2. l_k <- width
3. **for**[1] all the randomly selected set of $(n-2)$ numbers less than l_k
4. X <- {0, set of numbers, l_k}
5. Calculate difference set S for X

---

[1] Bold signifies the use of keywords.

6. **if** S is same as L
7. **return** the solution set X

11.4.2 Improved Naïve Algorithm

In brute force algorithm, elements were picked irrespective of being present in the set L. While computing pairwise differences, difference of each element with 0 must have been calculated, and therefore, it can be concluded that X will be a subset of L. An improved brute force algorithm for PDP optimizes the earlier algorithm to some extent by only considering elements that occur in L. In basic terms, the algorithm works by picking exhaustive subsets of cardinality $n - 2$ (since 0 and width are obvious elements of solution) from input set L. If the calculated differences of each pair of numbers from any subset matches with all the elements of set L, that particular subset becomes one of the solutions for the given input. Pseudocode for the same can be found later.

11.4.2.1 Pseudocode—Improved Naïve Algorithm

1. *Improved_ Naïve _Algorithm* (L, n)
2. M <- width
3. **for** every randomly selected set of $(n - 2)$ numbers from set L
4. X <- $\{0, x_2, ..., x_{n-1}, M\}$
5. Calculate difference set S from X
6. **if** S is same as L
7. **return** the solution set X
8. output "no solution"

Even though the new algorithm improves the running time of brute force significantly by only selecting elements that are in set L, it is still impractical for applications in the real world. Large sizes of input set result in worse algorithmic complexity.

11.4.3 Branch-and-Bound Algorithm

Branch and bound refers to a class of algorithm that is used for optimally solving combinatorial problems. This algorithm does the same by forming a set X and adding elements to it if they satisfy certain conditions. As seen in both of the earlier exhaustive searches, every element selected is independent of the previously added elements. This algorithm focuses on examining the previously added elements before adding a new element to the solution set. Initially, a set X with only element 0 is declared. We proceed by adding the width of set L to X and remove it from L. Taking the present highest element from set L, check whether its pairwise distances with elements of X exist in X. If they do, then the particular element is added to set X and the algorithm proceeds by repeating the steps until L is empty. If they don't, then the next highest element is selected and the earlier steps are repeated.

11.4.3.1 Pseudocode—Branch-and-Bound Algorithm

1. Solution set **X** = $\{0\}$
2. Find width in **L** and place it in **X**, **X** = $\{0, width\}$
3. Check **if** the pairwise differences of the element selected with X_i exists in **L**
4. When it does, remove the distances calculated from **L**
Repeat until **L** is empty.

Running time by using this technique is optimized to a limit, but this algorithm does not always lead to required answers, and even in the cases in which it does, it is only able to provide one solution set. Thus, this algorithm fails to provide homometric results.

11.4.4 Skiena's Backtracking Algorithm

In 1994, Skiena and Sundaram (1994) devised a practical algorithm that solved PDP in a limited bound of time. He used the earlier approach along with backtracking to produce all results, which optimized the running time by a considerable amount. This algorithm aims at finding all solutions by exploiting all possible paths in the search space tree using depth first search and backtracks if it produces the results or there is no branch left. Starting with eliminating the width of set L and adding it to the solution set X, this algorithm further evaluates the following condition. If $L = \{1, 1, 2, 3, 4, 7, 9, 10, 10, 11, 11, 11, 12, 13, 13, 14, 14, 20, 21, 24, 25\}$, we remove 25 from L and append it to X. Now, the highest element from L is picked and its difference with the elements of X is calculated. In case of the mentioned example, 24 is selected. If each of the resulting differences appears in L, the element is added to the solution set X, and the differences mentioned earlier are removed from L. Elements 1 and 24 are removed from L, and 24 is added to the set X. If the element fails to comply, its complement is processed through the same conditions if it exists in L; otherwise, the next highest element is evaluated. If the complement fulfils the condition, its differences are removed from L and the element is added to X. While performing these steps, 20 does not comply, and the next highest (i.e., 14) is evaluated. The algorithm backtracks if the condition is not satisfied by either of the element and its complement if one exists. This process is repeated until the cardinality (n) of solution set X satisfies the constraint $^nC_2 = k$, where k is the number of elements in L. The resulting set X thus will be the required solution. The pseudocode of the Skiena algorithm (Agarwal et al., 2018) is provided later as Pseudocode 4.

One more important conclusion that Skiena derived was about the number of solutions for a certain dataset. According to this, there is an upper bound to the number of solutions that can be obtained for a particular dataset. This bound being $\frac{1}{2}n^{1.2324827}$, which means the solutions to the set L with n elements will always be less than or equal to $\frac{1}{2}n^{1.2324827}$ (Lemke et al., 2003; Bannai et al., 1983; Agarwal et al., 1989). Also, in case of the cardinality of set L reaching infinity, there is a lower bound, i.e., the solutions to a set L with n elements will always be greater than or equal to $\frac{1}{2}n^{0.8107144}$ (Lemke et al., 2003). These results are of importance, as they can help reduce the time taken by algorithm for some cases.

There were limited drawbacks to this algorithm, until someone proved that this particular algorithm takes exponential running time for some instances of input. Zhang (1994), through his research, generated such datasets for which the algorithmic complexity of Skiena's algorithm (Skiena and Sundaram, 1994) became exponential. These datasets are popularly known as Zhang datasets or hard instances of data. Skiena's algorithm fails for these datasets, as they lead to wrong directions resulting in excessive backtracking.

11.4.4.1 Pseudocode—Skiena's Backtracking Algorithm

INPUT: L (pairwise distances set)
OUTPUT: all possible solution set X whose pairwise distances corresponds to L.

1. *place (L,X)*
2. y = **max** (L)
3. **if (**y-X$_i$**) in** L
4. add y in X
5. **for** i **in** (0,len(X))
6.   remove (y-X$_i$) from L
7. *place (L, X)*
8. remove y from X
9. **for** i **in** (0, len(X))
10.   add (y-X$_i$) in L
11. comp = width-y
12. **if abs**(comp-X$_i$) **in** L
13. add comp in X
14. **for** i **in** (0,len(X))
15.   remove **abs**(comp-X$_i$) from L
16. *place (L,X)*
17. remove comp from X
18. **for** i **in**(0,len(X))
19.   add **abs** (comp-X$_i$) from L
20. **return**

11.4.5 Modern PDP Algorithms

With the surge in technology and its ease of use, researchers are gaining motivation to use a wide variety of tools for solving problems of computational biology. Here, we discuss two modern algorithms that have improved the running time of Skiena's algorithm (Skiena and Sundaram, 1994) with the help of breadth first search. These algorithms provide results for Zhang data (Zhang, 1994) with accuracy and minimal time.

11.4.5.1 The Breadth First Search Algorithm

Prior to the mentioned algorithm (Abbas and Bahig, 2016), Depth First Search was widely used to solve PDP. This algorithm shifts our focus to Breadth First Search, as it reduces the time complexity. For instance, L = {42, 42, 42, 42, 84, 84, 84, 126, 126, 4,748, 4,790, 4,832, 4,832, 4,874, 4,874, 4,874, 4,916, 4,916, 4,958, 4,958, 5,000}. We begin with initializing an auxiliary set X with 0 width, deleting width from L. A copy of the resultant L is made in L$_1$. After that, we pick the highest element and its complement simultaneously for further evaluation. In the mentioned example, 4,958 and 42 are selected, and their difference with each element present in auxiliary X is calculated. If all these differences exist in auxiliary set L$_1$, the corresponding element is added to auxiliary set X, and the differences are removed from auxiliary L$_1$. Each step leads to two subbranches that run simultaneously, as shown in Figure 11.4. These steps are repeated until L$_1$ becomes empty. This algorithm improves at a point where the two simultaneous branches have exactly the same auxiliary L and auxiliary X. Then, one of these branches is terminated to stop repetition of further steps, which reduces the search space tree. In Figure 11.4, the red bold crosses depict the earlier condition. After the insertion of 4,958 in one of the branches, when 42 enters, we get similar auxiliary L and auxiliary X to those of the other branch, i.e., where 4,958 is inserted after 42. Either of the two branches is terminated.

The pseudocode for the algorithm is given by Abbas and Bahig (2016) later.

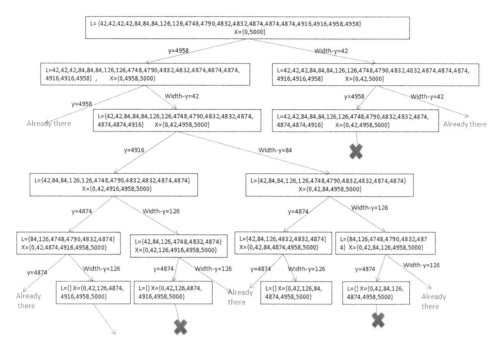

FIGURE 11.4
Working of BFS algorithm.

11.4.5.1.1 Pseudocode—The Utility Function

BEGIN
1. Initialize the set S with empty
2. Delete the maximum element from the set L and assign it to the element width
3. Assign the set (0, width) to the set X
4. Add the set L to the list L_1
5. Add the set X to the list Aux_X
6. **while** the list L_1 is not empty do:
7.   *GenerateNextLevel* (L_1, Aux_X, S)
8. **end while**
END

11.4.5.1.2 Pseudocode—Generate_Next_Level Function

Procedure Generate_Next_Level (L_1, Aux_X, S)
BEGIN
1. Initialize the auxiliary lists AL_D and ALx with empty
2. **while** the list L_1 is not empty **do**
3. Remove the first element from L_1 and store it to D
4.   Remove the first element from Aux_X and store it to X
5. **if** the set D is empty then
6. **if** the set X does not exist in the set S then
7. Add the set X to the set S
8. Continue // take a new iteration
9. **end if**

10. **end if**
11. Find the maximum element from the set D and assign it to the element y
12. **if** the set Δ (y,X) is a subset of set then
13.   Add the element y to the set X
14. Remove the elements of set Δ (y, X) from D
15. **if** set X does not exist in the list ALx, then
16. Add the set X to the list ALx
17.   Add the act to the list AL_D
18. **end if**
19. Remove the element from the set X
20. Add the elements of the set Δ (y, X) to D
21. **end if**
22. **if** the set Δ (width-y,X) is a subset of set D, then
23. Add the element width y to the set X.
24. Remove the elements of the set Δ (width-y,X) from D
25. **if** the set X does not exist in the list ALx, then
26. Add the set X to the list AL_X
27. Add the set D to the list AL_D
28. **end if**
29. **end if**
30. **end while**
31. Assign the list $A1_X$ to Aux_X and Al_D to L_1
END

11.4.5.2 *The Space-Optimized Breadth First Search Algorithm*

This particular algorithm aims at optimizing the space complexity of the BFS approach mentioned earlier. This algorithm uses the earlier BFS algorithm for building the solution. While creating the solution tree for PDP, it runs until it reaches a specific level α. In the level α, the algorithm builds the remainder subtrees individually using BFS algorithm. Also the worst case complexity of this algorithm is $M(\alpha) = O(n^2 2^\alpha) + O(n^2 2^{n-\alpha})$ (Abbas and Bahig, 2016). As a result, this particular algorithm is faster than previous algorithms mentioned in this section. The main advantages can be inferred as the optimized memory complexity, because of the use of pruning and the considerably reduced time complexity.

The pseudocode for the algorithm is given by Abbas and Bahig (2016) later.

11.4.5.2.1 *Pseudocode—Optimized BFS Algorithm*
BEGIN
    1. Initialize the set S with empty
    2. Delete the maximum element from the set L and assign it to the element width.
    3. Assign the set (0 width) to the set X
    4. Add the set L to the list L_1
    5. Add the set X to the list Aux_X
    6. *Find_α_M(N, α_M)*
    7. **for** i = 0 to α_{M-1} **do**
    8.   *GenerateNextLevel(L_1,Aux_X,S)*
    9. **end for**
    10. **for** each element D in the list L_1,**do**
    11. Assign the set eD to eL_1

12.   Assign the set eX to eAux_X
13. **while** the list eL_1 is not empty **do**
14. *GenerateNextLevel($eL_1,eAux\_X,S$)*
15.   **end while**
16. **end for**
END

11.4.5.2.2 Pseudocode—Find_α_M Function

Procedure Find_α_M (N, α_M)
BEGIN

1. $n = \dfrac{1+\sqrt{1+8N}}{2}$

2. $\alpha = \alpha_M = 1$
3. $M_{min} = n^2(2^\alpha + 2^{n-\alpha})$
4. **for** $\alpha = 2$ to n **do**
5. $M = n^2(2^\alpha + 2^{n-\alpha})$
6. **if** $M < M_{min}$ **then**
7. $M_{min} = M$
8. $\alpha_M = \alpha$
9. **end if**
10. **end for**
END

11.4.6 Computational Results

Figure 11.5 depicts the comparison between the Skiena algorithm and the BFS algorithm using random dataset. Figure 11.6 depicts the comparison between the Skiena algorithm and the BFS algorithm using Zhang datasets using data from Tables 11.1 and 11.2.

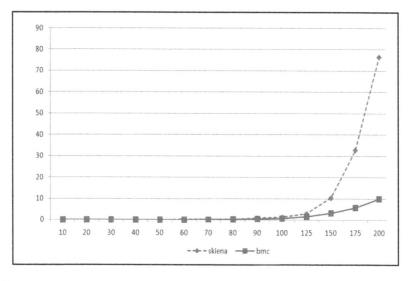

FIGURE 11.5
Graph on a random dataset.

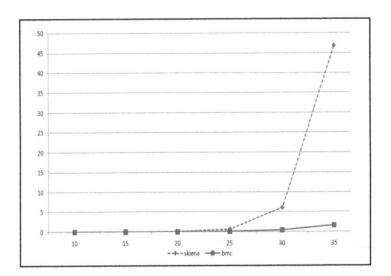

FIGURE 11.6
Graph on a Zhang dataset.

TABLE 11.1

For Random Dataset

N	Running Time of Brute Force Algorithm	Running Time of Skiena	Running Time of BFS Algorithm
10	∞	0.001106	0.001735
20	∞	0.005475	0.005829
30	∞	0.010242	0.010167
40	∞	0.019162	0.023423
50	∞	0.056081	0.04805
60	∞	0.141685	0.093598
70	∞	0.19791	0.160909
80	∞	0.33618	0.264709
90	∞	0.89527	0.429201
100	∞	1.29773	0.638853
125	∞	2.94528	1.54352
150	∞	10.3142	3.16611
175	∞	32.819	5.84061
200	∞	76.4913	9.91247

TABLE 11.2

For Zhang Dataset

n	Running Time of Brute Force Algorithm	Running Time of Skiena	Running Time of BFS Algorithm
10	∞	0.001727	0.004734
15	∞	0.008376	0.010727
20	∞	0.06794	0.034063
25	∞	0.67977	0.116555
30	∞	6.11509	0.428135
35	∞	46.8763	1.628660

11.5 Conclusion

In this chapter, we learnt about the renowned PDP, its applications in fields of bioinformatics such as DNA sequencing and genome cloning and the development of various algorithms to solve the problem. A detailed analysis of the best algorithms of their respective times is provided. Beginning with the naïve approach followed by the branch-and-bound algorithm, we find out that both take huge amount of time to obtain all the sets possible and hence are not feasible for use. Skiena proposed a backtracking algorithm that works well for random datasets but takes an exponential time for solving Zhang instances of data. The modern algorithms use a combination of data structures and complex mathematics and are robust in cases of random datasets. Among all the vivid solutions that exist for PDP, the algorithm proposed by Skiena is considered the most practical solution and is widely used till date. Proved to be NP-hard in cases of erroneous data, the question to PDP's computation complexity is not yet answered. Though, over time, there have been significant improvements in the procedures being proposed, the problem to solve the PDP still remains.

References

Abbas, M. M., & Bahig, H. M. (2016). A fast exact sequential algorithm for the partial digest problem. *BMC Bioinformatics, 17*(19), 510.

Agarwal, H., Prakash, S., Agarwal, U., Biswas, P., & Dawn, S. (2018). CPDP: A connection based PDP algorithm. *Fifth International Conference on parallel, Distributed and Grid Computing*, India.

Agarwal, P. K., Sharir, M., & Shor, P. (1989). Sharp upper and lower bounds on the length of general Davenport-Schinzel sequences. *Journal of Combinatorial Theory, Series A, 52*(2), 228–274.

Ahrabian, H., Ganjtabesh, M., Nowzari-Dalini, A., & Razaghi-Moghadam-Kashani, Z. (2013). Genetic algorithm solution for partial digest problem. *International Journal of Bioinformatics Research and Applications, 9*(6), 584–594.

Bahig, H. M., Abbas, M. M., & Mohie-Eldin, M. M. (2017, April). Parallelizing partial digest problem on multicore system. In *International Conference on Bioinformatics and Biomedical Engineering* (pp. 95–104). Springer, Cham.

Baker, M. (2011). Gene-editing nucleases. *Nature Methods, 9*, 23–26.

Bannai, E., Bannai, E., & Stanton, D. (1983). An upper bound for the cardinality of an s-distance subset in real Euclidean space, II. *Combinatorica, 3*(2), 147–152.

Bellon, B. (1988). Construction of restriction maps. *Bioinformatics, 4*(1), 111–115.

Blazewicz, J., Burke, E., Kasprzak, M., Kovalev, A., & Kovalyov, M. (2007). Simplified partial digest problem: Enumerative and dynamic programming algorithms. *IEEE/ACM Transactions on Computational Biology and Bioinformatics (TCBB), 4*(4), 668–680.

Błażewicz, J., Formanowicz, P., Kasprzak, M., Jaroszewski, M., & Markiewicz, W. T. (2001). Construction of DNA restriction maps based on a simplified experiment. *Bioinformatics, 17*(5), 398–404.

Bullough, R. K. (1961). On homometric sets. I. Some general theorems. *Acta Crystallographica, 14*(3), 257–268.

Cieliebak, M., & Eidenbenz, S. (2004, April). Measurement errors make the partial digest problem NP-hard. In *Latin American Symposium on Theoretical Informatics* (pp. 379–390). Springer, Berlin, Heidelberg.

Dakic, T. (2000). *On the Turnpike Problem*. British Columbia: Simon Fraser University.

Daurat, A., Gérard, Y., & Nivat, M. (2005). Some necessary clarifications about the chords' problem and the partial digest problem. *Theoretical Computer Science, 347*(1–2), 432–436.

Dear, P. H. (2001). *Genome Mapping*. eLS. John Wiley & Sons Ltd, Chichester. https://www.els.net. Nature Publishing Group, London, UK, 1–7.

Dix, T. I., & Kieronska, D. H. (1988). Errors between sites in restriction site mapping. *Bioinformatics, 4*(1), 117–123

Fitch, W. M., Smith, T. F., & Ralph, W. W. (1983). Mapping the order of DNA restriction fragments. *Gene, 22*(1), 19–29.

Fomin, E. (2018). A simple approach to the reconstruction of a set of points from the multiset of pairwise distances in n^2 steps for the sequencing problem: III. Noise inputs for the beltway case. *Journal of Computational Biology, 26*(1), 68–75.

Ganjtabesh, M., Ahrabian, H., & Dalini, A. N. (2012). Molecular solutions for double and partial digest problems in polynomial time. *Computing and Informatics, 28*(5), 599–618.

Hall, M. (1956). A survey of difference sets. *Proceedings of the American Mathematical Society, 7*(6), 975–986.

He, X., Hull, V., Thomas, J. A., Fu, X., Gidwani, S., Gupta, Y. K., ... Xu, S. Y. (2015). Expression and purification of a single-chain Type IV restriction enzyme Eco94GmrSD and determination of its substrate preference. *Scientific Reports, 5,* 9747.

Jones, N. C., Pevzner, P. A., & Pevzner, P. (2004). *An Introduction to Bioinformatics Algorithms*. MIT Press, Cambridge, MA.

Karp, R. M., & Newberg, L. A. (1995). An algorithm for analysing probed partial digestion experiments. *Bioinformatics, 11*(3), 229–235.

Lemke, P. & Werman, M. (1988). *On the complexity of inverting the autocorrelation function of a finite integer sequence, and the problem of locating n points on a line, given the* $\binom{n}{2}$ *unlabelled distances between them.* Preprint 453, Institute for Mathematics and its Application (IMA).

Lemke, P., Skiena, S. S., & Smith, W. D. (2003). Reconstructing sets from interpoint distances. In: Aronov, B., Basu, S., Pach, J., Sharir, M. (eds.) *Discrete and Computational Geometry* (pp. 597–631). Springer, Berlin, Heidelberg.

Narayanan, P. (2006). *Bioinformatics: A Primer*. New Age International. ISBN 10: 8122416101, ISBN 13: 9788122416107.

Newberg, L. A., & Naor, D. (1993). A lower bound on the number of solutions to the probed partial digest problem. *Advances in Applied Mathematics, 14,* 172–183.

Pääbo, S. (2001). The human genome and our view of ourselves. *Science, 291*(5507), 1219–1220.

Pandurangan, G., & Ramesh, H. (2002). The restriction mapping problem revisited. *Journal of Computer and System Sciences, 65*(3), 526–544.

Patterson, A. L. (1935). A direct method for the determination of the components of interatomic distances in crystals. *Zeitschrift für Kristallographie-Crystalline Materials, 90*(1–6), 517–542.

Rhee, G. (1988). DNA restriction mapping from random-clone data, Report Number: WUCS-88-18. All Computer Science and Engineering Research.

Skiena, S. S., & Sundaram, G. (1994). A partial digest approach to restriction site mapping. *Bulletin of Mathematical Biology, 56*(2), 275–294.

Stefik, M. (1978). Inferring DNA structures from segmentation data. *Artificial Intelligence, 11*(1–2), 85–114.

Sur-Kolay, S., Banerjee, S., Mukhopadhyaya, S., & Murthy, C. A. (2009). The double digest problem: Finding all solutions. *International Journal of Bioinformatics Research and Applications, 5*(5), 570–592.

Venter, J. C., Adams, M. D., Sutton, G. G., Kerlavage, A. R., Smith, H. O., & Hunkapiller, M. (1998). Shotgun sequencing of the human genome. *Science, 280*(5369), 1540–1542.

Zhang, Z. (1994). An exponential example for a partial digest mapping algorithm. *Journal of Computational Biology, 1*(3), 235–239.

12

Deep Learning for Next-Generation Healthcare: A Survey of State-of-the-Art and Research Prospects

Ankita Verma and Deepti Singh

Jaypee Institute of Information Technology

CONTENTS

12.1 Introduction

With the technological enhancement in the area of medical diagnosis and biomedical studies, there is a massive influx of complex, high-dimensional, heterogeneous, and irregular data, such as medical imaging, genomics, electronic health records (EHRs), speech, and sensory data (Jensen & Brunak, 2012; Murdoch & Detsky, 2013; Luo et al., 2016). Further, the apposite investigation of health informatics data is crucial for *precision medicine*, which ensures a timely and precise treatment that is tailored according to individual characteristics given to each patient. Pragmatic applications of sophisticated data mining and machine learning techniques can contribute to solve diagnostic and prognostic problems in the medical domain (Obermeyer & Emanuel, 2016; Byrne, 2017). This field has garnered worthy of attention from the research community as well as industries.

IBM's Watson Health[1] is continuously contributing toward healthcare by clinical decision making, automated drug discovery, and specialized assistance to oncologists. Google's DeepMind[2] has also ventured into the domain of healthcare applying machine learning techniques for precision medicine, tumor detection, and analysis of voluminous patient medical records for accelerating treatment. Catalyst.ai and healthcare.ai[3] are the novel models that incorporate machine learning technologies for transcending from reactive to predictive medical treatment. Moreover, the domain of healthcare is still open to novel challenges for the machine learning researcher sowing to its inherent complexity.

For the advancements in the smart healthcare systems, it is necessary to identify the potential problems or healthcare issues for which relevant data is acquired. Subsequently, machine learning algorithms are applied to reveal some of the hidden insights which are then analyzed for proper medical treatment or any such task. However, it is crucial that we measure the effectiveness of the prediction by any groundtruth or benchmark. Figure 12.1 shows the process flow adopted when the machine learning algorithms are applied in healthcare systems. In this context, extraction and identification of relevant features has an important part in the effectiveness of machine learning algorithms. In the domain of health informatics with such a complex data, feature engineering becomes a labor-intensive task on which the success of the entire intelligent system is heavily dependent (Bengio et al., 2013). However, deep learning, which derives its theoretical foundation from artificial neural networks (ANNs), has merged the feature engineering step into the learning process (Bengio, 2009). It attempts to discover informative feature representation from raw data automatically, without the aid of any human intervention (Schmidhuber, 2015; LeChun et al., 2015). This underpins the unprecedented success of deep learning in the area of health informatics, especially for the tasks like clinical imaging (Brosch et al., 2013; Prasoon et al., 2013; Yoo et al., 2014), disease diagnosis (Liu et al, 2014; Cheng et al., 2016a; Esteva et al., 2017), automated drug discovery (Mamoshina et al., 2016; Chen et al., 2018), efficient analysis of EHRs (Nguyen et al., 2017).

This chapter aims to focus upon some of the important applications using deep learning algorithms for the development of smart healthcare systems. We begin by providing a brief introduction of deep neural networks (DNNs) with their architectural description in Section 12.2. The next section will provide a consolidated review of the forthcoming

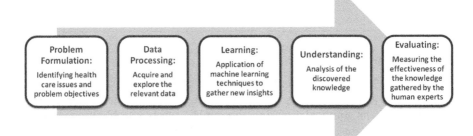

FIGURE 12.1
Machine learning algorithm life cycle in healthcare.

---

[1] https://www.ibm.com/watson/health/.
[2] https://deepmind.com/applied/deepmind-health/.
[3] https://www.healthcatalyst.com/.

and recent applications of deep learning in health informatics. We will then conclude this chapter with underlying challenges of the domain with future research prospects.

12.2 Deep Learning

Seminally, deep learning can be regarded as the enhancement and upgradation in the traditional neural network by the addition of more than two hidden layers and a sophisticated learning algorithm to learn parameters. DNNs are best known for discovering multiple-level feature representations. Within these feature representations, lower-level features were abstracted to provide more complex higher-level features (LeChun et al., 2015). As this abstraction or representation can be learned solely from the data, deep learning models facilitate the feature learning procedure and, thus, have achieved remarkable performance in various domains of artificial intelligence (Collobert & Weston, 2008; Karpathy & Fei-Fei, 2015; Hinton et al., 2012; Silver et al., 2016; Sutskever et al., 2011; Szegedy et al., 2013; Taigman et al., 2014; Zhang & Zong, 2015). In a nutshell, the two key features of deep learning algorithms are listed as follows:

- Machine learning techniques consisting of multiple layers or stages of nonlinear information transformation units.

- Efficient supervised as well as unsupervised feature learning at successive level of abstraction.

In the subsequent sections, we will discuss the motivation and the basic architecture of various deep learning models.

12.2.1 Motivation

The initial architecture of the deep learning model is inspired from cells that are present in cats' visual cortex (Hubel & Wiesel, 1962). Visual cortex consists of simple as well as complex cells. In response to some properties of the visual input, simple cells were fired. However, the complex cells are responsible for the perceptual invariance due to which visual inputs are identified invariant to the size, orientation, rotation, or contrast. Generally, complex cells are constructed from the naïve responses of simple cells. This inspires the basic architecture of the deep learning model, where each successive layer is responsible for learning more complex features from the previous lower-level features and creating a level of abstraction of the input data to be processed.

Moreover, in the last few years, the unprecedented growth of deep learning-based solutions for various problems in a variety of domains is underpinned by the following factors:

- The availability of massive processing capability at hand due to the technological advancements in central processing units, multicore computing, graphics processing units , and cloud computing.

- The gigantic amount of data at our disposal is to train DNNs.

- Novel learning algorithms are developed to train DNNs so that they can learn the weights efficiently for different types of architecture of DNNs (Hinton & Salakhutdinov, 2006; Vincent et al., 2010; Nair & Hinton, 2010; Srivastava et al., 2014; Ioffe & Szegedy, 2015).

12.2.2 Deep Learning Framework

A perceptron network is one of the earliest proposed ANNs that comprises a single-layer architecture with one input layer and one output layer for processing units. These processing units are also known as perceptron. Each perceptron transforms the weighted sum of all the inputs by applying an activation function to it. It is a binary classification model capable of segregating linearly separable data. Each perceptron transforms the weighted sum of all the inputs by applying an activation function to it. It is a binary classification model capable of segregating linearly separable data. Figure 12.2a represents the architecture of a single-layer neural network. To mitigate the issue of classification of complex data patterns, we need to add one or more hidden layers

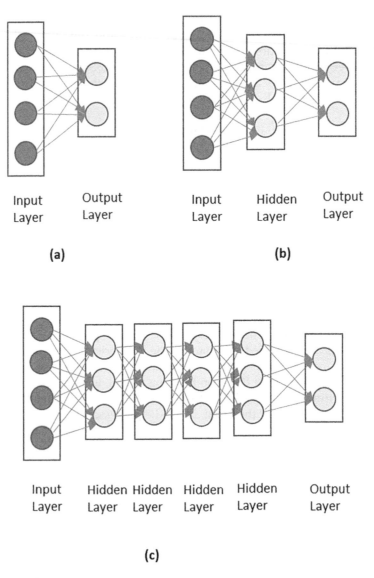

FIGURE 12.2
Feed-forward networks: (a) single-layer perceptron, (b) multilayer perceptron, and (c) deep neural network.

between input and output layers, and this gives rise to the multilayer perceptron model. In the generalized architecture of multilayer perceptron, all the layer nodes are fully connected to all the other successive layer nodes, but connection between the same layer nodes is not possible. Information flow in such type of network is toward the output layer from input layer via hidden layers, and there is no connection through which the output of the network is fed back. Thus, the network with such property is best recognized as feed-forward network. Figure 12.2b shows the basic architecture of a multilayer neural network.

As proved by Hornik (1991), a multilayer network comprising only one hidden layer behaves like a universal approximator, under the assumption that there are enough hidden units and the activation function is bounded and nonconstant. However, as the network is fully connectionist, the parameters (weights) to be learned are very large in number. It was observed that adding more hidden layers with fewer hidden units can solve complex problems with the same accuracy, and reduced parameters were required to be trained. This sets the stage for DNNs, which processes the raw input via multiple layers. Each of these layers comprises nonlinear processing units and has an abstract representation of data. Figure 12.2c represents the "deep architecture" of DNN.

12.2.3 Deep Learning Models

In this section, the focus is upon understanding the basic architecture and characteristics of some of the deep learning approaches.

12.2.3.1 Stacked Autoencoders

A neural network in which there are equal units in the input layer and output layer and only one hidden layer with a lesser number of hidden units is known as autoencoder (Bourlard&Kamp, 1988). Figure 12.3a represents an autoencoder. This neural network outputs the reconstructed approximation of the input data. Since the count of units in the hidden layer is lesser when compared with units in the input layer, a network can be employed to achieve lower-dimensional embedding of input data samples. To increment the representational power of autoencoders, many autoencoders were stacked in a way that the output of the hidden units of one autoencoder becomes the input of the next

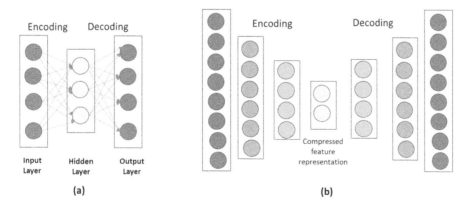

FIGURE 12.3
(a) Autoencoder and (b) deep autoencoder network.

autoencoder. Such configuration is known as deep or stacked autoencoder, as presented in Figure 12.3b (Bengio et al., 2007). For the training of such network, naive backpropagation algorithm does not perform well. So, to overcome this issue, a pretraining step is done first, in which greedy layerwise training on the network is performed to achieve appropriate initial weights for the backpropagation algorithm. In the pretraining step, training of each hidden layer is done separately by taking as input the output of the previous hidden layer in an unsupervised learning fashion.

12.2.3.2 Deep Belief Network

A restrictive Boltzmann machine (RBM) is a stochastic neural network consisting of a visible layer and a hidden layer (Ackely et al., 1986). There is a symmetric connection between every unit of the hidden layer and every unit of the visible layer, but there is no connection among the units of the identical layer, as shown in Figure 12.4a. It is a generative model capable of generating observed input observations from the hidden representation. The RBMs were stacked together to configure a deep belief network (DBN) in which there is a visible layer followed by a sequence of hidden layer (Hinton et al., 2006). The lower layers of DBN are connected via asymmetric connections, and only the topmost layers have the symmetric connections, as shown in Figure 12.4b. The DBN is trained by first pretraining the network with an unsupervised greedy layerwise strategy followed by fine-tuning of learned parameters. This is all done by applying wake–sleep algorithm (Hinton et al., 1995) with the target outputs.

12.2.3.3 Deep Boltzmann Machine

This is another deep learning model in which RBMs are piled up hierarchically. Deep Boltzmann machine (DBM) also has a visible layer followed by a sequence of hidden layers having symmetric connections among the units of successive layers, as shown in Figure 12.4c (Salakhutdinov & Hinton, 2009). It is a robust model due to the inclusion of information from both upper and lower layers. However, the inference from this network is time consuming.

12.2.3.4 Recurrent Neural Network

A special category of neural network that is ableto process the data stream is known as recurrent neural network (RNN) (Williams & Zipser, 1989). In certain applications like

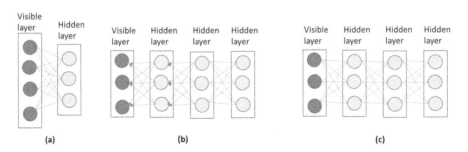

FIGURE 12.4
(a) Restricted Boltzmann machine, (b) deep belief network (DBN), and (c) deep Boltzmann machine (DBM).

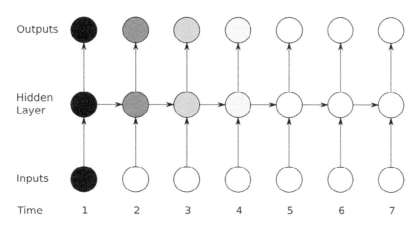

FIGURE 12.5
The recurrent neural network.

natural language processing, DNA sequencing, and speech recognition, analysis of sequence of data becomes crucial as the spatial organization of data is to be taken into consideration to make complete sense. RNN takes as input the current perceived training sample as well as the training sample perceived in the recent past.

As represented in Figure 12.5, the output of the hidden layer unit at "t" timestamp depends on the input at "t" timestamp and the output of the hidden layer unit in the preceding 't–1' timestep. Since the weights and bias are same for all time steps, the number of trainable parameters is less in RNNs. However, in the case of long-term dependency, the learning of RNN suffers from vanishing gradient problem, where gradient tends to zero, and exploding gradient problem, where the gradients end up to a very large problem (Bengio et al., 1994). A specific version of RNN is known as long short-term memory, which alleviates the vanishing gradient drawback (Hochreiter & Schmidhuber, 1997).

12.2.3.5 Convolutional Neural Networks

A neural network that is encouraged from the visual cortex of the cat is well suited to capture spatial and structural information in the data, known as convolutional neural network (CNN) (LeCun et al., 1998). CNN finds its successive application in image processing, computer vision (Krizhevsky et al., 2012; Szegedy et al., 2015), speech recognition (Trigeorgis et al., 2016), and text processing (Jaderberg et al., 2014). CNN is based on the convolutional operation that detects the local pattern in data using learnable local filter matrices. The model aims to learn more abstract features that are transitional invariant from the local patterns or low-level features. The basic model of CNN comprises a convolutional layer that performs convolution operation with a set of filters, followed by the pooling layer that performs downsampling for dimensionality reduction, and in some cases, an additional layer of activation function—rectified linear unit for introducing nonlinearity in the obtained feature maps.

These steps are performed for feature extraction and may be repeated multiple times to obtain a hierarchical abstract feature map. These feature maps are then passed through a completely connected layer of neurons for the classification task (as shown in Figure 12.6). The CNN is trained via backpropagation algorithm, but requires a large number of labeled samples.

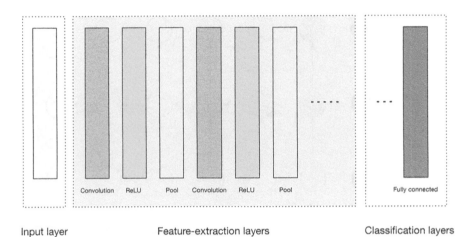

Input layer   Feature-extraction layers   Classification layers

FIGURE 12.6
Basic architecture of CNN.

12.3 Application of Deep Learning in Healthcare Systems

In the past decade, due to the easy access to multimodal data, the importance of data analytics in healthcare systems has increased tremendously. This has encouraged many researchers in the healthcare industry to come up with various machine learning, data-driven models in healthcare systems. In the earlier section, the discussion is about various deep learning models, their evolution from ANNs, and their different utilities in healthcare industry. Deep learning has become a significant tool for machine learning, capable to broaden the scope of artificial intelligence in healthcare systems. Figure 12.7 shows the top five key areas of deep learning in healthcare systems.

The following subsections focus on some of the significant applications of deep learning in health informatics. The key areas include medical imaging, bioinformatics, medical e-health records, and health monitoring.

12.3.1 Medical Imaging

One of the most active areas of study is medical imaging, where various techniques are imposed to generate visual illustrations of a body's interior. Further, these visual illustrations help to perform clinical examination and medical interference. Other than medical imaging, machine learning concepts are also applied in the areas of radiomics and computer-aided diagnosis (Suzuki, 2017). However, the traditional learning approaches are dependent on the relevant feature identification and selection that are often supervised by human experts. Moreover, the model learned via a certain handcrafted, predefined feature cannot be used in case of some small modifications in image features. As deep learning automatically detects the relevant features, it has vast varieties of applications in medical imaging.

Deep learning has a huge impact on the research work going on in the field of medical imaging. To support this fact, we can name some prominent applications like automatic detection of objects, detecting abnormalities in the given image, image classification, segmentation, registration, and many more. One significant characteristic of the deep learning

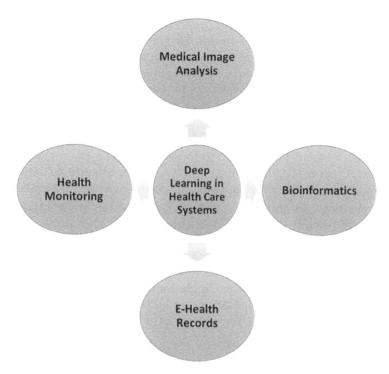

FIGURE 12.7
Key areas of deep learning in healthcare systems.

approach is to get a large set of labeled datasets as input so as to get more efficient results in disease detection and classification tasks. Following are some of the tasks performed in medical imaging:

- Classification: (Image classification and object/lesion classification). Image classification has as input a set of medical images that needs to be classified in different categories, whereas in an object or lesion classification, a small part of an image is to be classified (Miranda et al., 2016). Some of the classification tasks that are performed using deep learning are classifying Alzheimer's patients based on magnetic resonance imaging (MRI), classifying lung diseases via computed tomography (CT) images (Anthimopoulos et al., 2016), tuberculosis manifestation classification via X-ray images (Cao et al., 2016), and classifying skin cancer clinical images (Esteva et al., 2017). Some methods are proposed using stacked autoencoders and RBM, but most of the significant works have adopted CNN as the deep learning model.

- Computer-aided detection: The detection of concerned anatomical objects, such as organs, suspicious regions, lesions, and abnormalities, is a crucial part of medical diagnosis (Pham et al., 2000; Schwing & Zheng, 2014; Girshick et al., 2016). Deep learning-based approaches were utilized in detecting pulmonary nodules (Ciompi et al., 2015; Setio et al., 2016), lymph nodes (Roth et al., 2016), detecting sclerotic bone metastasis (Roth et al., 2015), and brain tumor identification (Pereira et al., 2016).

- Registration: Registration is a vital preprocessing step of transforming a set of images to be aligned in the same coordinate system. Few of the proposed methods employ deep learning models to compute the similarity between images for transformation (Wu et al., 2013; Miao et al., 2016; Simonovsky et al., 2016). Another line of work uses deep regression networks for learning the transformation parameters directly (Miao et al., 2016; Yang et al., 2016).

- Content-based image retrieval: Retrieving images based on few specific properties like color, shape, texture, and composition needs a specific technique. Content-based image retrieval techniques are focused on doing these tasks (Smeulders et al., 2000; Anavi et al., 2016). It is generally used for identifying similar cases in the past and thereby determining necessary course of action to be taken.

- Image generation and enhancement: Few deep learning models were proposed to enhance the quality of images, data augmentation, and image normalization enhancement (Yasmin et al., 2012; Bahrami et al., 2016).

Table 12.1 provides a brief information about more specific applications under medical imaging. This table enlists few significant applications in medical imaging, types of input data processed to approach these applications, and different deep learning models used in specific applications along with few relevant works in that application.

12.3.2 Bioinformatics

Bioinformatics is the study of gene–gene interactions and proteins with the aim of prognosis and diagnosis of diseases. Bioinformatics basically focuses on three areas: genomics (the study of structure, function, and evolution of genes), pharmacogenomics (the study of

TABLE 12.1

Deep Learning in Medical Image Analysis

Application	Input Data	Base Model	References
3D brain reconstruction	MRI/functional MRI, fundus images, Positron emission tomography (PET) scans	Deep autoencoders	Shan and Li (2016); Mansoor et al. (2016)
Neural cells classification	MRI/fMRI, fundus images, PET scans	CNN	Havaei et al. (2016); Jiang et al. (2015); Kleesiek et al. (2016); Nie et al. (2016); Suk et al. (2014)
Brain tissues classification	MRI/fMRI, fundus images, PET scans	DBN	Kuang and He (2014); Li et al. (2015)
Tissue classification	X-ray images, MRI images, CT scan images, microscopy fundus images, hyperspectral images, endoscopy images	Convolution DBN	Brosch et al. (2013); Zhen et al. (2016)
Organ segmentation	X-ray images, MRI images, CT scan images, microscopy fundus images, hyperspectral images, endoscopy images	CNN	Avendi et al. (2016); Xu et al. (2016)
Tumor detection	X-ray images, MRI images, CT scan images, microscopy fundus images, hyperspectral images, endoscopy images	DNN	Lerouge et al. (2015); Rose et al. (2010); Wang et al. (2016); Zhou and Wei (2016)
Cell clustering	MRI/CT images, endoscopy images, microscopy fundus images, X-ray images, hyperspectral images	Deep autoencoder	Avendi et al. (2016)

drug's effect on an individual based on genes), and epigenomics (the study of higher-level processes like protein formation and interactions). There has been a rapid adoption of deep learning in bioinformatics field.

One of the major tasks in genomics is the study of internal structure of high-dimensional and a continuous larger growing dataset, e.g., RNA measurements and DNA sequencing. To attain this task, deep learning models prove to be an excellent choice. It enables automatic selection of important features out of the input biological dataset and higher level of accuracy over traditional machine learning approaches (Ibrahim et al., 2014; Alipanahi et al., 2015).

Many other bioinformatics applications like cancer diagnosis (Fakoor et al., 2013), gene selection/classification (Ibrahim et al., 2014), RNA binding protein (Quang et al., 2014), and drug design (Ramsundar et al., 2015) have been benefited by using deep learning architectures. However, choosing the best model architectures is a bit tricky here. It needs a lot of proficiency in both computer science and biology. Also, deep learning approaches do not support a standard way of building statistical significance, and this leads to a limitation in case of forthcoming outcome assessments.

Table 12.2 provides a brief information on different applications under bioinformatics. This table contains an application column enlisting the names of some significant applications in bioinformatics and input data column providing the types of input data processed to approach these applications.

Another important column in Table 12.2 is the base model that enlists different deep learning models used in specific applications. And lastly, a reference column enlists the reference/s containing detailed information on each of the listed application.

TABLE 12.2

Deep Learning in Bioinformatics

Application	Input data	Base Model	References
Predicting chromatin marks	DNA sequences	CNN	Zhou and Troyanskaya (2015)
Learning sequence specificities of DNA and RNA binding proteins	DNA sequences RNA sequences	CNN	Alipanahi et al. (2015)
Prediction of protein backbones	Protein sequences	Stacked sparseautoencoder	Lyons et al. (2014)
Cancer diagnosis and classification	Gene expression data, micro RNA, microarray data	Deep autoencoders and stacked sparseautoencoder	Fakoor et al. (2013)
Gene selection and classification	Gene expression,micro RNA,microarray data	DBN	Ibrahim et al. (2014); Quang et al. (2014)
DNA methylation	Genes/RNA/DNA sequences	DNN	Angermueller et al. (2017)
Drug design	Molecule compounds	DNN	Chen et al. (2018); Ramsundar et al. (2015)
RNA binding protein	Genes/RNA/DNA sequences	DNN	Zhang et al. (2015)
Compound protein interaction	Protein structures Molecule compounds	DBN	Tian et al. (2016)

12.3.3 Medical e-Health Records

Due to the advancement of technology, there has been a drastic change in the process of maintaining medical records of patients. EHRs have made a revolution in the health-care industry by making faster accessibility of data in a more organized way. A lot of prediction models have been built using deep learning, which processes huge volumes of aggregated EHRs, including both structured and unstructured data (Cheng et al., 2016b).

These predictive models can predict a variety of diseases like heart failure, chronic obstructive pulmonary disease, etc. Apart from disease prediction, it can also perform automatic assignment of diagnosis to patient from their clinical records. Table 12.3 provides a brief information on different applications under e-health records. This table contains application column enlisting the names of some significant applications of e-health records and an input data column providing the types of input data processed to approach these applications. Another important column in the table is the base model that enlists different deep learning models used in specific applications. And lastly, a reference column enlists the reference/s containing detailed information on each of the listed application.

12.3.4 Health Monitoring

Manufacturing industry has been largely revolutionized by the technology advancement like Internet of Things and other big data techniques. In any computer network, there is a huge amount of data gathered from different connected machines. This big machinery data can be fully utilized by converting it into some meaningful information. Health monitoring using machinery data can be analyzed from different perspectives using various deep learning models. Table 12.4 provides a brief information on the different applications under health monitoring. This table contains an application column enlisting the names of some significant application in health monitoring and an input data column providing the types of input data processed to approach these applications. Another important column in the table is the base model that enlists different deep learning models used in specific applications. And lastly, a reference column enlists the references containing detailed information on each of the listed application.

TABLE 12.3

Deep Learning in Medical e-Health Records

Application	Input Data	Base Model	References
Predictive analysis of heart failures due to congestion and pulmonary disease	Longitudinal EHRs	CNN	Liu et al. (2014)
Diagnosis learning in pediatric intensive unit care	Clinical measurements of patients	RNN	Lipton et al. (2015)
Medicine prediction	Patient historical data records	RNN	Pham et al. (2016)
Future clinical events prediction	Patient clinical records data	Stacked denoising autoencoder (AE)	Miotto et al. (2016)
Automatic diagnosis assignment to patients	Patient clinical records data	Restricted Boltzmann machine	Liang et al. (2014)

TABLE 12.4

Deep Learning in Health Monitoring

Application	Input Data	Base Model	References
Estimation of energy expenditure using wearable sensors	Sensor data	CNN	Nweke et al. (2018); Zhu et al. (2015)
Predicting the quality of sleep from physical activity wearable data during awake time	Actigraphy sensor data	CNN	Sathyanarayana et al. (2016)
Human activity recognition to detect freezing of gait	Wearable sensor data	RNN, CNN	Hammerla et al. (2016)
Identification of photoplethysmography signals	Wearable biosensor data	Restricted Boltzmann machine	Jindal et al. (2016)

12.4 Challenges and Future Research Prospects

From the recent works in deep learning, it has been observed that there is a major improvement in multiple artificial intelligence tasks when compared with traditional machine learning techniques. However, there have been a lot of uncertainties about deep learning practices providing a complete solution for a problem. Let us discuss these challenges one by one.

i. High variety of data: In the healthcare systems, it has been observed that there is a major influx of a variety of data (structured or unstructured) (Kruse et al., 2016). Some of the data is simply the medical reports by doctors, and some are in the form of images like MRI, CT scan, X-ray images, etc. With an increase in data, it becomes challenging to decide on the levels in deep learning architecture about which feature needs to be fused or integrated. There is a lot of research work carried out on this issue.

ii. Data security and privacy issues: To get good results while solving different research problems in healthcare, we require a huge and high-quality labeled dataset. Several attempts have been made by various big players in healthcare industry to collaborate with different hospitals and medical research labs to do secure sharing of patient data. But still, there is a lot of trouble in covering the gap between these two parties (Kruse et al., 2016; Kostkova et al., 2016).

iii. Lack in getting training samples for the learning model: There are a lot of complexities involved in deep learning models. For training these models, large number of input data is required. Many organizations have already started maintaining their medical data online. But still, there is a lack of availability of disease-specific data. More efforts need to be done to make these medical records more structured and informative so that this data can be used as input for training deep learning models (Ravi et al., 2017).

iv. Feature improvement: Representation of appropriate feature spaces for data and feature engineering are often major application-specific challenges (Miotto et al., 2017). To characterize each patient effectively, a greater number of features are required. There is plenty of unstructured data available on various social media platforms. Integrating this data from various platforms and further integrating all to make a better feature-enriched dataset will definitely improve the performance of deep learning models.

v. Domain complexity: Healthcare domain is far more complex when compared with other application domains of deep learning like speech recognition, sentiment analysis, etc. (Liang et al., 2014). There are various body parts and a huge variety of diseases identified in healthcare domain. To acquire good domain knowledge in this field, one needs to dedicate enough time. A researcher has to do a lot of discussions with medical experts to understand the underneath concepts of healthcare issue to be worked upon.

All these challenges provide various opportunities for future work.

12.5 Conclusions

With the vast amount of biomedical data at our disposal, it becomes crucial that proper and effective analysis of such data is performed to accomplish numerous tasks like prognosis and later on diagnosis of various diseases, precision medicine, as well as holistic healthcare. However, clinical data are usually heterogeneous, complex, noisy, and unstructured, thereby causing difficulty in practical implication of various machine learning approaches. Deep learning provides a sophisticated data representation as well as novel learning algorithms that can scale up to huge volume of data. Because of the availability of huge computational resources and bulk of labeled data for training and free implementation packages for various algorithms, there has been a boom in practical implication of deep learning techniques in various healthcare-related tasks. Nonetheless, there are still certain open challenges such as volume and quality of available clinical data, the underlying complexity of the medical domain, and interpretation and justification of the predictive results. These open the novel research prospects for applying deep learning in healthcare systems.

References

Ackely, D., Hinton, G. E., & Sejnowski, T. J. (1986). Learning and relearning in Boltzmann machines. *Parallel Distributed Processing: Explorations in the Microstructure of Cognition, 1,* 282–317.

Alipanahi, B., Delong, A., Weirauch, M. T., & Frey, B. J. (2015). Predicting the sequence specificities of DNA-and RNA-binding proteins by deep learning. *Nature Biotechnology, 33*(8), 831.

Anavi, Y., Kogan, I., Gelbart, E., Geva, O., & Greenspan, H. (2016). Visualizing and enhancing a deep learning framework using patients age and gender for chest X-ray image retrieval. In *Medical Imaging 2016: Computer-Aided Diagnosis* (Vol. 9785, p. 978510). International Society for Optics and Photonics.

Angermueller, C., Lee, H., Reik, W., & Stegle, O. (2017). Accurate prediction of single-cell DNA methylation states using deep learning. *BioRxiv,* 055715. doi:10.1186/s13059-017-1189-z.

Anthimopoulos, M., Christodoulidis, S., Ebner, L., Christe, A., & Mougiakakou, S. (2016). Lung pattern classification for interstitial lung diseases using a deep convolutional neural network. *IEEE Transactions on Medical Imaging, 35*(5), 1207–1216.

Avendi, M. R., Kheradvar, A., & Jafarkhani, H. (2016). A combined deep-learning and deformable-model approach to fully automatic segmentation of the left ventricle in cardiac MRI. *Medical Image Analysis, 30,* 108–119.

Bahrami, K., Shi, F., Rekik, I., & Shen, D. (2016). Convolutional neural network for reconstruction of 7T-like images from 3T MRI using appearance and anatomical features. In *Deep Learning and Data Labeling for Medical Applications* (pp. 39–47). Springer, Cham.

Bengio, Y. (2009). Learning deep architectures for AI. *Foundations and Trends® in Machine Learning*, 2(1), 1–127.

Bengio, Y., Courville, A., & Vincent, P. (2013). Representation learning: A review and new perspectives. *IEEE Transactions on Pattern Analysis and Machine Intelligence*, 35(8), 1798–1828.

Bengio, Y., Lamblin, P., Popovici, D., & Larochelle, H. (2007). Greedy layer-wise training of deep networks. In *Advances in Neural Information Processing Systems* (pp. 153–160).

Bengio, Y., Simard, P., & Frasconi, P. (1994). Learning long-term dependencies with gradient descent is difficult. *IEEE Transactions on Neural Networks*, 5(2), 157–166.

Bourlard, H., & Kamp, Y. (1988). Auto-association by multilayer perceptrons and singular value decomposition. *Biological Cybernetics*, 59(4–5), 291–294.

Brosch, T., Tam, R., & Alzheimer's Disease Neuroimaging Initiative. (2013). Manifold learning of brain MRIs by deep learning. In *International Conference on Medical Image Computing and Computer-Assisted Intervention* (pp. 633–640). Springer, Berlin, Heidelberg.

Byrne, M. D. (2017). Machine learning in health care. *Journal of PeriAnesthesia Nursing*, 32(5), 494–496.

Cao, Y., Garcia, L. L., Curioso, W. H., Liu, C., Liu, B., Brunette, M. J.,…Garavito, E. S. (2016). Improving tuberculosis diagnostics using deep learning and mobile health technologies among resource-poor and marginalized communities. In *2016 IEEE First International Conference on Connected Health: Applications, Systems and Engineering Technologies (CHASE)* (pp. 274–281). IEEE, Washington, DC.

Chen, H., Engkvist, O., Wang, Y., Olivecrona, M., & Blaschke, T. (2018). The rise of deep learning in drug discovery. *Drug Discovery Today*, 23(6), 1241–1250.

Cheng, J. Z., Ni, D., Chou, Y. H., Qin, J., Tiu, C. M., Chang, Y. C.,…Chen, C. M. (2016a). Computer-aided diagnosis with deep learning architecture: Applications to breast lesions in US images and pulmonary nodules in CT scans. *Scientific Reports*, 6, 24454.

Cheng, Y., Wang, F., Zhang, P., & Hu, J. (2016b). Risk prediction with electronic health records: A deep learning approach. In *Proceedings of the 2016 SIAM International Conference on Data Mining* (pp. 432–440). Society for Industrial and Applied Mathematics, FL.

Ciompi, F., de Hoop, B., van Riel, S. J., Chung, K., Scholten, E. T., Oudkerk, M.,…van Ginneken, B. (2015). Automatic classification of pulmonary peri-fissural nodules in computed tomography using an ensemble of 2D views and a convolutional neural network out-of-the-box. *Medical Image Analysis*, 26(1), 195–202.

Collobert, R., & Weston, J. (2008). A unified architecture for natural language processing: Deep neural networks with multitask learning. In *Proceedings of the 25th International Conference on Machine Learning* (pp. 160–167). ACM, Helsinki, Finland.

Esteva, A., Kuprel, B., Novoa, R. A., Ko, J., Swetter, S. M., Blau, H. M., & Thrun, S. (2017). Dermatologist-level classification of skin cancer with deep neural networks. *Nature*, 542(7639), 115.

Fakoor, R., Ladhak, F., Nazi, A., & Huber, M. (2013). Using deep learning to enhance cancer diagnosis and classification. In *Proceedings of the International Conference on Machine Learning* (Vol. 28). ACM, New York.

Girshick, R., Donahue, J., Darrell, T., & Malik, J. (2016). Region-based convolutional networks for accurate object detection and segmentation. *IEEE Transactions on Pattern Analysis and Machine Intelligence*, 38(1), 142–158.

Hammerla, N. Y., Halloran, S., & Ploetz, T. (2016). Deep, convolutional, and recurrent models for human activity recognition using wearables. arXiv preprint arXiv:1604.08880.

Havaei, M., Guizard, N., Larochelle, H., & Jodoin, P. M. (2016). Deep learning trends for focal brain pathology segmentation in MRI. In Holzinger, A.(ed.) *Machine Learning for Health Informatics* (pp. 125–148). Springer, Cham.

Hinton, G. E., & Salakhutdinov, R. R. (2006). Reducing the dimensionality of data with neural networks. *Science*, 313(5786), 504–507.

Hinton, G. E., Dayan, P., Frey, B. J., & Neal, R. M. (1995). The "wake-sleep" algorithm for unsupervised neural networks. *Science*, 268(5214), 1158–1161.

Hinton, G. E., Osindero, S., & Teh, Y. W. (2006). A fast learning algorithm for deep belief nets. *Neural Computation*, 18(7), 1527–1554.

Hinton, G., Deng, L., Yu, D., Dahl, G. E., Mohamed, A. R., Jaitly, N., & Kingsbury, B. (2012). Deep neural networks for acoustic modeling in speech recognition: The shared views of four research groups. *IEEE Signal Processing Magazine*, 29(6), 82–97.

Hochreiter, S., & Schmidhuber, J. (1997). Long short-term memory. *Neural Computation*, 9(8), 1735–1780.

Hornik, K. (1991). Approximation capabilities of multilayer feed forward networks. *Neural Networks*, 4(2), 251–257.

Hubel, D. H., & Wiesel, T. N. (1962). Receptive fields, binocular interaction and functional architecture in the cat's visual cortex. *The Journal of Physiology*, 160(1), 106–154.

Ibrahim, R., Yousri, N. A., Ismail, M. A., & El-Makky, N. M. (2014). Multi-level gene/MiRNA feature selection using deep belief nets and active learning. In *Engineering in Medicine and Biology Society (EMBC), 36th Annual International Conference of the IEEE, 2014* (pp. 3957–3960). IEEE, Chicago, IL.

Ioffe, S., & Szegedy, C. (2015). Batch normalization: Accelerating deep network training by reducing internal covariate shift. arXiv preprint arXiv:1502.03167.

Jaderberg, M., Vedaldi, A., & Zisserman, A. (2014). Deep features for text spotting. In *European Conference on Computer Vision* (pp. 512–528). Springer, Cham.

Jensen, L. J., & Brunak, S. (2012). Mining electronic health records: Towards better research applications and clinical care. *Nature Reviews Genetics*, 13(6), 395.

Jiang, B., Wang, X., Luo, J., Zhang, X., Xiong, Y., & Pang, H. (2015). Convolutional neural networks in automatic recognition of trans-differentiated neural progenitor cells under bright-field microscopy. In *Fifth International Conference on Instrumentation and Measurement, Computer, Communication and Control (IMCCC), 2015* (pp. 122–126). IEEE, Qinhuangdao, China.

Jindal, V., Birjandtalab, J., Pouyan, M. B., & Nourani, M. (2016). An adaptive deep learning approach for PPG-based identification. In *IEEE 38th Annual International Conference of the Engineering in Medicine and Biology Society (EMBC), 2016* (pp. 6401–6404). IEEE, Orlando, FL.

Karpathy, A., & Fei-Fei, L. (2015). Deep visual-semantic alignments for generating image descriptions. In *Proceedings of the IEEE Conference on Computer Vision and Pattern Recognition* (pp. 3128–3137). Boston, MA.

Kleesiek, J., Urban, G., Hubert, A., Schwarz, D., Maier-Hein, K., Bendszus, M., & Biller, A. (2016). Deep MRI brain extraction: A 3D convolutional neural network for skull stripping. *NeuroImage*, 129, 460–469.

Kostkova, P., Brewer, H., de Lusignan, S., Fottrell, E., Goldacre, B., Hart, G.,...Ross, E. (2016). Who owns the data? Open data for healthcare. *Frontiers in Public Health*, 4, 7.

Krizhevsky, A., Sutskever, I., & Hinton, G. E. (2012). Imagenet classification with deep convolutional neural networks. In *Advances in Neural Information Processing Systems* (pp. 1097–1105).

Kruse, C. S., Goswamy, R., Raval, Y., & Marawi, S. (2016). Challenges and opportunities of big data in health care: A systematic review. *JMIR Medical Informatics*, 4(4), e38.

Kuang, D., & He, L. (2014). Classification on ADHD with deep learning. In *International Conference on Cloud Computing and Big Data (CCBD), 2014* (pp. 27–32). IEEE, Wuhan, China.

LeCun, Y., Bengio, Y., & Hinton, G. (2015). Deep learning. *Nature*, 521(7553), 436.

LeCun, Y., Bottou, L., Bengio, Y., & Haffner, P. (1998). Gradient-based learning applied to document recognition. *Proceedings of the IEEE*, 86(11), 2278–2324.

Lerouge, J., Herault, R., Chatelain, C., Jardin, F., & Modzelewski, R. (2015). IODA: An input/output deep architecture for image labeling. *Pattern Recognition*, 48(9), 2847–2858.

Li, F., Tran, L., Thung, K. H., Ji, S., Shen, D., & Li, J. (2015). A robust deep model for improved classification of AD/MCI patients. *IEEE Journal of Biomedical and Health Informatics*, 19(5), 1610–1616.

Liang, Z., Zhang, G., Huang, J. X., & Hu, Q. V. (2014). Deep learning for healthcare decision making with EMRs. In *IEEE International Conference on Bioinformatics and Biomedicine (BIBM), 2014* (pp. 556–559). IEEE, Belfast, UK.

Lipton, Z. C., Kale, D. C., Elkan, C., & Wetzel, R. (2015). Learning to diagnose with LSTM recurrent neural networks. arXiv preprint arXiv:1511.03677.

Liu, S., Liu, S., Cai, W., Pujol, S., Kikinis, R., & Feng, D. (2014). Early diagnosis of Alzheimer's disease with deep learning. In *IEEE 11th International Symposium on Biomedical Imaging (ISBI), 2014* (pp. 1015–1018). IEEE, Beijing, China.

Luo, J., Wu, M., Gopukumar, D., & Zhao, Y. (2016). Big data application in biomedical research and health care: A literature review. *Biomedical informatics insights, 8,* 1–10.

Lyons, J., Dehzangi, A., Heffernan, R., Sharma, A., Paliwal, K., Sattar, A.,…Yang, Y. (2014). Predicting backbone Cα angles and dihedrals from protein sequences by stacked sparse auto-encoder deep neural network. *Journal of Computational Chemistry, 35*(28), 2040–2046.

Mamoshina, P., Vieira, A., Putin, E., & Zhavoronkov, A. (2016). Applications of deep learning in biomedicine. *Molecular Pharmaceutics, 13*(5), 1445–1454.

Mansoor, A., Cerrolaza, J. J., Idrees, R., Biggs, E., Alsharid, M. A., Avery, R. A., & Linguraru, M. G. (2016). Deep learning guided partitioned shape model for anterior visual pathway segmentation. *IEEE Transactions on Medical Imaging, 35*(8), 1856–1865.

Miao, S., Wang, Z. J., & Liao, R. (2016). A CNN regression approach for real-time 2D/3D registration. *IEEE Transactions on Medical Imaging, 35*(5), 1352–1363.

Miotto, R., Li, L., Kidd, B. A., & Dudley, J. T. (2016). Deep patient: An unsupervised representation to predict the future of patients from the electronic health records. *Scientific Reports, 6,* 26094.

Miotto, R., Wang, F., Wang, S., Jiang, X., & Dudley, J. T. (2017). Deep learning for healthcare: Review, opportunities and challenges. *Briefings in Bioinformatics, 19*(6), 1236–1246.

Miranda, E., Aryuni, M., & Irwansyah, E. (2016). A survey of medical image classification techniques. In *International Conference on Information Management and Technology (ICIMTech),* (pp. 56–61). IEEE, Bandung, Indonesia.

Murdoch, T. B., & Detsky, A. S. (2013). The inevitable application of big data to health care. *JAMA, 309*(13), 1351–1352.

Nair, V., & Hinton, G. E. (2010). Rectified linear units improve restricted Boltzmann machines. In *Proceedings of the 27th International Conference on Machine Learning (ICML-10)* (pp. 807–814). IEEE, Haifa, Israel.

Nguyen, P., Tran, T., Wickramasinghe, N., & Venkatesh, S. (2017). Deepr: A convolutional net for medical records. *IEEE Journal of Biomedical and Health Informatics, 21*(1), 22–30.

Nie, D., Zhang, H., Adeli, E., Liu, L., & Shen, D. (2016). 3D deep learning for multi-modal imaging-guided survival time prediction of brain tumor patients. In *International Conference on Medical Image Computing and Computer-Assisted Intervention* (pp. 212–220). Springer, Cham.

Nweke, H. F., Teh, Y. W., Al-Garadi, M. A., & Alo, U. R. (2018). Deep learning algorithms for human activity recognition using mobile and wearable sensor networks: State of the art and research challenges. *Expert Systems with Applications, 105,* 233–261.

Obermeyer, Z., & Emanuel, E. J. (2016). Predicting the future—Big data, machine learning, and clinical medicine. *The New England Journal of Medicine, 375*(13), 1216.

Pereira, S., Pinto, A., Alves, V., & Silva, C. A. (2016). Brain tumor segmentation using convolutional neural networks in MRI images. *IEEE Transactions on Medical Imaging, 35*(5), 1240–1251.

Pham, D. L., Xu, C., & Prince, J. L. (2000). Current methods in medical image segmentation. *Annual Review of Biomedical Engineering, 2*(1), 315–337.

Pham, T., Tran, T., Phung, D., & Venkatesh, S. (2016). Deepcare: A deep dynamic memory model for predictive medicine. In *Pacific-Asia Conference on Knowledge Discovery and Data Mining* (pp. 30–41). Springer, Cham.

Prasoon, A., Petersen, K., Igel, C., Lauze, F., Dam, E., & Nielsen, M. (2013). Deep feature learning for knee cartilage segmentation using a triplanar convolutional neural network. In *International Conference on Medical Image Computing and Computer-Assisted Intervention*(pp. 246–253). Springer, Berlin, Heidelberg.

Quang, D., Chen, Y., & Xie, X. (2014). DANN: A deep learning approach for annotating the pathogenicity of genetic variants. *Bioinformatics, 31*(5), 761–763.

Ramsundar, B., Kearnes, S., Riley, P., Webster, D., Konerding, D., & Pande, V. (2015). Massively multi-task networks for drug discovery. arXiv preprint arXiv:1502.02072.

Ravı, D., Wong, C., Deligianni, F., Berthelot, M., Andreu-Perez, J., Lo, B., & Yang, G. Z. (2017). Deep learning for health informatics. *IEEE Journal of Biomedical and Health Informatics, 21*(1), 4–21.

Rose, D. C., Arel, I., Karnowski, T. P., & Paquit, V. C. (2010,). Applying deep-layered clustering to mammography image analytics. In *Biomedical Sciences and Engineering Conference (BSEC), 2010* (pp. 1–4). IEEE, Oak Ridge, TN.

Roth, H. R., Lu, L., Liu, J., Yao, J., Seff, A., Cherry, K.,…Summers, R. M. (2016). Improving computer-aided detection using convolutional neural networks and random view aggregation. *IEEE Transactions on Medical Imaging, 35*(5), 1170–1181.

Roth, H. R., Yao, J., Lu, L., Stieger, J., Burns, J. E., & Summers, R. M. (2015). Detection of sclerotic spine metastases via random aggregation of deep convolutional neural network classifications. In Yao, J., Glocker, B., Kinder, T., Li, S. (eds.) *Recent Advances in Computational Methods and Clinical Applications for Spine Imaging* (pp. 3–12). Springer, Cham.

Salakhutdinov, R., & Hinton, G. (2009). Deep Boltzmann machines. In *Artificial Intelligence and Statistics* (pp. 448–455).

Sathyanarayana, A., Joty, S., Fernandez-Luque, L., Ofli, F., Srivastava, J., Elmagarmid, A.,…Taheri, S. (2016). Correction of: Sleep quality prediction from wearable data using deep learning. *JMIR Mhealth and Uhealth, 4*(4), e125.

Schmidhuber, J. (2015). Deep learning in neural networks: An overview. *Neural Networks, 61*, 85–117.

Schwing, A. G., & Zheng, Y. (2014). Reliable extraction of the mid-sagittal plane in 3D brain MRI via hierarchical landmark detection. In *IEEE 11th International Symposium on Biomedical Imaging (ISBI), 2014* (pp. 213–216). IEEE, Beijing, China.

Setio, A. A. A., Ciompi, F., Litjens, G., Gerke, P., Jacobs, C., Van Riel, S. J.,…van Ginneken, B. (2016). Pulmonary nodule detection in CT images: False positive reduction using multi-view convolutional networks. *IEEE Transactions on Medical Imaging, 35*(5), 1160–1169.

Shan, J., & Li, L. (2016). A deep learning method for microaneurysm detection in fundus images. In *IEEE First International Conference on Connected Health: Applications, Systems and Engineering Technologies (CHASE), 2016* (pp. 357–358). IEEE, Washington, DC.

Silver, D., Huang, A., Maddison, C. J., Guez, A., Sifre, L., Van Den Driessche, G.,…Dieleman, S. (2016). Mastering the game of Go with deep neural networks and tree search. *Nature, 529*(7587), 484.

Simonovsky, M., Gutiérrez-Becker, B., Mateus, D., Navab, N., & Komodakis, N. (2016). A deep metric for multimodal registration. In *International Conference on Medical Image Computing and Computer-Assisted Intervention* (pp. 10–18). Springer, Cham.

Smeulders, A. W., Worring, M., Santini, S., Gupta, A., & Jain, R. (2000). Content-based image retrieval at the end of the early years. *IEEE Transactions on Pattern Analysis & Machine Intelligence, 22*(12), 1349–1380.

Srivastava, N., Hinton, G., Krizhevsky, A., Sutskever, I., & Salakhutdinov, R. (2014). Dropout: A simple way to prevent neural networks from overfitting. *The Journal of Machine Learning Research, 15*(1), 1929–1958.

Suk, H. I., Lee, S. W., Shen, D., & Alzheimer's Disease Neuroimaging Initiative. (2014). Hierarchical feature representation and multimodal fusion with deep learning for AD/MCI diagnosis. *NeuroImage, 101*, 569–582.

Sutskever, I., Martens, J., & Hinton, G. E. (2011). Generating text with recurrent neural networks. In *Proceedings of the 28th International Conference on Machine Learning (ICML-11)* (pp. 1017–1024). Washington, DC.

Suzuki, K. (2017). Overview of deep learning in medical imaging. *Radiological Physics and Technology, 10*(3), 257–273.

Szegedy, C., Liu, W., Jia, Y., Sermanet, P., Reed, S., Anguelov, D.,…Rabinovich, A. (2015). Going deeper with convolutions. In *Proceedings of the IEEE Conference on Computer Vision and Pattern Recognition* (pp. 1–9). Boston, MA.

Szegedy, C., Toshev, A., & Erhan, D. (2013). Deep neural networks for object detection. In *Advances in Neural Information Processing Systems* (pp. 2553–2561).

Taigman, Y., Yang, M., Ranzato, M. A., & Wolf, L. (2014). Deepface: Closing the gap to human-level performance in face verification. In *Proceedings of the IEEE Conference on Computer Vision and Pattern Recognition* (pp. 1701–1708).

Tian, K., Shao, M., Wang, Y., Guan, J., & Zhou, S. (2016). Boosting compound-protein interaction prediction by deep learning. *Methods*, *110*, 64–72. Columbus, OH.

Trigeorgis, G., Ringeval, F., Brueckner, R., Marchi, E., Nicolaou, M. A., Schuller, B., & (2016) Adieu features? end-to-end speech emotion recognition using a deep convolutional recurrent network. In *2016 IEEE International Conference on Acoustics, Speech and Signal Processing (ICASSP)* (pp. 5200–5204). IEEE.

Vincent, P., Larochelle, H., Lajoie, I., Bengio, Y., & Manzagol, P. A. (2010). Stacked denoising autoencoders: Learning useful representations in a deep network with a local denoising criterion. *Journal of Machine Learning Research*, *11*(Dec), 3371–3408.

Wang, J., MacKenzie, J. D., Ramachandran, R., & Chen, D. Z. (2016). A deep learning approach for semantic segmentation in histology tissue images. In *International Conference on Medical Image Computing and Computer-Assisted Intervention* (pp. 176–184). Springer, Cham.

Williams, R. J., & Zipser, D. (1989). A learning algorithm for continually running fully recurrent neural networks. *Neural Computation*, *1*(2), 270–280.

Wu, G., Kim, M., Wang, Q., Gao, Y., Liao, S., & Shen, D. (2013). Unsupervised deep feature learning for deformable registration of MR brain images. In *International Conference on Medical Image Computing and Computer-Assisted Intervention* (pp. 649–656). Springer, Berlin, Heidelberg.

Xu, T., Zhang, H., Huang, X., Zhang, S., & Metaxas, D. N. (2016, October). Multimodal deep learning for cervical dysplasia diagnosis. In *International Conference on Medical Image Computing and Computer-Assisted Intervention* (pp. 115–123). Springer, Cham.

Yang, X., Kwitt, R., & Niethammer, M. (2016). Fast predictive image registration. In *Deep Learning and Data Labeling for Medical Applications* (pp. 48–57). Springer, Cham.

Yasmin, M., Sharif, M., Masood, S., Raza, M., & Mohsin, S. (2012). Brain image enhancement-A survey. *World Applied Sciences Journal*, *17*(9), 1192–1204.

Yoo, Y., Brosch, T., Traboulsee, A., Li, D. K., & Tam, R. (2014). Deep learning of image features from unlabeled data for multiple sclerosis lesion segmentation. In *International Workshop on Machine Learning in Medical Imaging* (pp. 117–124). Springer, Cham.

Zhang, J., & Zong, C. (2015). Deep neural networks in machine translation: An overview. *IEEE Intelligent Systems*, *30*(5), 16–25.

Zhang, S., Zhou, J., Hu, H., Gong, H., Chen, L., Cheng, C., & Zeng, J. (2015). A deep learning framework for modeling structural features of RNA-binding protein targets. *Nucleic Acids Research*, *44*(4), e32.

Zhen, X., Wang, Z., Islam, A., Bhaduri, M., Chan, I., & Li, S. (2016). Multi-scale deep networks and regression forests for direct bi-ventricular volume estimation. *Medical Image Analysis*, *30*, 120–129.

Zhou, J., & Troyanskaya, O. G. (2015). Predicting effects of noncoding variants with deep learning–based sequence model. *Nature Methods*, *12*(10), 931.

Zhou, Y., & Wei, Y. (2016). Learning hierarchical spectral–spatial features for hyperspectral image classification. *IEEE Transactions on Cybernetics*, *46*(7), 1667–1678.

Zhu, J., Pande, A., Mohapatra, P., & Han, J. J. (2015). Using deep learning for energy expenditure estimation with wearable sensors. In *17th International Conference on e-Health Networking, Application & Services (HealthCom), 2015* (pp. 501–506). IEEE, Boston, MA.

13

Applications of Protein Nanoparticles as Drug Delivery Vehicle

Reema Gabrani, Ritu Ghildiyal, Neetigyata Pratap, Garima Sharma, and Shweta Dang
Jaypee Institute of Information and Technology

CONTENTS

13.1 Introduction

"Proteome" is a broad term used for proteins derived from the entire genome of an organism and its modification system, whereas "Proteomics" refers to the comprehensive study of specific proteome, their variations and modifications, along with their interacting partners and networks, to understand cellular processes (Abhilash, 2009). "Clinical proteomics" is a subdivision of proteomics that involves the application of proteomic technologies for the identification of specific biomarkers signature present in the clinical specimens such as blood, tissues, and cells of patients. These biomarkers are usually helpful in the diagnosis of particular disease and toward the development of personalized therapy/treatment (Zhou et al., 2016). Nowadays, protein-based therapeutics has revolutionized the area of nanomedicine. Protein-based diagnostics have become an important tool in management of many diseases like cancer, autoimmune diseases, and infectious diseases, as these proteins have been involved in certain biological pathways. Proteins can act as enzymes, antibodies, and hormones and are involved in storage, transportation of molecules, energy balance as well as repair, maintenance, and development. Moreover, several biological pathways depend on protein–protein interactions which can be targeted via developing agonist peptides and proteins. Advancement in protein as therapeutics comprises innovative manufacturing technologies, process control, and protein characterization (Vaishya et al., 2015). Over the past years, effective medication against complicated situations has been developed, but simultaneously, it is observed that they are linked to numerous side effects (Rizvi & Saleh, 2018). Furthermore, the problem of poor bioavailability and high dosage requirement of proteins and peptides has been addressed by nanotechnology. Nanoparticle (NP)-based therapeutics have much advantage over traditional drugs.

Nanoencapsulation, ionic gelation, and ultrasonication methods are the main methods that are generally used for the preparation of protein NPs. Targeted drug delivery is one of the most studied and advanced methods to deliver drug into a system. Targeted drug delivery not only helps in increasing the efficacy of the drug but also helps to minimize the possible side effects of the drug. Researchers have been continuously focusing toward a specific target due to the emergence of various diseases involving complex pathways. Delivering drug specific to the target site assists in improving the probability to treat disease. Entrapping the drug molecules into nanocarriers specifically and delivering it to the target site are major advancements, which have been made possible due to the presence of NPs. Generally, NPs are molecules of sizes ranging from 1 to 100nm.NPs have much great surface area per unit volume, which makes it more active than other molecules. NPs can be formed by a variety of materials and can have different properties depending on the coating or material used.

In the field of biomedical and material sciences, proteins exhibit potential applications, as it possesses amphiphilic properties suitable for NPs. Generally, NPs synthesized from natural proteins possess biodegradable and metabolizing properties that can be easily modified during its binding with the target. NPs can be synthesized from both water-soluble proteins like bovine serum albumin (BSA) and water-insoluble proteins like zein and gladin (Lohcharoenkal, Wang, Chen, & Rojanasakul, 2014). Nanotechnology is giving a basic platform for research to overcome the drawbacks associated with the current applications of proteins and peptides. They are also reported for crossing the blood–brain barrier safely and hence are suitable for neurologic diseases (Rizvi & Saleh, 2018). NP technologies show a promising result in promoting the efficacy of drugs.

NPs of proteins/peptides are rising as a new approach in disease diagnosis and treatment. Before developing a therapeutic peptide/protein, complete and in-depth knowledge of stability of peptide in biological environment and its interactions with the biological surrounding are indeed necessary. There is an exponential increment in the development of nanoencapsulated peptides, and it is reported that more than 1,000 nanoencapsulated peptides are present in clinical phases (Yadav, Kumari, & Yadav, 2011).

13.2 Characterization of Protein NPs

Various NPs have been developed that efficiently deliver the drug molecule to the target site and are able to circulate in the blood stream for longer periods of time to deliver its effects. NPs are thus modified along with their particle size and surface charge to provide maximum efficacy to the drug molecule. There are many factors like diameter of nanocarriers, surface properties, and particle morphology that play a crucial role in increasing the effectiveness of NPs carrying drugs. Protein-based NPs (PBNs) have several advantage over other nanocarriers like reduced toxicity, enhanced bioavailability, and controlled release of drug for longer durations (Elaissari, 2017). The complications related to drug resistance in the body are overcome by the use of PBNs. Small doses of PBNs are enough for the enhanced action and hence show better rate of dissolution. Along with all these properties, route of drug delivery is an important aspect, as it is vital to preserve/protect the drug during the whole journey of delivery into the system. Drug should be intact with no chemical modification during delivery. PBNs can be incorporated through oral administration, vascular administration, and inhalation. Choice of effective route of administration, matrix constitution, and size of PBNs affect the properties of PBNs and its performance (Elaissari, 2017; Verma, Gulati, Kaul, Mukherjee, & Nagaich, 2018).

It has been reported that the size of NPs plays an important role in the successful delivery of the drug. The size of NPs varies depending on the target site and the drug carrier molecule. Size of polymeric NPs varies from 10 to 1,000 nm, which shows biodegradable and biocompatible properties (Bhatia, 2016).

13.3 General Protein Used for Preparation of NPs

In the biomedical field, proteins have been potentially used for the preparation of NPs (Figure 13.1). PBNs are particularly interesting, because they are relatively safe and easy to prepare, and their size distribution can be easily monitored. Proteins are easy to modify and incorporate potential functional groups. Some of the proteins that can be consumed daily like albumin, soy protein, and milk protein can be used for the preparation of PBNs and are widely reported for the treatment of diseases like cancer.

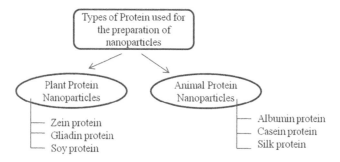

FIGURE 13.1
Types of protein used as carrier for the preparation of NPs.

13.3.1 Albumin

The osmotic pressure inside the blood vessels is maintained by albumin. It also helps in the transportation of nutrients and binding with drug molecules. Egg white (ovalbumin), BSA, and human serum albumin (HSA) are rich in albumin and can be obtained from these sources. Albumin is becoming the choice for the preparation of NPs, as it is highly soluble in water as well as salt solutions, biodegradable, and stable at a pH range of 4–9. These NPs are easily prepared and have thiol, amino, and carboxyl functional groups for the modification during the preparation to obtain high-efficient NPs (Lohcharoenkal et al., 2014).

Property of albumin to get accumulated in tumor cells makes it a potential carrier. For treatment of breast cancer, albumin-bound paclitaxel (Abraxane, ABI-008) got an approval from the Food and Drug Administration (FDA) (Cucinotto et al., 2013). Still many clinical trials are currently going on for albumin-bound nanocarrier system. In a randomized, phase III study of metastatic breast cancer, NP albumin-bound (nab)-paclitaxel was found to have improved efficacy and safety compared with conventional, solvent-based paclitaxel. Preliminary data also suggest roles for nab-paclitaxel as a single agent and in combination therapy for first-line treatment of metastatic breast cancer as well as other solid tumors, including non-small-cell lung cancer, ovarian cancer, and malignant melanoma. Then biotechnology promises to have a broad utility in cancer therapy, and clinical trials are underway using nab formulations of other water-insoluble anticancer agents such as docetaxel and rapamycin. Also, albumin-bound rapamycin (ABI-009) is still in a clinical trial for the treatment of nonhematologic malignancies since 2008. Recently, cationic BSA-based novel siRNA delivery system has been developed for therapy of metastatic lung cancer (Han, Wang, Zhang, Gong, & Sun, 2014). The preparation of cationic serum albumin is simple, and the modification with its cationic group allows control of the protein's pI and surface charge for optimized drug delivery (Lohcharoenkal et al., 2014; Vaishya et al., 2015).

13.3.2 Gelatin and Elastin

Collagen that is present in the skin and bones is hydrolyzed and can be converted to different forms of gelatin: gelatin A and gelatin B. US FDA has approved gelatin as a safe molecule for its use in pharmaceutical field and drug formulations, as it is biodegradable, nontoxic, and has chemically modified properties. Gelatin is rich in glycine, proline, and alanine, whose ionizable functional groups enable it to modify chemically during the development of NPs. Cross-linking of gelatin NPs (GNPs) can be done by the addition of cross-linking agents like glutaraldehyde, which enhanced the integrity of GNPs. Cross-linking plays an important role, as it directly depends on the controlled release of drug. All these properties make gelatin a suitable and potential molecule for NPs.

Elastin constitutes a connective tissue that is responsible for the flexibility in body/tissues. It is also used for efficient drug delivery systems (Lohcharoenkal et al., 2014).

13.3.3 Gliadin and Legumin

For oral administration, gliadin is used for drug delivery as it is a gluten protein and possesses bioadhesive properties. It has bioadhesive properties due to its neutral amino acids and shows interaction with intestinal mucosa by hydrogen bonding, and lipophilic amino acids make it suitable for the development of mucoadhesive NPs. The amine and disulfide groups of gliadin protein get attached with the mucin and hence are highly preferred for the synthesis of NPs used for the treatment of gastrointestinal tract. This kind of bioadhesion property can be utilized for the release of anticancer drug in case of colon cancer. The targeted delivery of anticancer drug cyclophosphamide has been delivered by gliadin. In pea seeds, legumin is the storage protein and hence is a good source of sulfur. Therefore, this protein can form NPs due to the self-assembly after the cross-linking process (Lohcharoenkal et al., 2014).

13.3.4 Zein

This protein contains amino acids like proline and glutamine and is usually obtained from the endosperm of corn kernel. The protein exhibits hydrophobic properties, due to which it is used for coating purpose and hence in the preparation of NPs. It is an FDA-approved protein used in the drugs development containing ivermectin, coumarin, and 5-fluorouracil (5-FU) encapsulated in zein, which has been reported in several studies and has demonstrated the suitability of zein in a drug delivery system (Marini et al., 2014).

13.3.5 Soy and Milk Protein

This protein exhibits great nutritional values and are a rich source of plant protein. Soy base NP can be prepared by desolvation or simple coacervation method. Nowadays, NPs of milk protein are getting more attention as the milk has unique properties. Milk contains β-lactoglobulin (BLG) and casein proteins. BLG possesses disulfide and thiol groups that help it to preserve it from peptic and chymotryptic degradation. BLG is a good and effective polymer for PBNs, as it is easily available in milk and has gelling properties. Casein is also used in delivery system and is reported to have particle sizes ranging from 100 to 200 nm. Casein-formed micelles help in the inheritance of calcium by offsprings from mothers. Micelles are formed through hydrophobic interactions, in which the size can be altered depending on temperature, pH, pressure, ionic strength, and other environmental conditions (Lohcharoenkal et al., 2014).

13.3.6 Whey Proteins

During the formation of NPs, drugs get encapsulated in the hydrogels of whey proteins. For the lipophilic compounds, BLG proved to be a suitable carrier in drug delivery (Verma et al., 2018).

13.4 Factors Affecting Protein NP Preparation

PBNs are directly and indirectly influenced by the physical and chemical properties of proteins like composition, solubility and surface properties of protein and drug properties (Figure 13.2). Protein composition affects the NPs on the basis of the type of protein source (animal protein or plant protein) used in the formulation. Even, a change in composition of protein's fraction during the preparation of NPs shows a considerable change in the characteristics of NPs. Storp, Engel, Boeker, Ploeger, and Langer (2012) studied about the size of HSANP, influenced by the starting batch composition, and reported that the higher amount of albumin increased the size of NP. Furthermore, the solubility of protein

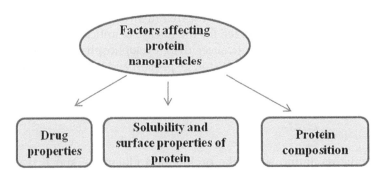

FIGURE 13.2
Factors affecting the preparation of PBN.

is another major characteristic that influences the properties of NP and has an important basis to decide the method of preparation of NP. The choice of preparation of PN depends on the solubility in aqueous solvents, nonaqueous solvents as well as polarity of solvents. Duclairoir, Orecchioni, Depraetere, Osterstock, and Nakache (2003) reported that the solubility of gliadin is influenced by the size of gliadin NPs.

During the preparation of PBNs, the surface of protein gets modified, which eventually alters the properties of PBNs. Proteins have many functional groups like amine, carboxyl, and thiol groups present on its surface, which can be modified, resulting in the conformational changes to enhance biodistribution, biocompatibility, drug loading, and stability of PBN. Cross-linkers like glutaraldehyde and polymers like polyethylene glycol are exploited to attach to the surface of protein which alters the properties of PBNs and increases its half-life. Modification of protein via attachment of these functional groups to the surface also enhances their interaction with the biological membranes. Characterization of NPs can be done by spectroscopic analysis, in which the chemical composition of NP surface is analyzed by X-ray photoelectron spectroscopy and the detection of a specific molecule/functional group is identified by Raman spectroscopy. Moreover, the knowledge of interaction of biopolymers can be studied by infrared spectroscopy. Moreover, the properties of drugs also influence PBNs, as either the drug is surrounded by NP or bonded with protein NP. Drugs have some physicochemical properties like solubility, log P, and molecular weight, which are directly related to the loading rate of drug inside PBNs. It is reported that for GNPs, hydrophilic drugs have shown immense encapsulation efficiency than hydrophobic drugs (Tarhini et al., 2018).

13.5 Technique for the Preparation of Protein NPs

Different methods are used for the preparation of nanocarriers. Many methods were previously reported, which are now being modified to improve the overall efficacy of particle formation. The preparation methods target in improving entrapment efficiency, size distribution, and stability of NPs. They can decrease the toxicity of formulation and can idealize the release of drug from the particle (Tarhini et al., 2018; Verma et al., 2018).

During the preparation of PBNs, some parameters like force of attraction and repulsion should be balanced, and have low intramolecular hydrophobic interactions. Unfolded protein may expose the functional groups like disulfides and thiol groups, which makes them

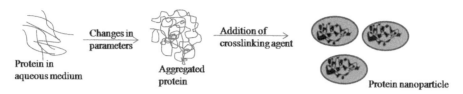

FIGURE 13.3
Preparation of polymeric nanoparticles by coacervation/desolvation method.

highly active. During NP preparation, protein's composition, concentration, pH conditions, and the type of solvent influence the properties of NPs. NPs are stabilized by adding surfactants. Methods like coacervation/desolvation and emulsion based are generally used for the formation of NPs (Greenwood et al., 2017).

13.5.1 Coacervation/Desolvation Method

This is the most extensively used method for the preparation of NPs. This method analyzes the properties of a protein that shows a varied range of solubility depending on solvents (Figure 13.3). Solvent polarity, ionic strength, presence of electrolytes, and pH are the general parameters that have an effect on the solubility of protein. The addition of organic solvents and dissolving agent leads to phase separation and conformation changes, respectively, in protein structure, resulting in protein precipitation. In coacervate, the size of the NPs formed can be controlled by the aforementioned parameters. Cross-linking agents like glyoxal and glutaraldehyde are used to stabilize the protein NPs and reduce enzymatic degradation and drug release from NPs. Organic solvents like acetone and ethanol play a crucial role, as they are used for the precipitation of prepared NPs. Studies showing the effect of various factors in the formation of albumin NP have been reported. Use of acetone as an antisolvent resulted in smaller albumin NPs, whereas ethanol leads to bigger NPs. The ratio of antisolvent and solvent directly influences the size of NPs as an increased ratio is inversely proportional to smaller size. Moreover, Storp et al. reported the importance of pH conditions before the desolvation steps, as it affects the HSA NPs. High pH conditions resulted in smaller size, and he reported that the pH conditions must be very different to the pI of protein so that the protein can deaggregate. To promote protein agglomeration, neutralization of the charges present on the surface of protein can be achieved by high salt concentration, which results in the small size of NPs (Lohcharoenkal et al., 2014; Rai, Jenifer, Theaj, & Upputuri, 2017).

13.5.2 Emulsion/Solvent Extraction

An aqueous solution of proteins is prepared followed by emulsification in oil. The process of emulsification is obtained using a high-speed homogenizer, which leads to the formation of NPs at the water–oil interphase. Ultrasonic shears can also be used instead of homogenizer to achieve the process. To stabilize the surface of formed NPs, surfactants like phosphatidylcholine are added followed by the removal of oil phase. The oil phase can be separated by an organic solvent (Figure 13.4). This method has been widely reported for the formation of albumin and whey protein NPs. It is reported that olive oil phase has been utilized for the preparation of HSA NP. Here, phosphatidylcholine present in the aqueous solution of protein acts as a surfactant, in which olive oil was added gradually followed by continuous stirring and ultrasonication. Furthermore, addition of glutaraldehyde to the

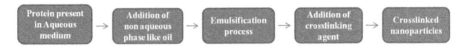

FIGURE 13.4
Preparation of polymeric nanoparticles by emulsion/solvent extraction method.

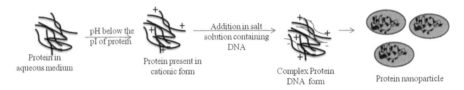

FIGURE 13.5
Preparation of polymeric nanoparticles by complex coacervation.

emulsion resulted in the size of NPs ranging from 100 to 800 nm. The size of NPs depends on the ratio of protein concentration and phase volume as high ratio results in the large size of NPs (Lohcharoenkal et al., 2014).

13.5.3 Complex Coacervation

A complex coacervation method is highly suitable for the preparation of NPs (NPs comprise DNA) used in gene therapy. The proteins contain a number of functional groups which helps to make the protein either cationic or anionic on the basis of pH and pI of protein. Protein is present in cationic form if the pH lies below the pI of protein and anionic if the pH lies above the pI of protein. The DNA gets entrapped in the NP by coacervation, with the help of interaction between the charged protein and other electrolytes present (Figure 13.5). DNA, endolysomotropic agents, and drugs can be encapsulated within the protein matrix during the process of coacervation. GNPs containing DNA have been produced by salt-induced coacervation. The positive charge of gelation at pH 5 is responsible for the coacervate–DNA complex, and the salts present are responsible for the desolvation process of electrolytes that give rise to the formation of NPs. Consequently, the generated NPs are stabilized by the addition of cross-linkers (Lohcharoenkal et al., 2014).

13.5.4 Electrospray

PBNs can also be prepared by this new technique, which is extensively utilized for the synthesis of gliadin and elastin-like peptide NPs. Here, the emitter emits the protein solution through the nozzle, and a high voltage is applied against this jet stream resulting in the formation of aerosolized liquid droplets of PBNs which are then collected. This method is highly efficient for loading therapeutics drugs and nucleic acids to nanocarriers (Cheng et al., 2017; Lohcharoenkal et al., 2014).

13.6 Toxicity of NPs

In the process of obtaining ideal nanocarriers, obstacles related to the toxic effects are always considered as a priority to be overcome. It is reported in the preliminary studies that NPs either directly or indirectly affect the biological environment (Bundschuh et al., 2018). NPs believed to show their effects at the cellular, subcellular, tissue, organ, and protein levels are essential to remove/lower down the toxicity related to NPs. NPs are proved to be safe and efficient during small-scale production so that NPs can be prepared in large scale in the field of pharmaceutics. Usually, the toxicity generated due to the physical and chemical properties of drug, nucleic acid, and protein are related to size, purity, electronic property or crystallinity, inorganic or organic surface coatings, solubility, shape, and aggregation behavior. To check the toxicity, a large number of standardized *in vitro* and *in vivo* assays have been exploited. Both *in vivo* and *in vitro* studies have advantages, as *in vitro* studies can be performed repeatedly, which helps to generate robust results as it is easy to perform and reduce the chance of animal handling (Zaman, Ahmad, Qadeer, Rabbani, & Khan, 2014). Many clinical trials are being carried out to check the effects of certain nanocarriers. During cancer chemotherapy, liposomal doxorubicin is used, which is a FDA-approved formulation associated with some side effects. Several studies have been conducted for liposomal doxorubicin, which shows that it is less toxic than other second-line chemotherapy regimens for ovarian cancer. It has been reported that side effects like skin, hypersensitivity reactions, and severe myelosuppression occur with the use of liposome NPs (Pisano et al., 2013). A study reported that asthenia and hand–foot syndrome were adverse side effects of liposomal doxorubicin during phase II trial of ovarian cancer. This phenomenon was observed in 41.6% of patients. Other adverse side effects were also observed: nausea (38.2%), neutropenia (37.1%), stomatitis (34.8%), rash (28.1%), mucositis (21.3%), vomiting (19.1%), anorexia (13.5%), and diarrhea (12.4%) (Iwamoto, 2013).

MTT assay (3-[4, 5-dimethylthiazol-2-yl]-2-5 diphenyltetrazolium bromide) is one of the widely used assay to determine cell viability. Cell membrane integrity is determined by performing lactate dehydrogenase assay. Gao et al. (2013) treated colon cancer with doxorubicin by preparing star-shaped poly(caprolactone)–poly(ethylene glycol) (PCL/PEG) micelles as a delivery system which showed less cytotoxicity with elimination of symptoms of hemolysis.

Inside the body, the primary site of interaction of nanocarriers is the cell membrane where they initially attach and alter the concentration of charge present on the surface and eventually perturbs the lipid phosphobilayer. Toxic effects have also been observed in membrane proteins where ion channels have an important role in molecular transport and transmembrane signaling. Nanomaterial can also put forth their effects at genetic level, as they bind directly or indirectly to DNA and damage it through inflammatory response or by promoting oxidative stress. Some nanocarriers have also been reported to damage the neuronal cells. Phase I clinical trial of albumin nanocarrier-bound paclitaxel related with hypersensitivity reactions and neuropathy are ongoing (Cucinotto et al., 2013).

13.7 Protein NP as Diagnostic Tool

Proteins and peptides provide an important biomarker and correlate with the actual changes in the cell. The proteins get altered under various physiological and diseased conditions, and their profile provides an important indication of pathological conditions. The amino acid sequence of the protein, known as primary structure, provides the framework for the secondary structure, wherein peptide folds as α-helices or β-strands and further attains a three-dimensional native structure. Nanotechnology-based methods provide an increased level of sensitivity and accuracy in detection of diseases. Nanoscience develops an interest in researchers to focus on biomedical-based detection and therapeutic tools (Estrada & Champion, 2015).

In general, nanobiotechnology can be defined as the intersection of nanotechnology and biotechnology. In the era of nanotechnology, researchers use nanotools to overcome the limitations that have been reported for current therapeutic as well as diagnostics. Protein NPs are made up of various metallic like copper-, gold-, silver-, and platinum-based nanoscale particles generally having a constant 3D structure. The exposed functional group of proteins on the surface of NP are used for imaging to detect various diseases. When compared with the synthetic nanomaterial, PBNs have higher biocompatibility and also have *in vivo* clinical applications (Lohcharoenkal et al., 2014).

For detection of several cancers at their early stages, NPs fully loaded with peptides get attached to the tumor, and the release of high concentration of biomarkers helps in the detection of tumors at its early stage. The same happens in the detection of oral cancer where carbon-and gold-based NPs detects the indicative protein at a very early stage and provides accurate results in a very less time, which can improve the prognosis for cancer patients.

The recent studies of Li et al. (2015) have showed that the super paramagnetic iron oxide NPs associated with the conjugate of folate–BSA can be used for early diagnosis of tumor by image contrasting.

Early and exact diagnosis of tumor is difficult due to false and irrelevant signals of positron emission tomography in combination with computed tomography. This problem can be overcome using metal NPs that are compatible to our system; on the other hand, these are expensive. The specificity of this technique can be enhanced by coupling NPs to the antibodies for the targeted marker. Membrane-bound Hsp70 plays an important role in by fulfilling all criteria of a suitable marker. The antibodies against Hsp70 bound with gold NPs can be easily detected (Kimm et al., 2015).

Autoimmune diseases are diseases that arise from an abnormal immune response of the body against substances and tissues generally present in the human body. According to statistics, autoimmune disease is one of the top ten leading causes of death in female and children. The National Institutes of Health estimates up to 23.5 million Americans suffer from autoimmune disease and that the prevalence is on the rise. According to researchers, 80–100 autoimmune disorders have been identified. Protein NPs play an important role in the diagnosis of various autoimmune disorders (Miller et al., 2012).

Proteinticles are self-assembled nanoscale proteins having a constant structure and surface topology that occur naturally. Proteinticles can also be modified by adding a speci-fied C- or N- terminus similar to chemically synthesized PBNs. Many of the proteinticles are used for diagnosis of human autoimmune and infectious diseases by recognizing the specific antibodies on the surface of cells. Laboratory detection of myelin oligodendro-cyte glycoprotein and antigenic peptides from hepatitis C virus on the surface of protein-ticles have already been tested, which shows 100% accuracy (Lee et al., 2013). Haidar and Tabrizian (2007) reported an ultrasensitive protein nanoprobe system that is able to detect Type I diabetes at an early stage. In diabetes Type I, 65 kDa glutamate decarboxylase-specific autoantibody remains as an early marker that can be detected by a supramolecular protein NP (Haidar & Tabrizian, 2007; Lee et al., 2013).

Transferrin receptor 1 (TfR1), one of the known receptors, is overexpressed by various tumor tissues, and heavy chain ferritin, which is an iron storage protein, has the ability to bind these TfR1. Therefore, scientists developed a strategy to visualize cancer cells using iron oxide NPs encapsulated in a recombinant human heavy-chain ferritin. These NPs get attached with the overexpressed TfR1 and catalyzed the reaction in which peroxide substrate gets oxidized and assist in the differentiation between normal and cancer cells (Fan et al., 2012).

Matrix metalloproteinase 2 (MMP-2) is also recognized as a potential target for the diagnosis of metastatic cancer. CTT peptides that bind to MMP-2 were conjugated to naturally occurring shock protein nanocages through genetic modification and were used in the detection of cancer cells using near infrared rays (Kawano et al., 2015).

13.8 Protein NPs as Therapeutics

Apart from diagnosis, protein NPs have been most extensively used as delivery vehicles for various drugs. The conventional methods of therapy of cancer include surgery, radiation, chemotherapy, and immunotherapy, but researchers are making efforts in nanotechnology-based therapeutic agents to cure diseases. The conventional drug delivery systems are highly linked with a number of hurdles like poor specificity, high toxicity, and induction of drug resistance. Due to side effects of conventional therapies, research is going to develop NPs (<100 nm) as carriers that are biodegradable and biocompatible to avoid preferably reticuloendothelial system and increase the circulation time. So, continuous research has been putting its efforts to improve the effectiveness of NPs to cure cancer and other diseases (Din et al., 2017).

13.8.1 NPs for Anticancer Therapy

To treat cancer, anticancer drug should cross various barriers after administration and should reach the targeted tumor site. The administered drug should retain its activity while reaching the targeted site and maintain its activity to kill cancerous cells effectively with minimal side effects to normal cells. For long and desirable therapeutic effects, drugs inside the NP should be released in a controlled manner.

Undoubtedly, cancer is the major cause of human death and is considered as a complex disease because of the involvement of multiple cellular systems of the body. NPs have been developed for early diagnosis, prediction, prevention, and personalized therapy. These NPs can be developed by conjugating with other functional molecules. Targeted delivery of NPs directly interacts with the receptors of the cancerous cells (Tietze et al., 2015).

Several PBNs have been designed as a therapy for threatening diseases like cancer and autoimmune diseases. Preparation of PBNs for triple-negative breast cancer have been reported, in which angiopep-2 was used to create modified NPs by fabricating GNPs with doxorubicin-loaded dendrigraft polylysine (DGL) to obtain the final product as Angio-DOX-DGL-GNP. Its accumulation and potential ability to penetrate deep into the 4T1 breast cancer cell was examined. The results showed higher accumulation, as angiopep-2 was able to bind low-density lipoprotein receptors and related proteins that were overexpressed by triple-negative breast cancer, and the penetration was enhanced when these particles come in contact with MMP-2, as it helped in the reduction of large size particles (Hu, Chun, Wang, He, & Gao, 2015). Maiolino et al. (2015) developed hyaluronan and polyethyleneimine-linked biodegradable NPs of poly(lactic-co-glycolic) acid (PLGA) for the delivery of anticancer drug doctexel and proved it to be a novel method to target CD44 cytokine, which is overexpressed in lung cancer. Therefore, it also helped in treating cancer without affecting the normal cells

(Maiolino et al., 2015). Similarly, silk fibroin (SF) protein-based biomacromolecule was used to create NPs for targeted drug delivery due to its ability to bind to various drug molecules like paclitaxel, and controlled drug release has been reported to have superior antitumor efficacy on gastric cancer *in vivo* when administered loco regionally (Chen, Shao, & Chen, 2011). The floxuridine-loaded SF NPs have been prepared and observed to adhere to HeLa cells more easily as compared to free drug. These kinds of PBNs have a potential use in lymphatic chemotherapy (Yu et al., 2014). Apo transferrin and lactoferrin NPs were used for the targeted delivery of doxorubicin to treat hepatocellular carcinoma in rats. In the active tumor, the receptors of apo transferrin and lactoferrin protein molecules get overexpressed, which makes it a potential target for anticancerous therapy. The results concluded the increased efficacy and bioavailability of drug when administered with these NPs orally and intravenously (Golla, Cherukuvada, Ahmed, & Kondapi, 2012). Protein molecules like E_2 obtained from pyruvate dehydrogenase of certain bacteria like *Geobacillus stearothermophilus* have also been used to develop NPs that are functionalized with antibody fragment (anti-EGFR), encapsulating anticancer drug to target cancer cells overexpressed with epidermal growth factor receptor (EGFR) (Buecheler et al., 2015). In another finding, BSA- and HSA-based NPs were shown to reduce cancer by enhanced drug delivery. As conventional radiotherapy has been used for the treatment of cervical cancer, the problem of radio resistance comes into picture during long-term therapy. BSA NPs encapsulated with organic seleno compound (PSed) with folate showed enhanced levels of reactive oxygen species, VEGF/VEGFR2 inactivation, and DNA damage repair, thus making its potential use in radiotherapy (Zhou et al., 2016). Magnetic NPs coated with BSA and linked to a peptide by glutaric aldehyde were used to encapsulate anticancer drug for diagnostic and therapeutic cancer (Niemirowicz et al., 2015). Kocbek, Cegnar, Kos, and Kristl (2007) studied PLGA immuno-NPs, which were used to target breast cancer cells by covalently or noncovalently attaching the monoclonal antibody to the surface of NP and can therefore be used for target delivery of small or large active substances.

13.8.2 NPs for Immunomodulation

Apart from cancer therapy and diagnosis, protein NPs are used in the detection and therapy of autoimmune diseases. In the case of type I diabetes, the insulin-producing β-cells in pancreas are destroyed by an autoimmune response. Herein, the scientists used an agonist peptide namely exendin-4, a glucagon-like peptide 1 (GLP1), which enhances the insulin production in pancreas. It has an antiapoptotic effect that was used to develop magnetic iron oxide NPs that target GLP1 receptors in pancreas and were used to imagine stages of disease and also potential therapeutics (Wang et al., 2014).

Inducing targeted immune tolerance is one of the methods to treat the autoimmune disease in which the immune response generated has been suppressed by certain peptides or protein. Hunter et al. (2014) demonstrated the use of PLGA NPs with myelin antigen-coupled particles for the treatment and prevention of encephalomyelitis.

Usually, immunosuppressive drugs have been used to control surplus immune responses, but nowadays antigen-specific immunological tolerance is being induced to control immune responses. Maldonadoa et al. (2014) developed synthetic and biodegradable NPs, encapsulating in them either a protein or a peptide antigen and an immunomodulator-like rapamycin, which helps generating antigen-specific immune tolerance. The results showed inhibition of CD4 and CD8 T-cell activation and hypersensitivity reaction, which are antigen specific, and an increase in regulatory cells along with long-lasting B-cell tolerance (Maldonado et al., 2014).

PBNs show enhanced activity against various infectious conditions. Development of vaccines for infectious diseases like malaria, Human immunodeficiency virus, and influenza were always related with major obstacles, so Doll et al. (2015) developed icosahedral self-assembling protein NPs that served as a vaccine platform for infectious diseases.

Porcine circovirus type II(PCV2) causing postweaning multisystemic wasting syndrome was targeted through nanobased techniques. An immunomagnetic nanobead created from a single domain of specific antibody have the capability to act with a capsid protein of PCV2 that is being conjugated to nanobeads for the detection and capturing of the virus in a complex clinical sample (Yang et al., 2015).

13.8.3 NPs for Ocular Disorders

Kim et al. (2015) reported the use of HSA NPs encapsulated with brimonidine (HSA-Br-NPs) and their effect on the retinal ganglion cells which exhibited a neuroprotective effect, as these NPs inhibited Aβ deposition. They have declared these NPs as safe and promising neuroprotective agents (Kim et al., 2015).

Millions of people are facing the problem of blindness globally. The current therapy of blindness and visual mutilation has certain limitations because of the peculiar structure of this organ to protect the inner part of eye. Therefore, nanoencapsulation of therapeutic potential protein and peptides acts as an emerging field. Nanoencapsulation helps therapeutic proteins for ocular delivery to overcome optical barriers, increase resident time, better performance, and increase in local drug level (Pescina et al., 2013).

13.8.4 NPs Reported for Other Therapies

To enhance the antileishmanial activity, GNPs encapsulated with 1, 2-diacyl-sn-glycero-3-phospho-1-serine loaded in amphotericin B was developed. It has been observed that increased concentration of AmB in the liver and spleen will elevate the activity of macrophages and reduce the cytotoxicity (Verma et al., 2018).

Chitosan NPs were used to encapsulate therapeutic proteins that bind to *Mycobacterium tuberculosis* CFO-10 and CFP-21 proteins, and the results showed increased bioavailability and decreased cytotoxicity. Chitosan has been proved biodegradable, biocompatible, and safe for humans and has been used in various drug delivery systems. Chemical functional groups present in chitosan makes it versatile for its application as an NP. Chitosan-derived NPs have been exploited for the treatment of several diseases like cancer, gastrointestinal diseases, and pulmonary diseases (Verma, Pandey, Chanchal, & Sharma, 2011).

Surface protein of *Plasmodium falciparum*, i.e., Pfs230, Pfs25, and Pfs48/45, were identified as target antigens for the development of vaccines. Pfs25 was extensively evaluated during preclinical trials. Malaria transmission-blocking vaccines is one way of controlling the transmission of virus as it generates immune responses that act on the different stages; therefore, scientists had created gold nanoparticles with codon-harmonized recombinant Pfs25 (CHrPfs25) from *Escherichia coli*, which has the ability to block transmission of virus via production of blocking antibodies (Kumar et al., 2015).

Moreover, the importance of integrin α1 and β3 factor for the differentiation of human alveolar epithelial stem cells has been revealed, as they are important factors for the induction of differentiation in human alveolar epithelial stem cells. Furthermore, integrin nanoparticles have been developed, which are effective as novel chronic obstructive pulmonary (COPD) treatment target compounds. COPD results in the collapse of alveoli, which is an irreversible condition in which there is an obstruction to airflow. Developed integrin nanoparticles have the capability to increase differentiation of human epithelial stem cells, as integrins have been reported as the factor responsible for the induction of differentiation (Horiguchi, Kojima, Sakai, Kubo, & Yamashita, 2014).

13.9 Conclusion

Proteins are the building blocks of human body. Protein plays an important role in vital cellular processes. Metabolism of protein indicates several processes inside the human body. Proteins are used as theranostic, which means that they can be used in diagnostics and therapeutics. However, due to some problems like poor bioavailability, degradation inside the digestive tract, and high dosages researchers explored the tool of nanoscience. Nanotechnology can be used as an arsenal to fight against several diseases with lots of advantages. As protein comes to nanoscale, it has the ability to cross any barrier, which is not possible with its native structure. Due to lack of specific target and improper biodistribution, it leads to high usage of the drug and hence causes side effects. Compatibility of proteins with the human body makes them suitable delivery vehicles for regular drugs. Attachment of site-specific antibody to the nanoparticle makes it convenient to deliver it in a site-specific manner like a post with address. According to the current situation of therapeutics, nanosized delivery containers are needed for controlled drug delivery. Major challenge in the field of diagnostics is early detection of tumor. Hence, use of nanosized proteins for bright field imaging of tumors with low false and negative signals can help in rapid and accurate diagnosis of tumors. Protein and peptide nanoparticles conjugated with BSA and other molecules are greatly utilized for the detection of early tumor. Development and improvement of NPs have shown a great impact for the treatment of life-threatening diseases. Furthermore, PBNs have good efficacy if administered via oral, nasal, ocular, and pulmonary route. Proteins like HSA, BSA, and many glycoproteins are used as nanotools to deliver drugs like paxicital, and doxorubicin against many tumors and breast cancer. NPs of SF protein have been used for delivery of molecules and the combination of drugs with significant release rate. Several studies have been reported in literature for the treatment of cancer. PLGA-based NPs show a great advantage in the therapy for immune-related diseases.

In future, nanoparticle-based therapy and early diagnosis will be further enhanced by designing more specific, compatible, and safe NPs of peptides and antibodies to identify and cure diseases, leading to the development of personalized therapy to improve health.

References

Abhilash, M. & Tech, B. (2009). Applications of proteomics. *The Internet Journal of Genomics and Proteomics*, 4(1), 1–11. doi:10.5580/1787.

Bhatia, S. (2016). Nanoparticles types, classification, characterization, fabrication methods and drug delivery applications. In *Natural Polymer Drug Delivery Systems* (1st ed., pp. 33–93). Springer International Publishing. doi:10.1007/978-3-319-41129-3.

Buecheler, J. W., Howard, C. B., de Bakker, C. J., Goodall, S., Jones, M. L., Win, T., … Lim, S. (2015). Development of a protein nanoparticle platform for targeting EGFR expressing cancer cells. *Journal of Chemical Technology and Biotechnology*, 90(7), 1230–1236. doi:10.1002/jctb.4545.

Bundschuh, M., Filser, J., Lüderwald, S., Mckee, M. S., Metreveli, G., Schaumann, G. E., … Wagner, S. (2018). Nanoparticles in the environment : Where do we come from, where do we go to ? *Environmental Sciences Europe, 30*(1), 6. doi:10.1186/s12302-018-0132-6.

Chen, M., Shao, Z., & Chen, X. (2012). Paclitaxel-loaded silk fibroin nanospheres. *Journal of Biomedical Materials Research Part A, 100*(1), 203–210. doi:10.1002/jbm.a.33265.

Cheng, D., Yong, X., Zhu, T., Qiu, Y., Wang, J., Zhu, H., … Xie, J. (2017). Synthesis of protein nanoparticles for drug delivery synthesis of protein nanoparticles for drug delivery. *European Journal of Biomedical Research, 2*(2), 8–11. doi:10.18088/ejbmr.2.2.2016.pp8-11.

Cucinotto, I., Fiorillo, L., Gualtieri, S., Arbitrio, M., Staropoli, N., Grimaldi, A., … Tagliaferri, P. (2013). Nanoparticle albumin bound paclitaxel in the treatment of human cancer: Nanodelivery reaches prime-time? *Journal of Drug Delivery, 2013*, 1–10. doi:10.1155/2013/905091.

Din, F. U., Aman, W., Ullah, I., Qureshi, O. S., Mustapha, O., Shafique, S., & Zeb, A. (2017). Effective use of nanocarriers as drug delivery systems for the treatment of selected tumors. *International Journal of Nanomedicine, 12*, 7291–7309. doi:10.2147/IJN.S146315.

Doll, T. A. P. F., Neef, T., Duong, N., Lanar, D. E., Shirley, A. M., & Burkhard, P. (2015). Optimizing the design of protein nanoparticles as carriers for vaccine applications. *Nanomedicine: Nanotechnology, Biology, and Medicine, 11*(7), 1705–1713. doi:10.1016/j.nano.2015.05.003.

Duclairoir, C., Orecchioni, A. M., Depraetere, P., Osterstock, F., & Nakache, E. (2003). Evaluation of gliadins nanoparticles as drug delivery systems: a study of three different drugs. *International Journal of Pharmaceutics, 253*(1–2), 133–144. doi:10.1016/S0378-5173(02)00701-9.

Elaissari, A. (2017). Protein-based nanoparticles: From preparation to encapsulation of active molecules. *International Journal of Pharmaceutics, 522*(1–2), 172–197. doi:10.1016/j.ijpharm.2017.01.067.

Estrada, L. P. H., & Champion, J. A. (2015). Biomaterials Science Protein nanoparticles for therapeutic protein delivery. *Biomaterials Science, 3*(6), 787–799. doi:10.1039/c5bm00052a.

Fan, K., Cao, C., Pan, Y., Lu, D., Yang, D., Feng, J., … Yan, X. (2012). Magnetoferritin nanoparticles for targeting and visualizing tumour tissues. *Nature nanotechnology, 7*(7), 459. doi:10.1038/NNANO.2012.209.

Gao, X., Wang, B.,Wei, X.,Rao, W.,Ai, F.,Zhao, F., … Wei, Y. (2013). Preparation, characterization and application of star-shaped PCL/PEG micelles for the delivery of doxorubicin in the treatment of colon cancer. *International Journal of Nanomedicine, 8*, 971–982. doi:10.2147/IJN.S39532.

Golla, K., Cherukuvada, B., Ahmed, F., & Kondapi, A. K. (2012). Efficacy, safety and anticancer activity of protein nanoparticle-based delivery of doxorubicin through intravenous administration in rats. *PLoS One, 7*(12). e51960. doi:10.1371/journal.pone.0051960.

Greenwood, J., Udenaes, M. H., Jones, H. C., Stitt, A. W., Vandenbrouke, R. E., Romero, I. A., … Khrestchatisky, M. (2017). Current research into brain barriers and the delivery of therapeutics for neurological diseases: A report on CNS barrier congress and their influence on leukocyte migration. *Fluids and Barriers of the CNS, 14*(1), 31 doi:10.1186/s12987-017-0079-9.

Haidar, Z. S., Tabrizian, M. (2007). Core – shell polymeric nanomaterials and their biomedical applications. In C. S. S. R. Kumar (Ed.), *Nanomaterials for the Life Sciences* (Vol. 10, pp. 285–309) Wiley-VCH Verlag GmbH & Co. KGaA: Weinheim. doi:10.1002/9783527610419.ntls0254.

Han, J., Wang, Q., Zhang, Z., Gong, T., & Sun, X. (2014). Cationic bovine serum albumin based self-assembled nanoparticles as siRNA delivery vector for treating lung metastatic cancer. *Small, 10*(3), 524–535. doi:10.1002/smll.201301992.

Horiguchi, M., Kojima, H., Sakai, H., Kubo, H., & Yamashita, C. (2014). Pulmonary administration of integrin-nanoparticles regenerates collapsed alveoli. *Journal of Controlled Release, 187*, 167–174. doi:10.1016/j.jconrel.2014.05.050.

Hu, G., Chun, X., Wang, Y., He, Q., & Gao, H. (2015). Peptide mediated active targeting and intelligent particle size reduction-mediated enhanced penetrating of fabricated nanoparticles for triple-negative breast cancer treatment. *Oncotarget, 6*(38), 41258–41274.

Hunter, Z., Mccarthy, D. P., Yap, W. T., Harp, C. T., Getts, D. R., Shea, L. D., & Miller, S. D. (2014). A biodegradable nanoparticle platform for the induction of antigen-specific immune tolerance for treatment of autoimmune disease. *ACS Nano, 8*(3), 2148–2160.

Iwamoto, T. (2013). Current topics challenges of drug delivery systems that contribute to cancer chemotherapy clinical application of drug delivery systems in cancer chemotherapy : Review of the efficacy and side effects of approved drugs. *Biological and Pharmaceutical Bulletin, 36*(5), 715–718.

Kawano, T., Murata, M., Piao, J. S., Narahara, S., … Hashizume, M. (2015). Systemic delivery of protein nanocages bearing CTT peptides for enhanced imaging of MMP-2 expression in metastatic tumor models. *International Journal of Molecular Sciences, 16*(1), 148–158. doi:10.3390/ijms16010148.

Kim, K. E., Jang, I., Moon, H., Kim, Y. J., Jeoung, J. W., Park, K. H., & Kim, H. (2015). Neuroprotective effects of human serum albumin nanoparticles loaded with brimonidine on retinal ganglion cells in optic nerve crush model. *Investigative Ophthalmology & Visual Science, 56*(9), 5641–5649. doi:10.1167/iovs.15–16538.

Kimm, M. A., Stangl, S., Schmid, T. E., Noël, P. B., Rummeny, E. J., & Multhoff, G. (2015). Imaging of Hsp70-positive tumors with cmHsp70. 1 antibody-conjugated gold nanoparticles. *International Journal of Nanomedicine, 10,* 5687–5700.

Kocbek, P., Cegnar, M., Kos, J., & Kristl, J. (2007). Targeting cancer cells using PLGA nanoparticles surface modified with monoclonal antibody. *Journal of Controlled Release, 120,* 18–26. doi:10.1016/j.jconrel.2007.03.012.

Kumar, R., Ray, P. C., Datta, D., Bansal, G. P., Angov, E., & Kumar, N. (2015). Nanovaccines for malaria using Plasmodium falciparum antigen Pfs25 attached gold nanoparticles. *Vaccine, 33*(39), 5064–5071. doi:10.1016/j.vaccine.2015.08.025.

Lee, E. B.,Seo, H. S.,Song, J. A.,Kwon, K. C.,Lee, E. J.,Kim, H. J., … Lee, E. B. (2013). Proteinticle engineering for accurate 3D diagnosis. *ACS Nano, 7*(12), 10879–10886. doi:10.1021/nn404325t.

Li, H., Yan, K., Shang, Y., Shrestha, L., Liao, R., Liu, F., … Xu, H. (2015). Folate-bovine serum albumin functionalized polymeric micelles loaded with superparamagnetic iron oxide nanoparticles for tumor targeting and magnetic resonance imaging. *Acta Biomaterialia, 15,* 117–126. doi:10.1016/j.actbio.2015.01.006.

Lohcharoenkal, W., Wang, L., Chen, Y. C., & Rojanasakul, Y. (2014). Protein nanoparticles as drug delivery carriers for cancer therapy. *BioMed Research International, 2014,* 12. doi:10.1155/2014/180549.

Maiolino, S., Russo, A., Pagliara, V., Conte, C., Ungaro, F., Russo, G., & Quaglia, F. (2015). Biodegradable nanoparticles sequentially decorated with Polyethyleneimine and Hyaluronan for the targeted delivery of docetaxel to airway cancer cells. *Journal of Nanobiotechnology, 13,* 29. doi:10.1186/s12951-015-0088-2.

Maldonado, R. A., Lamothe, R. A., Ferrari, J. D., Zhang, A., Rossi, R. J., Kolte, P. N., … Kishimoto, T. K. (2014). Polymeric synthetic nanoparticles for the induction of antigen-specific immunological tolerance. *Proceedings of the National Academy of Sciences of the United States of America, 112*(2), E156–E165. doi:10.1073/pnas.1408686111.

Marini, V. G., Martelli, S. M., Zornio, C. F., Caon, T., Simões, C. M., Micke, G. A., & Soldi, V. (2014). Biodegradable nanoparticles obtained from zein as a drug delivery system for terpinen-4-ol. *Química Nova, 37*(5), 839–843. doi:10.5935/0100-4042.20140135.

Miller, F. W., Alfredsson, L., Costenbader, K. H., Kamen, D. L., Nelson, L. M., Norris, J. M., & De Roos, A. J. (2012). Epidemiology of environmental exposures and human autoimmune diseases: Findings from a National Institute of Environmental Health Sciences Expert Panel Workshop. *Journal of Autoimmunity, 39*(4), 259–271. doi:10.1016/j.jaut.2012.05.002.

Niemirowicz, K., Prokop, I., Wilczewska, A. Z., Wnorowska, U., Piktel, E., Wątek, M., … Bucki, R. (2015). Magnetic nanoparticles enhance the anticancer activity of cathelicidin LL-37 peptide against colon cancer cells. *International Journal of Nanomedicine, 10,* 3843–3853. doi:10.2147/IJN.S76104.

Pisano, C., Cecere, S. C., Napoli, M., Di, Cavaliere, C., Tambaro, R., Facchini, G., … Pignata, S. (2013). Clinical Trials with pegylated liposomal doxorubicin in the treatment of ovarian cancer. *Journal of Drug Delivery, 2013,* 898146. doi:10.1155/2013/898146.

Rai, A., Jenifer, J., Theaj, R., & Upputuri, P. (2017). Nanoparticles in therapeutic applications and role of albumin and casein nanoparticles in cancer therapy. *Asian Biomedicine*, *11*(1), 3–20. doi:10.5372/1905–7415.1101.534.

Rizvi, S. A. A., & Saleh, A. M. (2018). Applications of nanoparticle systems in drug delivery technology. *Saudi Pharmaceutical Journal*, *26*(1), 64–70. doi:10.1016/j.jsps.2017.10.012.

Storp, B. V., Engel, A., Boeker, A., Ploeger, M., & Langer, K. (2012). Albumin nanoparticles with predictable size by desolvation procedure. *Journal of Microencapsulation*, *29*(2), 138–146. doi:10.3109/02652048.2011.635218.

Tarhini, M., Benlyamani, I., Hamdani, S., Agusti, G., Fessi, H., Elaissari, A. (2018). Protein-based nanoparticle preparation via nanoprecipitation method. *Materials*, *11*(3), 1–18. doi:10.3390/ma11030394.

Tietze, R., Zaloga, J., Unterweger, H., Lyer, S., Friedrich, R. P., Janko, C., & Alexiou, C. (2015). Magnetic nanoparticle-based drug delivery for cancer therapy. *Biochemical and Biophysical Research Communications*, *468*(3), 463–470. doi:10.1016/j.bbrc.2015.08.022.

Vaishya, R., Khurana, V., Patel, S., & Mitra, A. K.(2015). Long-term delivery of protein therapeutics, *Expert Opinion on Drug Delivery*, *12*(3), 415–440. doi:10.1517/17425247.2015.961420.

Verma, A. K., Pandey, R. P., Chanchal, A., & Sharma, P. (2011). Immuno-potentiating role of encapsulated proteins of infectious diseases in biopolymeric nanoparticles as a potential delivery system. *Journal of Biomedical Nanotechnology*, *7*(1), 63–64. doi:10.1166/jbn.2011.1202.

Verma, D., Gulati, N., Kaul, S., Mukherjee, S., & Nagaich, U. (2018). Protein based nanostructures for drug delivery. *Journal of Pharmaceutics*, 2018. doi:10.1155/2018/9285854.

Wang, P., Yoo, B., Yang, J., Zhang, X., Ross, A., Pantazopoulos, P., Moore, A.(2014). GLP-1R—Targeting magnetic nanoparticles for pancreatic islet imaging. *Diabetes*, *63*(5), 1465–1474. doi:10.2337/db13-1543.

Yadav, S. C., Kumari, A., & Yadav, R. (2011). Peptides Development of peptide and protein nanotherapeutics by nanoencapsulation and nanobioconjugation. *Peptides*, *32*(1), 173–187. doi:10.1016/j.peptides.2010.10.003.

Yang, S., Shang, Y., Wang, D., Yin, S., Cai, J., & Liu, X. (2015). Diagnosis of porcine circovirus type 2 infection with a combination of immunomagnetic beads, single-domain antibody, and fluorescent quantum dot probes. *Archives of Virology*, *160*(9), 2325–2334. doi:10.1007/s00705-015-2508-x.

Yu, S., Yang, W., Chen, S., Chen, M., Liu, Y., Shao, Z., & Chen, X. (2014). *RSC Advances*, 18171–18177. doi:10.1039/c4ra02113d.

Zaman, M., Ahmad, E., Qadeer, A., Rabbani, G., & Khan, R. H. (2014). Nanoparticles in relation to peptide and protein aggregation. *International Journal of Nanomedicine*, *9*(1), 899–912. doi:10.2147/IJN.S54171.

Zhou, L., Wang, K., Li, Q., Nice, E. C., Zhang, H., & Huang, C. (2016). Clinical proteomics-driven precision medicine for targeted cancer therapy: Current overview and future perspectives, *Expert Review of Proteomics*, *13*(4), 367–381. doi:10.1586/14789450.2016.1159959.

14

Exploring Food Domain Using Deep Neural Networks

Megha Rathi, Samyak Jain, and Uday Aggarwal

Jaypee Institute of Information Technology

CONTENTS

14.1 Introduction

Well-being and health are being considered as the topics of immense importance and essential factors associated with enhancement in the standard of life. Many people are turning their heads toward this important aspect of one's life. Food is the cornerstone of a person's lifetime. People have begun to be conscious about their dietary intake and just how nutritious or harmful a food item is, since an unhealthy diet leads to numerous diseases like heart diseases, diabetes, etc. Tagging of different food items accurately goes a long way to assist us in keeping good health.

Recently, convolutional neural network (CNN) have enjoyed substantial popularity for the task of image classification, ever since Krizhevsky et al. (2012) won the 2012 ImageNet Large-Scale Visual Recognition Challenge (ILSVRC). As a modification of the standard artificial neural network, CNN is distinguished by an exceptional network architecture comprising convolutional and pooling layers, which are interspersed to bring out and merge together local features from a two- or three-dimensional input (Liu et al., 2016).

Some other works in this domain are attentive on the design of a complete pipeline for diet monitoring in real time. Often, these systems exploit mobile application for food recognition, assessment, and logging. Examples of such systems are described in Kitamura et al. (2009), Kong and Tan (2012), Kawano and Yanai (2015), and in Zhu et al. (2010).

CNN, when juxtaposed to the traditional manually crafted feature extraction techniques, has an upper hand, since it can learn necessary features from images on its own.

In this chapter, our objective is to construct a multiclass classification model that is fast as well as accurate when there are a large number of classes (food categories).

The study was aimed to apply CNN with the use of data augmentation techniques to a set of five categories with a medium-scaled food image dataset.

14.2 Challenges

In the past few years, progress in image processing, deep learning, and CNNs have established themselves to be the state-of-the-art technology for image classification and recognition, including the issue of food item recognition. Researchers have worked on different aspects of food recognition system, but still there is a dearth of a good enough solution in terms of speed and accuracy for food identification and classification (Joutou & Yanai, 2009). Therefore, it is a challenging task to an extreme degree to precisely identify every food object, as many of the said objects may resemble each other in color or shape and may not be distinguishable even to the human eyes. Therefore, we propose that it would suffice to recognize a generalized version of a particular food item, based on which its dietary value can be approximately estimated, for instance, calories. It can provide people with necessary information and help them in planning their daily intake.

As the research scales more and more, the specific food items can also be encapsulated with specific or detailed information that were previously generalized (Hoashi et al., 2010).

The deep learning algorithms are designed to learn gradually through data. Large enough datasets are necessary to ensure that the deep learning network predicts accurately and delivers desired results. Deep learning mimics human mind, and as human brain requires lots of past events and experiences to assimilate and grasp information, similarly the equivalent neural networks require large volume of data. As the number of classes (food categories) increases, more and more data are needed for the machine to distinguish sufficiently enough between classes (He et al., 2014).

One other challenge is the necessity of a high-performance hardware. To perform a task of resolving a real-world problem, the system needs to be qualified with sufficient processing capacity, which generally comes from multicore high-performing Graphics Processing Units (GPUs) and interchangeable processing units. Otherwise, the training speed can be quite slow and the window for tweaking various hyperparameters for optimal performance of the network narrows down.

14.3 Related Work

Food object identification is one of the most active research topic in the domain of computer vision. Researchers have published numerous methods to solve this problem. The first issue is to dynamically observe the images that contain food objects

(Yanai & Kawano, 2015). This is an inevitable step for a preprogrammed food recognition and analysis system. Sometimes, it is sufficient to categorize a food picture when the primary goal is to determine images that comprise food for the target of assembling them into separate classes. In dietary assessment, it would help if one is able to figure out which food objects are in a picture. Additionally, the proposed work highlights the mixes for sustenance picture examination and an order approach in light of k-closest neighbors and vocabulary trees. The framework is assessed on a sustenance picture dataset comprising 1,453 pictures in 42 nourishment classifications procured by 45 members in normal eating circumstances.

The work done by Sun et al. (2008) proposes a technique that holds an alignment card as a kind of perspective; this card ought to be put beside the sustenance while catching the picture, with the goal that the measurements of nourishment are known. In any case, this card should dependably be available in the photograph when the client needs to utilize the framework. The downside is that the framework won't work without this card, which implies that, on account of removal or nonattendance of the card, the framework won't work.

Similar technique (Ahmad et al., 2014) utilizes the photograph of nourishment and bolsters that to a neural network created by specialists. In any case, the client must catch the photograph in an uncommon plate (for adjustment purposes), which won't be constantly conceivable; thus, the strategy may be hard to take after for the normal client.

14.4 Methodology

The research consists of two steps: identifying food from an image and converting the food identified into calories (He et al., 2014). We performed food image classification using CNN. The detailed steps are given in Figure 14.1.

14.4.1 Dataset

One of the dataset available publicly is Food-101, having 100 categories of food. Random forest algorithm has been used on that dataset to achieve an accuracy of 65% on

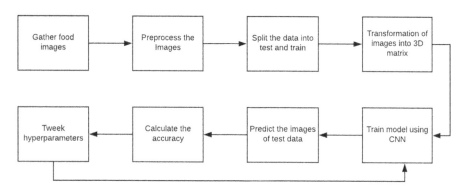

FIGURE 14.1
Our approach to the given problem.

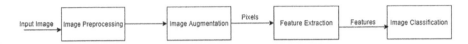

FIGURE 14.2
General steps in image recognition.

TABLE 14.1

Number of Images in Different Categories

Category	French Fries	Pizza	Hamburger	Cake	Waffles
Image Number	1,780	1,732	1,463	1,675	1,882

100 categories (Bossard et al., 2014). There are 1,000 pictures for each category, so in total, there are 100,000 images (Figure 14.2).

We have used five categories in our project, and the number of images in each category is described in Table 14.1. They are French fries, pizza, hamburger, cake, and waffles.

14.4.2 CNN Machine Learning Algorithm

Our network consists of four layers: two convolutional pooling and two fully connected layers, different from the final layer of output. Note that input is not considered as a layer. Convolutional layer has 32 kernels of size 3×3 of stride length 1 pixel, taking an input of size $100 \times 100 \times 3$, where 100×100 is the rescaled size of our images and 3 denotes the color aspect (RGB) of the image, then max pooling operation is done using pool size of 2×2.

The aforementioned layer has been repeated once more, where the kernels have been increased from 32 to 64 to get more filtered images for the fully connected layers.

Then, two fully connected layers are used with 128 and 90 neurons, respectively, and dropouts have been added 0.01 in between the dense layers to prevent overfitting by making the weights of some random neurons to zero so as to prevent overfitting on some particular neurons.

All the convolved 2D layers and other layers have an activation function of rectified linear unit.

The last layer is the output layer consisting of five neurons equivalent to the number of categories, and each neuron has an output of a probability corresponding to that particular neuron. The CNN predicts the category to be the one with the highest probability (Kagaya & Aizawa 2015). Figure 14.3 shows the detailed steps of our CNN architecture.

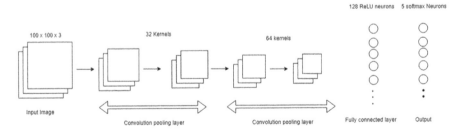

FIGURE 14.3
Architecture of our implementation of CNN.

Implementation of CNN was done using Keras package, which is a high-level abstraction of Tensorflow.

14.4.3 R Packages Used

Sections 14.4.3.1, 14.4.3.2 and 14.4.3.3 describe employed R packages of this research work.

14.4.3.1 *Keras*

Keras is a high-level abstraction of Tensorflow, which makes the implementation easier. Features including code can be run on a Central Processing Unit (CPU) or GPU. Application programming interface (API) is quick and easy to use and can run on multiple backends like CNTK, Theano, Tensorflow, etc.

14.4.3.2 *CARET*

Classification And REgression Training (CARET) package consists of a function that can be used to implement predictive models. The package contains tools for

- Data manipulation
- Features to be selected
- Resampling to tune model

14.4.3.3 *Shiny*

Shiny is a package of R used to implement server and ui part of the app. It brings together the frontend and backend. HTML, css, Javascript, Markdown, etc. are supported in Shiny.

14.5 Result

We first implemented the CNN not using data expansion techniques, and Figure 14.4 shows the accuracy and loss while training with 40 training epochs. Accuracy on test data was found out to be 82% compared with a training accuracy of 90%.

The results for each individual food category: food items such as pizza and French fries are being generalized well by the CNN in contrast to hamburger and waffles in which the CNN has difficulty in learning the features specific to these food items. The result accuracy for cake was intermediate, as shown in Figure 14.5.

Three different conventional algorithms, such as Support Vector Machine (SVM), K Nearest Neighbor (KNN), and random forest classification techniques, were used to train their respective models on a dataset of five categories, and their accuracy on the test images were recorded for the justification of using conventional neural networks. As is evident later (Figure 14.6), CNN far outperforms the traditional algorithms, which, without a doubt, proves its efficiency with respect to image classification.

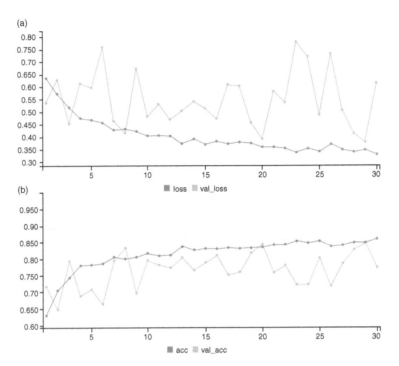

FIGURE 14.4
Loss (a) curves and accuracy (b).

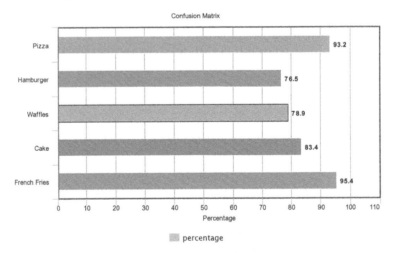

FIGURE 14.5
Individual accuracy for individual class.

14.6 User Interface

An easy-to-use interface is created for food recognition and calorie estimation. In today's era, a healthy diet is essential for a healthy life, and a proposed app is able to compute the total calorie intake so that one can control food consumption for a healthy lifestyle (Figures 14.7–14.9).

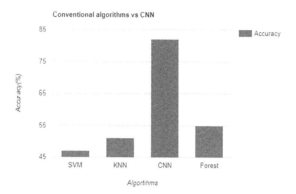

FIGURE 14.6
Comparison of accuracies of CNN with traditional image classification algorithms.

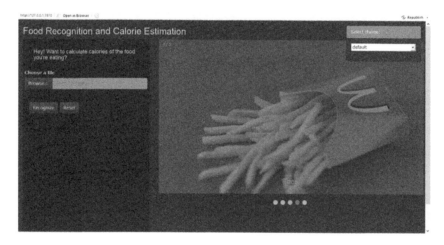

FIGURE 14.7
User interface.

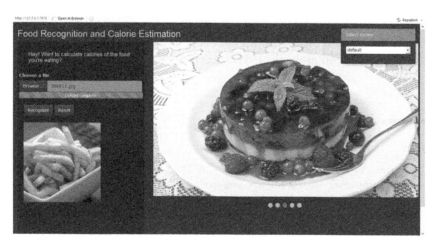

FIGURE 14.8
After the image has been uploaded.

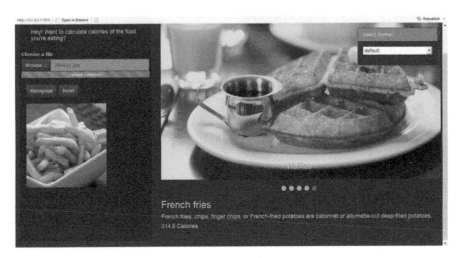

FIGURE 14.9
The results are displayed at the bottom of the main screen section.

14.7 Conclusion

To conclude, we successfully achieved good results by creating a neural network used to classify food images. A CNN model of four layers was put together to attain the test accuracy of 82%, which was best among other algorithms. The number of layers was determined by trial and error, taking into consideration CNNs with a different number of layers as well. The CNN model suffered from discernible high variance due to limitation of training data. This problem was addressed to an extent by enlarging the training data through image augmentation, which also improved the performance of the model considerably with an overall test accuracy to a level of over 88%. Training the neural nets with different number of epochs showed us the limitation for further improvement in test accuracy, which could also be achieved in some other ways like gathering more training data and optimizing the network architecture and hyperparameters of the neural net. It is not always the solution of increasing the number of epochs, because if it is done so in this case among the others, it would make the overfitting issue worse.

References

Ahmad, Z., Khanna, N., Kerr, D. A., Boushey, C. J., & Delp, E. J. (2014, February). A mobile phone user interface for image-based dietary assessment. In *Mobile Devices and Multimedia: Enabling Technologies, Algorithms, and Applications 2014* (Vol. 9030, p. 903007). International Society for Optics and Photonics.

Bossard, L., Guillaumin, M., & Van Gool, L. (2014, September). Food-101–mining discriminative components with random forests. In *European Conference on Computer Vision* (pp. 446–461). Springer, Cham, Munich, Germany.

He, Y., Xu, C., Khanna, N., Boushey, C. J., & Delp, E. J. (2014, October). Analysis of food images: Features and classification. In *IEEE International Conference on Image Processing (ICIP), 2014* (pp. 2744–2748). IEEE, Taipei, Taiwan.

Hoashi, H., Joutou, T., & Yanai, K. (2010, December). Image recognition of 85 food categories by feature fusion. In *IEEE International Symposium on Multimedia (ISM), 2010* (pp. 296–301). IEEE San Diego, CA, USA.

Hou, L., Wu, Q., Sun, Q., Yang, H., & Li, P. (2016, August). Fruit recognition based on convolution neural network. In *12th International Conference on Natural Computation, Fuzzy Systems and Knowledge Discovery (ICNC-FSKD), 2016* (pp. 18–22). IEEE, Kunming, China.

Joutou, T., & Yanai, K. (2009, November). A food image recognition system with multiple kernel learning. In *16th IEEE International Conference on Image Processing (ICIP), 2009* (pp. 285–288). IEEE, Cairo, Egypt.

Kagaya, H., & Aizawa, K. (2015, September). Highly accurate food/non-food image classification based on a deep convolutional neural network. In *International Conference on Image Analysis and Processing* (pp. 350–357). Springer, Cham, Waterloo, Canada.

Kawano, Y., & Yanai, K. (2015). Foodcam: A real-time food recognition system on a smartphone. *Multimedia Tools and Applications*, 74(14), 5263–5287.

Kitamura, K., Yamasaki, T., & Aizawa, K. (2009, October). FoodLog: capture, analysis and retrieval of personal food images via web. In *Proceedings of the ACM multimedia 2009 workshop on Multimedia for cooking and eating activities* (pp. 23–30). ACM, Beijing, China.

Kong, F., & Tan, J. (2012). DietCam: Automatic dietary assessment with mobile camera phones. *Pervasive and Mobile Computing*, 8(1), 147–163.

Krizhevsky, A., Sutskever, I., & Hinton, G. E. (2012). Imagenet classification with deep convolutional neural networks. In *Advances in Neural Information Processing Systems* (pp. 1097–1105).

Liu, C., Cao, Y., Luo, Y., Chen, G., Vokkarane, V., & Ma, Y. (2016, May). Deepfood: Deep learning-based food image recognition for computer-aided dietary assessment. In *International Conference on Smart Homes and Health Telematics* (pp. 37–48). Springer, Cham, Singapore.

Sun, M., Liu, Q., Schmidt, K., Yang, J., Yao, N., Fernstrom, J. D., ... Sclabassi, R. J. (2008, August). Determination of food portion size by image processing. In *Engineering in Medicine and Biology Society, 2008. EMBS 2008. 30th Annual International Conference of the IEEE* (pp. 871–874). IEEE.

Yanai, K., & Kawano, Y. (2015, June). Food image recognition using deep convolutional network with pre-training and fine-tuning. In *IEEE International Conference on Multimedia & Expo Workshops (ICMEW), 2015* (pp. 1–6). IEEE, San Diego, USA.

Zhu, F., Bosch, M., Woo, I., Kim, S., Boushey, C. J., Ebert, D. S., & Delp, E. J. (2010). The use of mobile devices in aiding dietary assessment and evaluation. *IEEE Journal of Selected Topics in Signal Processing*, 4(4), 756–766.

Index

A

Abdominal diseases and organ detection, 141
Accuracy, 2, 4–8, 22, 24–7, 29, 50–2, 59, 63, 65,
        128–32, 136, 141–4, 156, 160, 161, 163,
        172, 183, 189, 208, 218, 219, 221, 222, 224
Acquired immuno deficiency syndrome (AIDS),
        98
AdaBoost, 127–9
Adaboost random forest (ADBRF), 127, 128
ADC, *see* Apparent Diffusion Coefficient (ADC)
AIDS, *see* Acquired immuno deficiency
        syndrome (AIDS)
Air Pollution, 109, 110, 114, 122
Air Quality Index (AQI), 110, 111, 113, 114, 116,
        118–20, 122
Air quality prediction, 109–22
Algorithm, 2, 5–11, 18, 19, 23–6, 28, 29, 32, 34,
        42–4, 47, 50–3, 55–9, 63, 73, 76, 78, 112,
        127–30, 133, 136, 142, 153, 154, 156–9,
        161, 163, 167–77, 180, 181, 184, 185, 192,
        218–21, 223, 224
Alzheimer, 128, 139, 140, 187
Android, 31, 33, 34, 40, 42, 70–4, 76, 77, 79, 80
ANN, *see* Artificial neural network (ANN)
Antibiotics, 83, 84, 93, 97
Antifungal agents, 96–7
Antigens, 97, 98, 152, 211
Antimicrobial, 83, 84, 93–6, 100, 101
Antiparasitic, 99, 100
Apache Hadoop, 4
API, *see* Application Program Interface (API)
Apparent Diffusion Coefficient (ADC), 126
Apple Operating system (iOS), 34, 72
Application Program Interface (API), 70, 78, 79,
        221
Applications (apps), 4, 5, 7–9, 11, 31, 32, 34, 69–72,
        84, 100, 116, 130, 136, 138, 139, 143, 144,
        159, 165, 166, 170, 177, 179–81, 184, 186,
        188–90, 200, 208
AQI, *see* Air Quality Index (AQI)
Area under curve (AUC), 63, 99
Artificial neural network (ANN), 6–8, 55, 56,
        62, 63, 65, 112, 114, 116–18, 120, 122, 131,
        155, 217
Atmospheric Temperature, 113, 115, 116
AUC, *see* Area under curve (AUC)
Autoantibody, 208

Auto-encoder, 140–2, 183, 184
Autoimmune disorders, 208

B

Back-propagation algorithm, 184, 185
Backtracking, 169, 171, 177
Barcode Description, 41
Bayesian, 6–8, 18, 25, 112, 130
BBD, *see* Box Behnken Design (BBD)
β-lactoglobulin (BLG), 203
BFS, *see* Breadth first search (BFS)
Bias field, 127, 129
Big data, 1–11, 13, 190
Bioavailability, 83–5, 93, 99, 101, 200, 201,
        210–12
Biodegradable, 200–2, 209–11
Biofilm, 95, 96
Bioinformatics, 177, 186, 188–9
Biomarkers, 140, 200, 207, 208
Biomedical, 130, 192, 200, 201, 208
BLG, *see* β-lactoglobulin (BLG)
Block substitution matrix (BLOSUM), 153
Blood banks, 70, 71, 73–6, 78
BLOSUM, *see* Block substitution matrix
        (BLOSUM)
Bond length prediction, 153, 156
Bovine serum albumin (BSA), 200, 202, 208, 210,
        212
Box Behnken Design (BBD), 93
Braille keyboard, 32, 47
Brain abnormality, 140
Brain tumor segmentation (BRATS), 127, 128,
        131, 132, 138, 139
Branch & Bound, 170–1, 177
BRATS, *see* Brain tumor segmentation (BRATS)
Breadth first search (BFS), 169, 172–6
Breast cancer, 10, 18, 21, 22, 27, 50–2, 140, 143,
        202, 209, 210, 212
Breast Cancer Type 1 (BRCA1), 50
Breast Cancer Type 2 (BRCA2), 50
Brute force, 169, 170, 176
BSA, *see* Bovine serum albumin (BSA)

C

CAD, *see* Computer-aided diagnosis (CAD)
Calendar Plot, 120

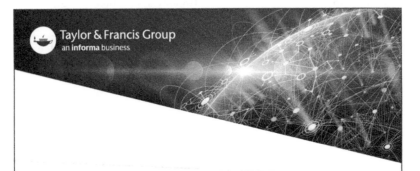

Printed and bound by CPI Group (UK) Ltd, Croydon, CR0 4YY

23/10/2024

01778253-0007